ESSENTIAL ATLAS OF
HEART DISEASES

Second Edition

NOTICE

Medicine is an ever-changing science. As new research and clinical experience broaden our knowledge, changes in treatment and drug therapy are required. The author and the publisher of this work have checked with sources believed to be reliable in their efforts to provide information that is complete and generally in accord with the standards accepted at the time of publication. However, in view of the possibility of human error or changes in medical sciences, neither the author nor the publisher nor any other party who has been involved in the preparation or publication of this work warrants that the information contained herein is in every respect accurate or complete, and they disclaim all responsibility for any errors or omissions or for the results obtained from use of the information contained in this work. Readers are encouraged to confirm the information contained herein with other sources. For example and in particular, readers are advised to check the product information sheet included in the package of each drug they plan to administer to be certain that the information contained in this work is accurate and that changes have not been made in the recommended dose or in the contraindications for administration. This recommendation is of particular importance in connection with new or infrequently used drugs.

ESSENTIAL ATLAS OF
HEART DISEASES

Second Edition

EDITOR–IN–CHIEF

EUGENE BRAUNWALD, MD, MD (HON), SCD (HON)
Distinguished Hersey Professor of Medicine
Harvard Medical School
Faculty Dean for Academics
Brigham and Women's Hospital
Massachusetts General Hospital
Vice President for Academic Programs
Partners Healthcare System
Boston, Massachusetts

CONTRIBUTING EDITORS

KENNETH L. BAUGHMAN, MD
Professor
Department of Medicine
Johns Hopkins School of Medicine
Chief of Cardiology
The Johns Hopkins Hospital
Baltimore, Maryland

EUGENE BRAUNWALD, MD, MD (HON), SCD (HON)
Distinguished Hersey Professor of Medicine
Harvard Medical School
Faculty Dean for Academics
Brigham and Women's Hospital
Massachusetts General Hospital
Vice President for Academic Programs
Partners Healthcare System
Boston, Massachusetts

WILLIAM VIRGIL BROWN, MD
Charles Howard Candler Professor of Medicine
Emory University
Chief of Medicine
Atlanta VA Medical Center
Atlanta, Georgia

ROBERT M. CALIFF, MD
Professor of Medicine
Duke University School of Medicine
Duke Clinical Research Institute
Durham, North Carolina

WILSON S. COLUCCI, MD
Professor of Medicine
Boston University
Chief, Cardiovascular Medicine
Boston University Medical Center
Boston, Massachusetts

ROBERT M. FREEDOM, MD
Professor of Pediatrics, Pathology, and Medical Imaging
University of Toronto
Head, Division of Cardiology
Hospital for Sick Children
Toronto, Ontario
Canada

SAMUEL Z. GOLDHABER, MD
Associate Professor of Medicine
Department of Medicine
Director, Venous Thromboembolism Research Group
Director, Cardiac Center's Anticoagulation Service
Brigham and Women's Hospital
Boston, Massachusetts

NORMAN K. HOLLENBERG, MD, PHD
Professor of Medicine
Department of Medicine
Harvard Medical School
Director of Physiologic Research
Brigham and Women's Hospital
Boston, Massachusetts

SHABUDIN H. RAHIMTOOLA, MB, FRCP, MACP, MACC
Distinguished Professor/ George C. Griffith
Professor of Cardiology
Department of Cardiology
Keck School of Medicine
University of Southern California
Los Angeles, California

MELVIN SCHEINMAN, MD
Professor of Medicine
Department of Medicine/Cardiac Electrophysiology
University of California San Francisco
San Francisco, California

WITH 130 CONTRIBUTORS

Developed by Current Medicine, Inc., Philadelphia

McGraw-Hill
Medical Publishing Division

New York Chicago San Francisco Lisbon
London Madrid Mexico City Milan New Delhi
San Juan Seoul Singapore Sydney Toronto

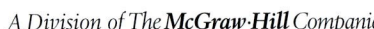

McGraw-Hill

A Division of The McGraw·Hill Companies

CURRENT MEDICINE

400 MARKET STREET, SUITE 700 • PHILADELPHIA, PA 19106

Developmental Editor .... *Teresa M. Giuliana*

Editorial Assistant .... *Annmarie D'Ortona*

Illustrator .... *Wieslawa Langenfeld*

Design .... *Christine Keller-Quirk*

Assistant Production Manager .... *Simon Dickey*

Indexing .... *Alexandra Nickerson*

Library of Congress Cataloging-in-Publication Data

Essential atlas of heart diseases / editor-in-chief, Eugene Braunwald ;
contributing editors, Walter H. Abelmann ... [et al.].-- 2nd ed.
        p. ; cm.
    Includes bibliographical references and index.
    ISBN 1-57340-163-3 (alk. paper)
    1. Heart--Diseases--Atlases.
    [DNLM: 1. Cardiovascular Diseases--Atlases. WG 17 E78 2000] I.
Title: Heart diseases. II. Braunwald, Eugene, 1929-
    RC682.E85 2000
    616.1'2--dc21

                                    00-047323

ISBN 0-07-137645-3

Printed in Singapore by Imago Productions (FE) Ltd.

10 9 8 7 6 5 4 3 2 1

The publisher wishes to acknowledge the contributions made by the many authors, whose images appear in this volume, to the original series.

PREFACE

Disorders of the cardiovascular system are the most common causes of death and serious morbidity in the industrialized world. In 1999, more than 40% of all deaths in the United States were attributed to cardiac and vascular diseases. These conditions accounted for almost 5 million years of potential life lost.

Despite these sobering statistics, progress in cardiovascular medicine has been immense, and is, in fact, accelerating. Our understanding of the pathobiology of most forms of heart disease has advanced steadily and there have been enormous advances in the diagnosis, treatment, and prevention of cardiovascular disorders. For example, during just one decade, from 1989 to 1999, the overall death rates from cardiovascular disease declined by 26% and death rates from acute myocardial infarction and stroke declined by 32%. Similar progress has been made in other major cardiovascular disorders, including hypertension, valvular and congenital heart disease, congestive heart failure, and the arrhythmias.

Physicians responsible for the care of patients with cardiovascular disease—both primary care physicians and specialists—now have available numerous publications for obtaining up-to-date information, including excellent journals and textbooks of every conceivable size, scope, and depth. In developing new strategies for transmitting information about these conditions, it is important to consider that cardiovascular medicine is the most "visual" of medical specialties. Cardiovascular diagnosis is based on the recognition and understanding of a variety of graphic waveforms, images, decision trees, and microscopic sections.

Treatment increasingly involves the intelligent use of algorithms, which are most effectively portrayed visually. Likewise, mechanical correction of cardiovascular disorders, whether catheter-based or surgical, can best be described pictorially. This *Essential Atlas of Heart Diseases* has been designed to provide a detailed and comprehensive visual exposition of all aspects of cardiovascular medicine. The *Essential Atlas* should be especially useful to primary care physicians as well as to specialists. The most important images from each volume in the *Atlas of Heart Diseases* series, accompanied by detailed captions written by the expert authors, were reviewed by their respective volume editors, who serve as chapter authors in this *Essential Atlas*.

Many people deserve credit for the successful completion of this ambitious effort. The expertise and hard work of the contributors and the devoted efforts of the volume editors naturally form the foundation of the *Essential Atlas of Heart Diseases*. Great credit is also due to Abe Krieger, President of Current Medicine, who conceived the project, and to Kathryn Saxon, who coordinated the efforts in my office.

All of us who have been engaged in this project hope that this *Essential Atlas* will be useful to physicians of all specialties who are responsible for the care of patients with cardiovascular disorders, to investigators and teachers of cardiovascular medicine, and ultimately to the millions of patients worldwide with disorders of the heart and circulation.

Eugene Braunwald, MD

CONTENTS

CHAPTER 10
COR PULMONALE, PRIMARY PULMONARY HYPERTENSION, AND CARDIAC TUMORS

Edited by Samuel Z. Goldhaber

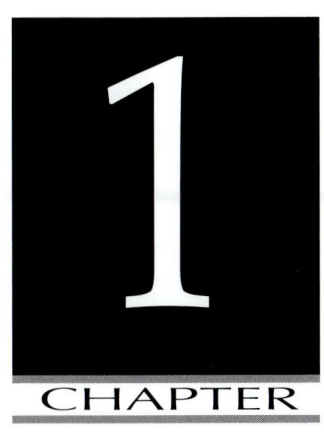

1 CHAPTER

ATHEROSCLEROSIS: RISK FACTORS AND TREATMENT

Edited by W. Virgil Brown

G.M. Anantharamaiah, H. Bryan Brewer, Jr., Alan Chait, David W. Garber,
Don P. Giddens, Seymour Glagov, Michael B. Gravanis, Jeffrey M. Hoeg,
Andreas R. Huber, Donald B. Hunninghake, Ngoc-Anh Le,
Sampath Parthasarathy, Michael E. Rosenfeld, Marschall S. Runge,
Jere P. Segrest, Christopher K. Zarins

FORMATION OF THE ATHEROSCLEROTIC PLAQUE

EARLY EVENTS IN THE INITIATION OF ATHEROSCLEROTIC LESIONS

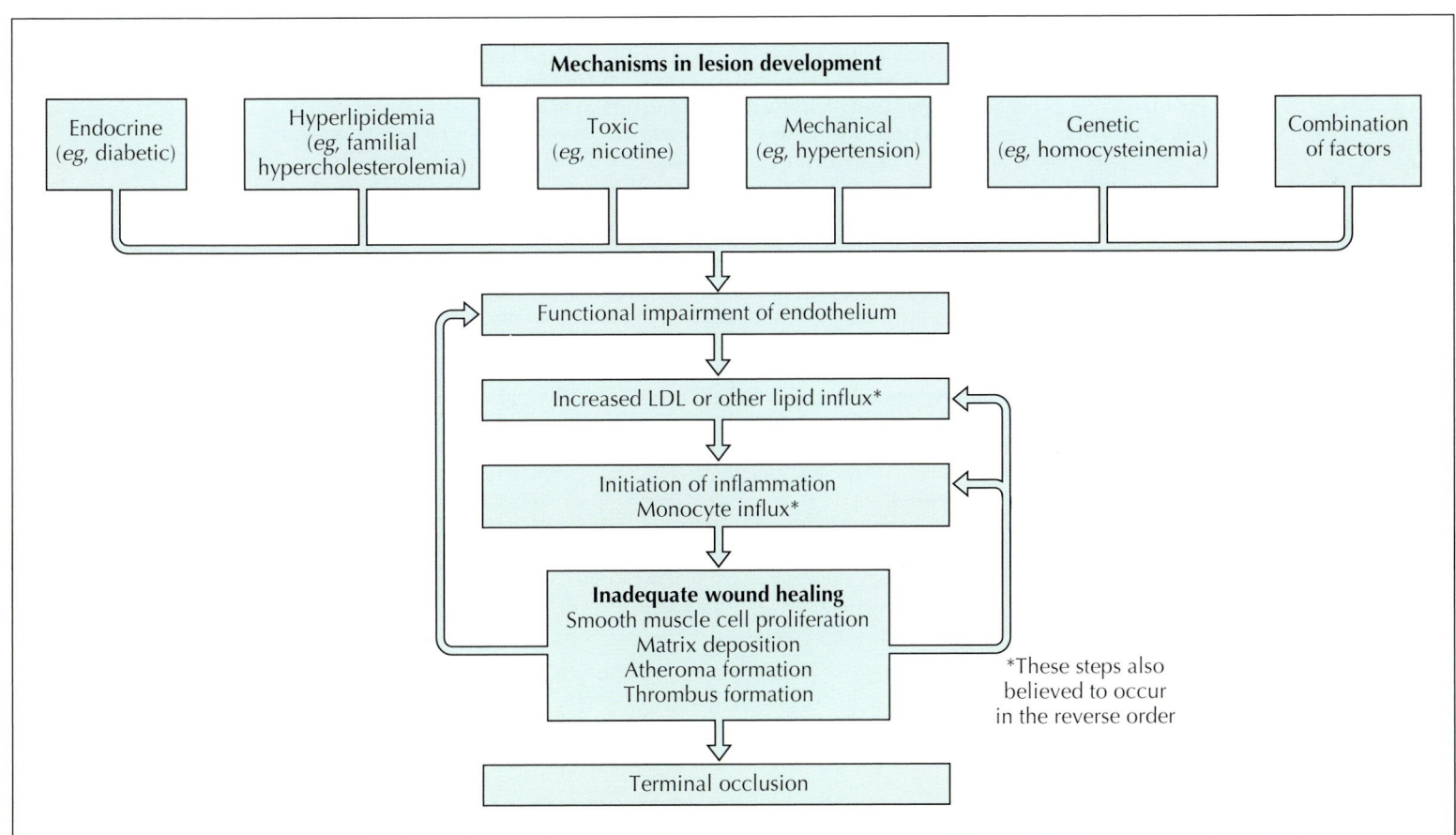

FIGURE 1-1. Mechanisms in arteriosclerotic lesion formation. Multiple risk factors and pathologic states have been correlated with early lesion formation and lesion progression. It is hypothesized that these factors all induce functional impairment of the arterial endothelium resulting in either increased lipid influx or initiation of an inflammatory vessel wall response. This process is propagated by additional accumulation of inflammatory cells such as monocytes within the vessel wall. Consequently, under persistence of the noxious agent(s), chronic inflammation persists, leading to inadequate wound healing. Ultimately terminal occlusion of the vessel by a thrombus occurs. LDL—low-density lipoprotein.

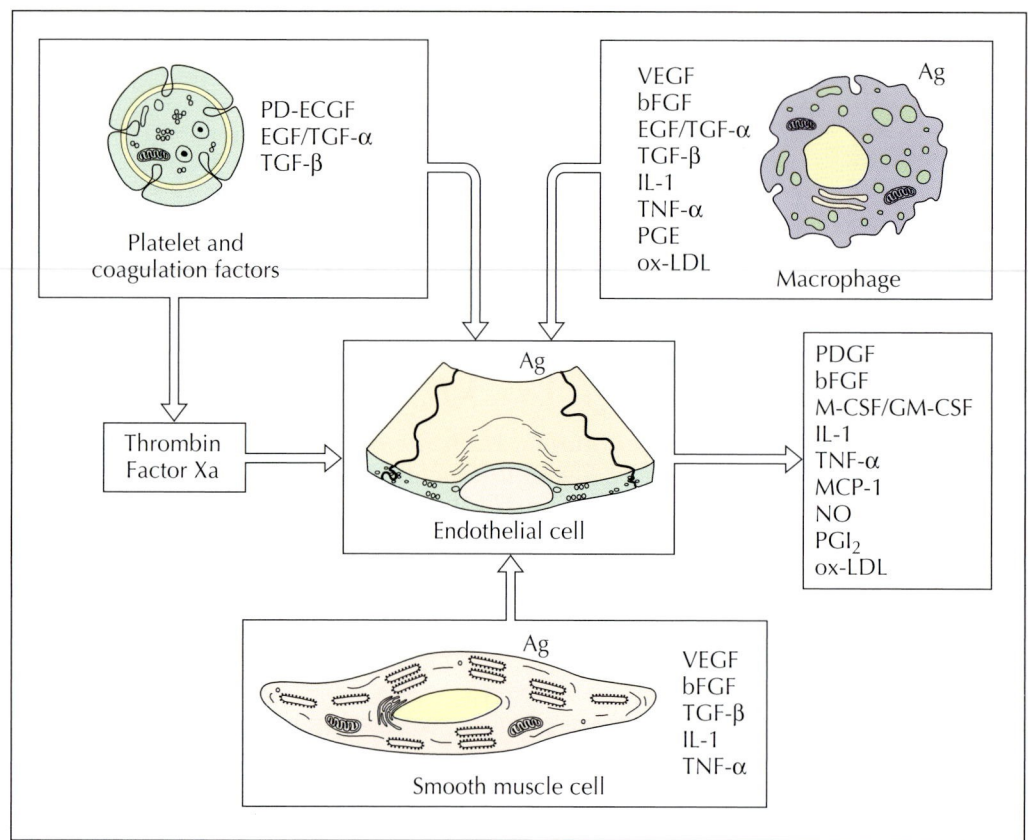

FIGURE 1-2. Platelet, macrophage, and smooth muscle products in the endothelial response to vascular injury. During atherogenesis, the endothelium interacts with macrophages, platelets, smooth muscle cells, and T lymphocytes. These interactions result in the expression and secretion of several potential mediators of vascular lesion formation. Macrophages produce endothelial mitogens including vascular endothelial growth factor (VEGF), fibroblast growth factor (FGF), interleukin-1 (IL-1), and transforming growth factor-α and -β (TGF-α, TGF-β). IL-1 and both TGF-α and TGF-β can inhibit endothelial proliferation and induce secondary gene expression by the endothelium of such growth factors as platelet-derived growth factor (PDGF) and other potential regulators of vascular lesion formation. TGF-β also induces synthesis and secretion of connective tissue by the endothelium.

The endothelium and macrophages can produce oxidized low-density lipoprotein (ox-LDL), causing further injury to endothelial cells. Platelets produce TGF-α, TGF-β, and platelet-derived endothelial cell growth factor (PD-ECGF), a potent mitogen. A procoagulant state of the endothelium can be stimulated by thrombin and factor Xa, present in plasma. Several of the same molecules formed by macrophages and platelets are also generated in the artery wall or in atherosclerotic lesions underlying the endothelium by smooth muscle cells. Endothelial cells in injured vessels express several growth-regulatory molecules, including those that cause connective tissue to proliferate (PDGF, bFGF, TGF-β) and those that induce secondary gene expression for PDGF in smooth muscle and endothelial cells. Further, endothelial cells produce macrophage colony stimulating factor (M-CSF), granulocyte macrophage-colony stimulating factor (GM-CSF), and ox-LDL, which are mitogenic and activating factors for underlying macrophages. Endothelial cells also provide potent chemotactic factors that affect leukocyte chemotaxis, including ox-LDL and monocyte chemotactic protein-1 (MCP-1), and modulate vasomotor tone through the formation of nitric oxide (NO) and prostacyclin (PGI₂).

Thus, multiple interactions among platelets, macrophages, and smooth muscle cells have been documented and are likely to provide the inflammatory and growth-promoting milieu necessary for repair of vascular injury. In abnormal arteries, it is likely these same mechanisms stimulate formation of pathologic vascular lesions. Ag—antigen; EGF—epidermal growth factor; PGE—prostaglandin E; TNF—tumor necrosis factor. (*Adapted from* Ross *et al.* [1].)

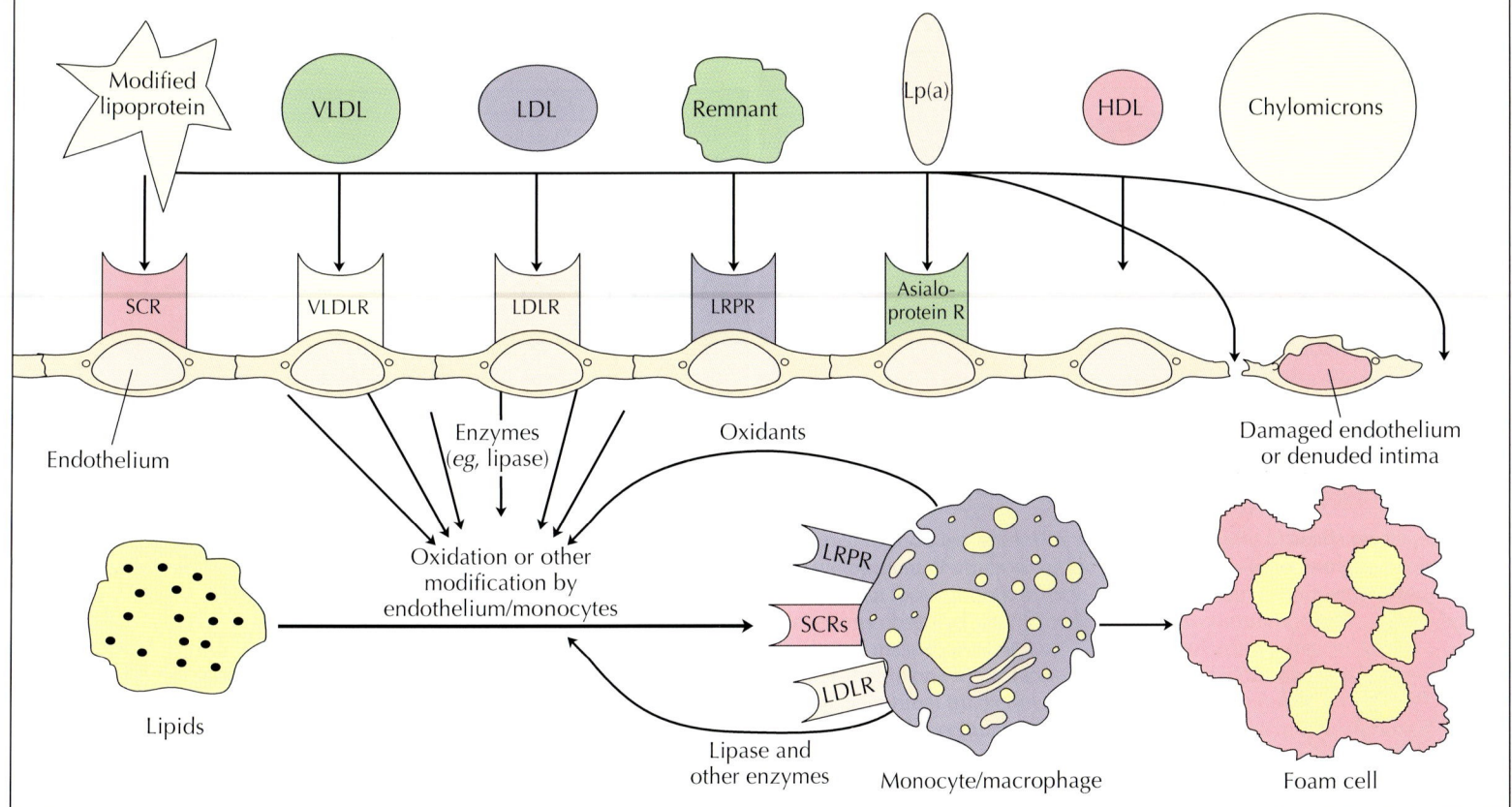

FIGURE 1-3. Postulated lipid entry mechanisms into macrophages. Many lipoproteins have been associated with arteriosclerosis. Foremost low-density lipoprotein (LDL), modified (*eg*, oxidized) LDL, lipoprotein (a) (Lp[a]), and other substances in the blood can be detected at high levels within the damaged vessel wall segments. Accumulation in the vessel wall may occur through diffusion either interjunctionally or in areas of denudation. In addition, a functionally impaired endothelium could mediate increased lipoprotein uptake via specific receptor-coupled pathways. To date, at least five lipoprotein receptors have been characterized in detail, including the two or more scavenger receptors (SCRs), LDL receptor (LDLR), very LDL receptor (VLDLR), LDL receptor related protein (LRPR), and asialoprotein receptor (R). Furthermore, lipoproteins captured in the subendothelial intimal space may be modified by oxidants or enzymes derived from either endothelial cells, monocytes, or smooth muscle cells leading to increased uptake into monocytes via the SCRs and, possibly, other receptors. With time, monocytes will develop into foam cells. HDL—high-density lipoprotein.

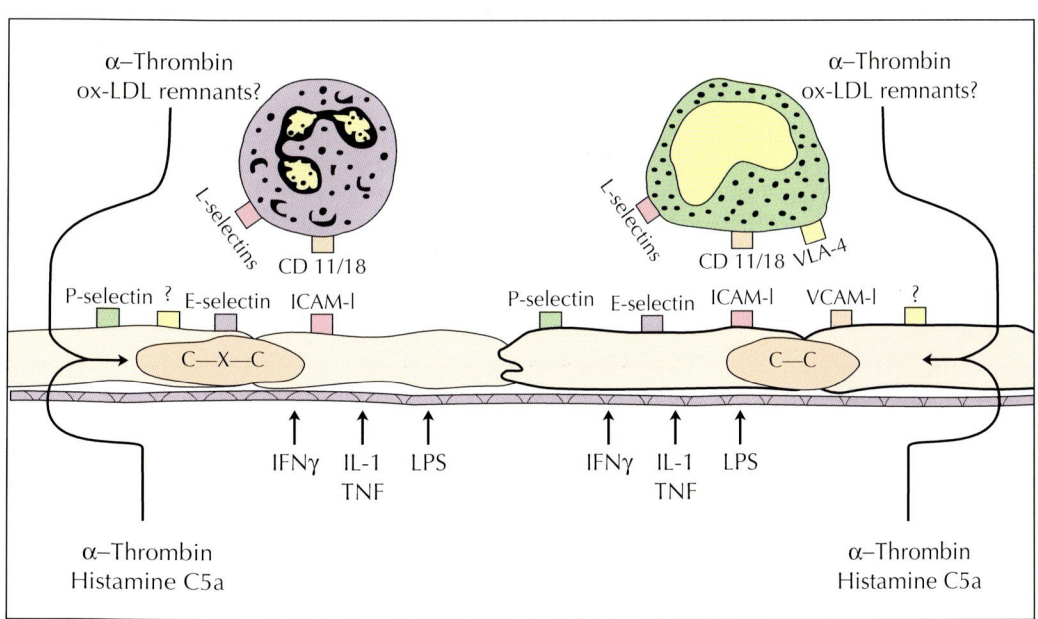

FIGURE 1-4. Regulation of leukocyte immigration into early lesions. Many proinflammatory cytokines such as interleukin-1 (IL-1), tumor necrosis factor (TNF), blood- and tissue-borne enzymes (*eg*, α-thrombin, histamine C5a), and oxidized low-density lipoproteins (ox-LDL) have the potential of inducing endothelial expression of a variety of adhesion molecules (*eg*, P-selectin, E-selectin, intercellular adhesion molecule-1 [ICAM-1], vascular cell adhesion molecule-1 [VCAM-1]), and secretion of chemokines. These factors contribute to activation of circulating leukocytes, expression of leukocyte adhesion molecules (L-selectins, CD11/18, and very late antigen-4 [VLA-4]) and subsequent interaction with the impaired ("inflamed") endothelium including adhesion and diapedesis. C-X-C—α-chemokines; C-C—β-chemokines; IFNγ—interferon-γ; LPS—lipopolysaccharide.

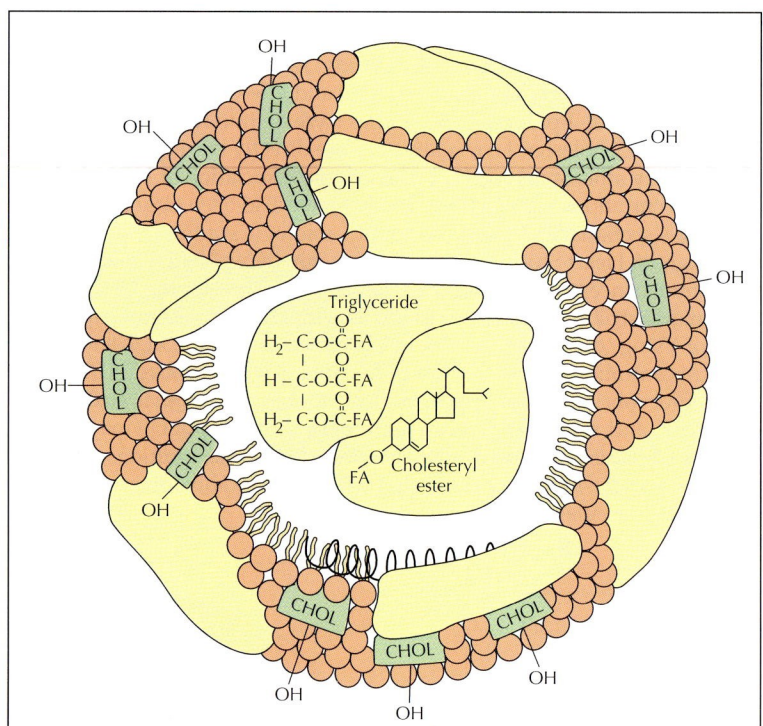

FIGURE 1-22. Schematic model of a plasma HDL particle. The surface of the lipoprotein particle is covered by phospholipids with the polar head groups of the phospholipids interacting with the aqueous environment. The protein components of the lipoprotein, designated apolipoproteins, and cholesterol (CHOL) are intercalated between the polar head groups of the phospholipids. The neutral lipids, cholesteryl esters and triglycerides, fill the core of the lipoprotein particle. Several different apolipoproteins are present on the lipoprotein particle. The apolipoproteins are associated with the lipoprotein particle by protein–protein as well as protein–lipid interactions. The apolipoprotein functions in lipoprotein metabolism as ligands for receptors, cofactors for enzymes, and structural proteins for lipoprotein particle biosynthesis [26].

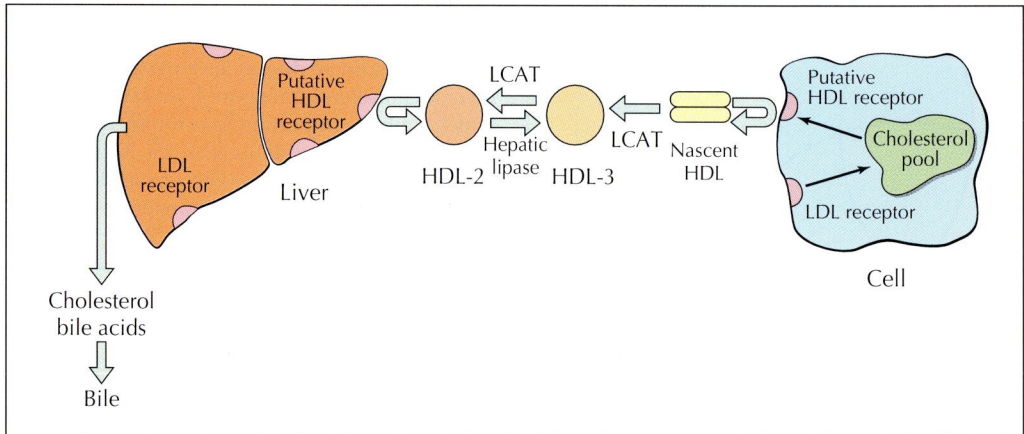

FIGURE 1-23. Schematic pathway of HDL and reverse cholesterol transport. The metabolism of all the plasma lipoproteins are interrelated and involve the interplay of lipolytic enzymes, apolipoproteins, receptors, and transfer proteins. Nascent HDLs, or pre β-HDLs, which are composed primarily of apo A-I phospholipid discs, are secreted from both the human intestine and liver. Nascent HDLs acquire excess cholesterol from peripheral cells, and lecithin-cholesterol acyltransferase (LCAT) catalyzes the esterification of lipoprotein cholesterol to cholesteryl esters. With the formation of cholesteryl esters, the nascent HDLs are converted to spherical lipoproteins with a hydrated density of HDL-3. HDL-3 particles are converted to the particles larger HDL-2 by the acquisition of lipids and apolipoproteins released during the stepwise delipidation and remodeling of the triglyceride-rich chylomicrons and VLDLs as well as by the esterification of the cholesterol removed from peripheral tissues. HDL-2 particles then interact with the liver and transfer HDL cholesterol to the hepatocyte where it can be converted to bile acids or secreted into the bile as cholesterol for removal from the body. HDL-2 is converted back to HDL-3 by the removal of phospholipids and triglycerides by hepatic lipase as well as by the transfer of cholesteryl esters into VLDL–intermediate-density lipoprotein (IDL)-LDL by the cholesteryl ester transfer protein (CETP) and by the transfer of cholesterol to the liver and other tissues. Thus, cholesterol may be transported back to the liver directly by HDL or following exchange to VLDL-IDL-LDL. A variable portion of tissue cholesterol has also been proposed to be transported to the liver by HDL particles containing apo E, which may interact with both the hepatic remnant and LDL receptors.

TREATMENT OF HYPOALPHALIPOPROTEINEMIA

- Beneficial lifestyle changes to increase plasma HDL levels
  - Exercise
  - Caloric restriction if the patient is not at ideal body weight
  - Stop cigarette smoking
- Drug treatment of hypoalphalipoproteinemia
  - Nicotinic acid
  - Fibrates
  - Statins
  - Bile sequestrants

FIGURE 1-24. Individuals with established coronary heart disease or an increased risk of cardiovascular disease based on family history or other clinical parameters should be considered for diet and lifestyle changes as well as drug treatment when appropriate. In addition, to specifically raise HDL, the use of agents such as statins to lower LDL cholesterol in a patient with reduced HDL cholesterol is useful. There are no definitive prospective studies to date that have established that raising HDL reduces the risk or decreases the progression of established atherosclerosis in patients with low HDL. Most experts believe that there is enough evidence to warrant drug treatment in those individuals with established disease or with a strong family history of cardiovascular disease cosegregating with low HDL.

TRIGLYCERIDE-RICH LIPOPROTEINS

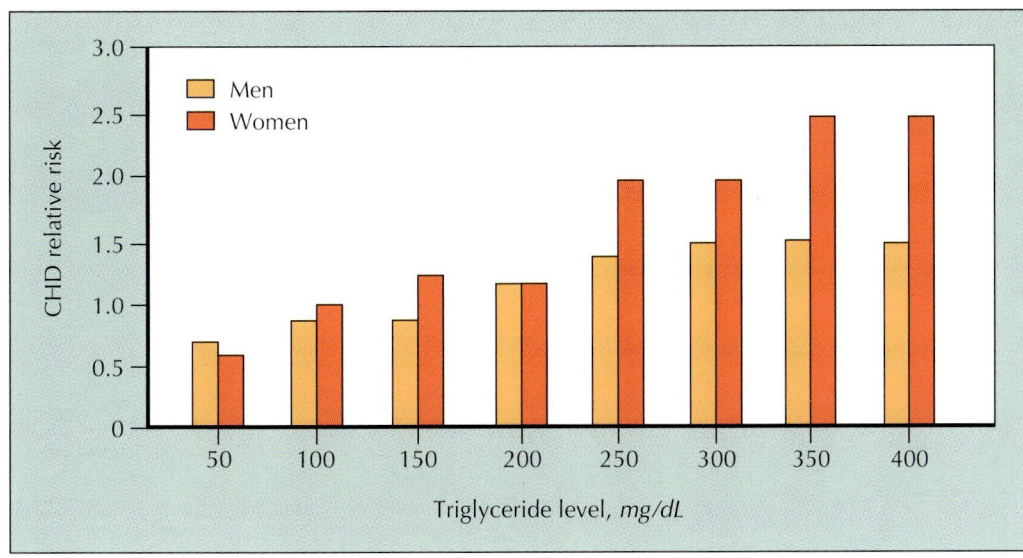

FIGURE 1-25. The incidence of coronary heart disease (CHD)–induced events, such as myocardial infarction and cardiac death, was found to be higher in both men and women with triglyceride levels above the mean for the population. The increase is most obvious as the baseline levels rise from approximately 150 to 350 mg/dL. This relationship of plasma triglycerides to risk of CHD is often stronger in women than in men, as was found in the Framingham Heart Study [19].

RISK FACTORS ASSOCIATED WITH PLASMA TRIGLYCERIDES

- Low HDL cholesterol
- Low apo A-I
- Increased LDL cholesterol
- Increased apo B
- Small dense LDL
- Glucose intolerance
  - Insulin resistance/hyperinsulinemia
  - Diabetes mellitus
- Obesity (abdominal obesity?)
- High blood pressure

FIGURE 1-26. Risk factors associated with increased plasma triglycerides include low high-density lipoprotein (HDL) cholesterol [27], low apolipoprotein A-I (apo A-I) [28], increased low-density lipoprotein (LDL) cholesterol, and small dense LDL particles [29]. In addition, glucose intolerance with insulin resistance and hyperinsulinemia or definite diabetes mellitus is frequently found [30,31]. Obesity is a common contributing factor to hypertriglyceridemia. The occurrence of intra-abdominal obesity, in particular, appears to be linked to glucose intolerance, high blood pressure, and the lipoprotein abnormalities noted above [32].

RISK OF CHD WITH INCREASING TRIGLYCERIDES

	RELATIVE RISK*	
	MEN	WOMEN
Univariate analysis	1.33	2.02
Adjusted for HDL cholesterol	1.24	1.57

*Risk ratio for CHD in middle-aged persons for each 100 mg/dL rise in serum triglycerides. Data based on meta-analysis of 14 prospective studies [35].

FIGURE 1-27. In recent meta-analyses of several observational studies, the simple measurement of total plasma triglycerides in men has been found to predict an increase in vascular events by 33% for each 100 mg/dL increase in the plasma concentration [33]. A similar rise in plasma triglycerides for women was associated with an increase in risk of coronary heart disease (CHD) by 100%. Men with plasma triglyceride levels of 300 mg/dL would be expected to have 66% more CHD than their counterparts with a plasma triglyceride level of 100 mg/dL. For women, a similar increase in plasma triglycerides would be expected to increase risk of CHD by fourfold.

There is a moderate, but highly significant, inverse relationship between plasma triglyceride and HDL cholesterol concentrations. When the risk associated with a rise in triglycerides from 100 to 300 mg/dL is adjusted for the lower HDL cholesterol, the residual effect is a 47% and 113% increased risk of CHD and in men and women, respectively. Furthermore, individuals with moderately elevated triglycerides (range, 200 to 500 mg/dL) often have higher LDL cholesterol levels; the adjustment for this relationship further reduces the risk that can be assigned specifically to elevations in triglycerides.

The usual daily fluctuations in human plasma levels are much greater for triglycerides than for cholesterol. This variation would significantly weaken any correlation of triglycerides with CHD risk. Few studies have accounted for the true biologic variation in triglycerides and, in fact, virtually all large studies have used single measures for statistical analyses. This may mean that the reported positive relationship between CHD risk and plasma triglycerides may be significantly stronger than current estimates [34].

SYNTHESIS AND METABOLISM OF CHYLOMICRONS AND VLDL

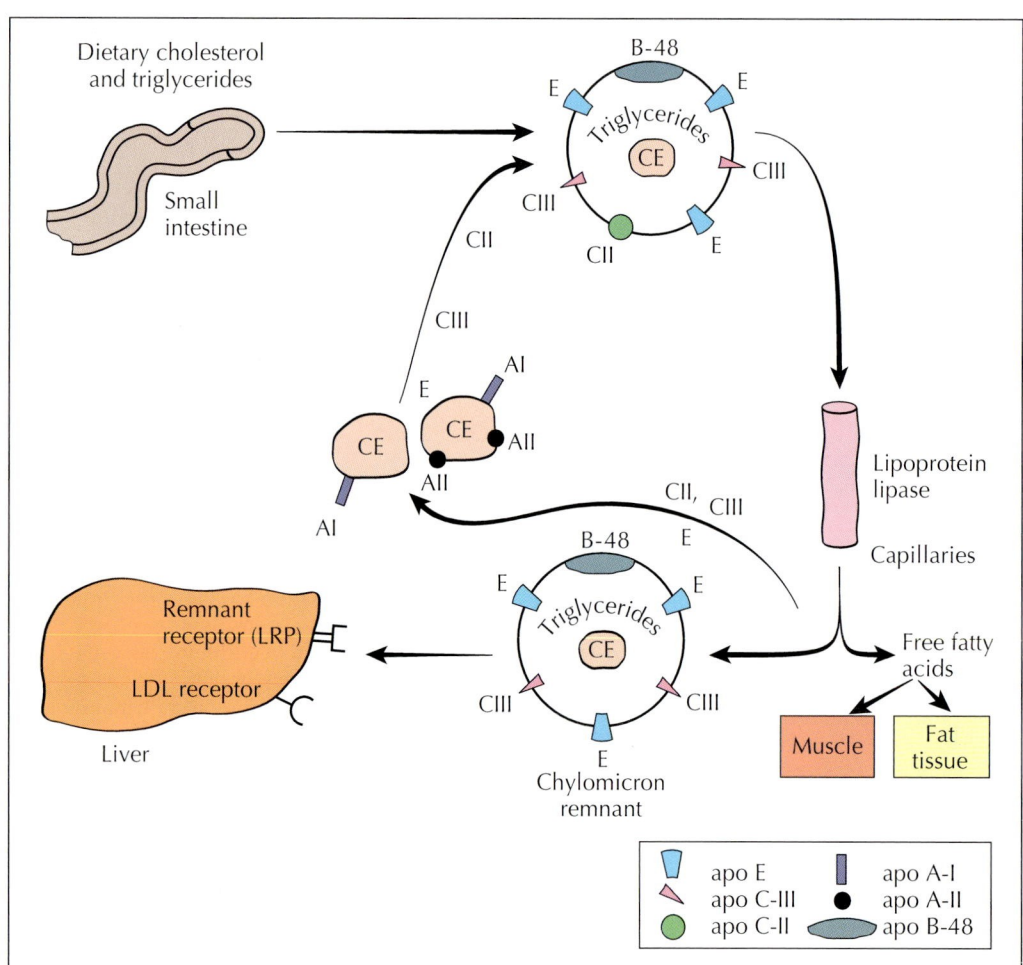

lipase. Apo C-III is a negatively charged protein of the same size that is believed to 1) stabilize the surface, preventing aggregation of lipid particles, and 2) inhibit uptake by cell surfaces, allowing preferential binding to lipoprotein lipase for hydrolysis at the capillary endothelial cell as mediated by apo C-II. The apo C-II and apo C-III proteins are released during lipase action to return to HDL [35].

A third protein, apo E, is also added to chylomicrons through transfer from HDL. Compared with apo C-II and C-III, a lesser amount of this is released from chylomicrons by lipoprotein lipase. Consequent to this enzyme action, remnant particles are generated that are relatively depleted in triglycerides, apo C-II, and apo C-III but relatively enriched in cholesteryl esters and apo E. A single copy of apo B-48 and many copies of apo E reside on this remnant particle. On circulation through the liver, there are at least two receptors that have high affinity for apo E; these include the LDL receptor and a larger protein referred to as the LDL-receptor related protein (LRP) [36]. Apo B-48 does not have a binding site for either of these receptors.

Uptake in the liver can be regulated by the numbers of apo E and apo C-III molecules. The greater the number of copies of apo E, the higher the affinity of the particle for liver cell surfaces, presumably due to multisite attachment. Increased quantities of apo C-III displace apo E to HDL and reduce the rate of uptake of remnants by the liver.

Hepatic triglyceride lipase is another enzyme on cell surfaces in Disse's spaces. This enzyme may further digest chylomicron remnant triglycerides and phospholipids. It also removes apo E from the surface of these particles [37]. Its role in the clearance of chylomicron remnant lipoprotein is not fully understood.

FIGURE 1-28. Chylomicron metabolism. Chylomicrons are formed in the intestinal epithelium after absorption of dietary cholesterol, as well as monoglycerides, fatty acids, and other hydrolytic products of dietary fats. The synthesis of apo B-48 and the transfer of newly synthesized triglycerides are two essential steps in the generation of chylomicrons. The gene for this protein generates mRNA, which is edited in the intestine to translate only 48% of the gene sequence. The liver lacks this editing system and uses the full transcript (100%) to secrete the entire protein, called apo B-100.

Several additional apolipoproteins are transferred from HDL to chylomicrons after arrival in the plasma. These include apo C-II, a small (9 kD) protein essential for activity of lipoprotein

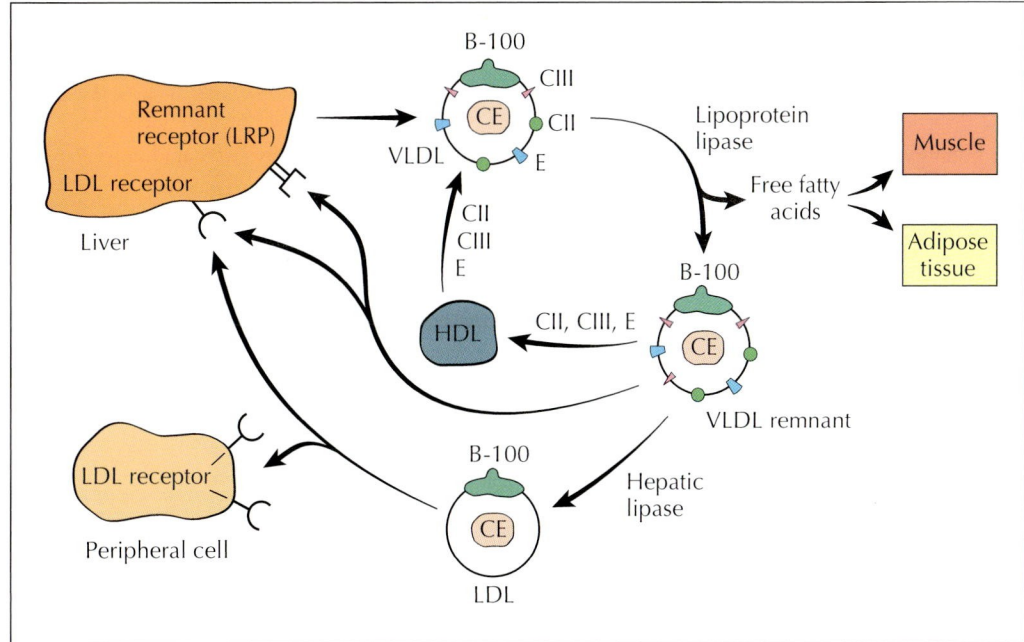

FIGURE 1-29. Metabolism of very low-density lipoproteins (VLDL). Triglyceride synthesis in the liver provides for efficient energy transfer into the plasma as VLDL. The VLDL particle is assembled by adding lipid to a large (550,000 D) protein, apo B-100. This protein is a full transcript of the apo B gene. Several copies of apo C-II, apo C-III, and apo E are also added in the liver cell, although additional copies of these latter proteins are transferred from HDL to the nascent VLDL after their arrival in the plasma. VLDLs follow a process similar to that discussed in Figure 1-28 for chylomicrons involving lipoprotein lipase and the generation of a remnant lipoproteins [35]. Major differences in

the fate of VLDL remnants as compared with chylomicron remnants are possible. VLDL remnants have available an additional binding site for the LDL receptor via apo B-100. However, they are taken up by liver cells less rapidly than are chylomicron remnants. This may be because of their containing fewer apo E molecules per particle—a function of their smaller size and surface area.

The VLDL remnant may alternatively be converted to LDL via the action of hepatic triglyceride lipase, which does not require the presence of apo C-II [38]. The LDL conversion is possible because apo B-100 can adopt a configuration that stabilizes a particle of the size and composition of LDL (apo B-48 does not appear capable of this function). Conversion of VLDL remnants involves removing most of the remaining triglyceride and leaving cholesteryl esters as the major core lipid. In addition, residual apo E, apo C-II, and apo C-III are removed. Most LDL in the plasma of humans appears to be derived from this pathway. Its clearance from the plasma is highly dependent on the LDL receptor because apo B-100 does not bind to the LDL-receptor related protein (LRP). Every cell in the normal human body is capable of expressing LDL receptors. However, most available LDL receptors occur on hepatocytes and, therefore, the liver removes 75% to 80% of LDL.

INHERITED SYNDROMES WITH HYPERTRIGLYCERIDEMIA

DYSBETALIPOPROTEINEMIA

Phenotype	Increased concentrations of VLDL and chylomicron remnants
	VLDL cholesterol/triglyceride >0.3 enriched in apo E rich β mobility on electrophoresis
Frequency	1/5000
Inheritance	Polygenic
Probable cause	Apo E defective (E2/E2)
Clinical consequence	Increased production of VLDL
	Increased CHD
	Tubero-eruptive xanthomata
	Palmar xanthomata

FIGURE 1-30. Dysbetalipoproteinemia is an uncommon disorder of remnant clearance caused by the superimposition of at least two common genetic traits. The first is a defective apo E molecule that has very low binding affinity for remnant receptors. There are three common alleles for apo E, two of which (E3 and E4) bind normally [39,40]. A third common allele, E2, results in a defective protein with weak binding affinity. Approximately 15% of the population has at least one defective allele, and approximately 1% is homozygous for this allele. Dysbetalipoproteinemia is usually a recessive trait (*ie*, requires two defective alleles). Other less common defective E proteins may have no affinity for the receptor and the clinical disorder may be expressed as a heterozygous

defect [40]. Marked elevations in remnants do not usually occur unless there is a concomitant overproduction of VLDL that is separately inherited. The coexistence of two traits, each of which exists in 1% to 2% of the population, gives the observed expression of one in 5000 to one in 10,000 persons.

The clinical diagnosis is suggested by elevations of cholesterol and triglycerides to approximately equivalent levels (250 to 800 mg/dL each). There are tubero-eruptive xanthomata on elbows (*see* Fig. 1-31), knees, or buttocks in 15% to 30% of patients, and some have planar xanthomata along the palmar creases [41].

The isolation of VLDL can confirm the diagnosis because the remnant particles are relatively rich in cholesterol and apo E, with lesser amounts of apo C-II and apo C-III. Consequently, the cholesterol-to-triglyceride mass ratio for isolated VLDL is greater than 0.3 as compared with a ratio of 0.2 obtained for normal VLDL. In addition, the isolated VLDLs have electrophoretic mobility comparable to β-globulins and LDL rather than normal pre-β mobility.

Atherosclerosis is prevalent in both peripheral arteries and in the coronary arteries of affected persons by midlife.

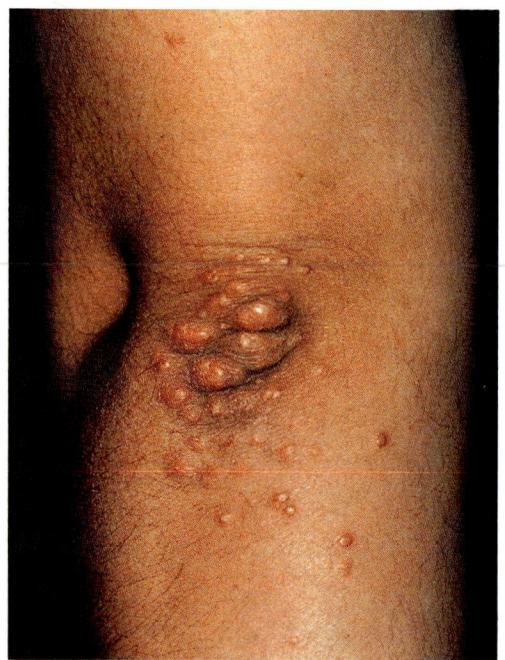

FIGURE 1-31. Tubero-eruptive xanthomata on the elbow of a patient with dysbetalipoproteinemia. (Courtesy of J. Davignon, MD, Montreal, Canada.)

FAMILIAL COMBINED HYPERLIPIDEMIA

Phenotype	Increased VLDL and/or LDL of normal composition; the dominant lipoprotein elevation may present as VLDL *or* LDL
Frequency	1%–2% of population
Inheritance	Autosomal dominant with expression in the third to fourth decade; first-degree relatives may show elevated VLDL and/or LDL
Probable cause	Overproduction of VLDL particles and consequent increased LDL production
Clinical consequences	Increased CHD

FIGURE 1-32. Familial combined hyperlipidemia is one of the most common forms of hypertriglyceridemia [42]. It is usually defined as the existence of elevated triglycerides or elevated LDL cholesterol (exceeding the 95th percentile for age and gender) with one or more first-degree relatives similarly affected. VLDL is normal in composition and has pre-β mobility on electrophoresis. Children usually have high values of triglycerides for their age but may not fully express the disorder until the fourth decade of life [43]. LDL may be only moderately elevated at times, particularly when the triglyceride level exceeds 400 mg/dL.

Overproduction of apo B-100 has been well demonstrated in several kindreds who meet the definition for this disorder [44,45]. The association with coronary heart disease (CHD) in the fifth through seventh decades is well established.

FAMILIAL HYPERTRIGLYCERIDEMIA

Phenotype	Increased VLDL with normal or low LDL; fasting chylomicrons occasionally present
Frequency	1/100
Inheritance	Autosomal dominant
Probable cause	Overproduction of triglycerides without incurred conversion of VLDL to LDL
Clinical consequences	No definite relation to CHD

FIGURE 1-33. Familial hypertriglyceridemia is characterized by increased plasma VLDL triglycerides and, in some cases, with triglycerides above 500 mg/dL, chylomicrons may be present in fasting plasma [44]. The total cholesterol may lie within normal limits because LDL cholesterol and HDL cholesterol are often at or below the lower limits of normal. Hepatic synthesis of triglyceride is increased, although the higher rate of VLDL particle production seen in familial combined hyperlipidemia is not observed [45,46]. The nascent VLDLs are presumed to be larger and relatively more triglyceride-rich than nascent particles.

HDL cholesterol is reduced and small dense LDL and HDL are usually present. The risk of coronary heart disease (CHD) may be only modestly increased, perhaps due to the low LDL cholesterol.

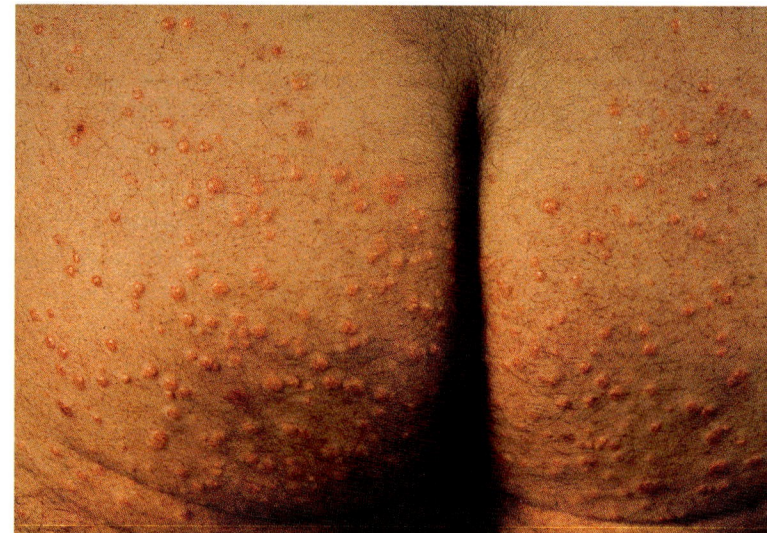

FIGURE 1-34. Eruptive xanthomata on the buttocks of a patient with familial hypertriglyceridemia and hyperchylomicronemic syndrome [47]. (*Courtesy of* J. Davignon, MD, Montreal, Canada.)

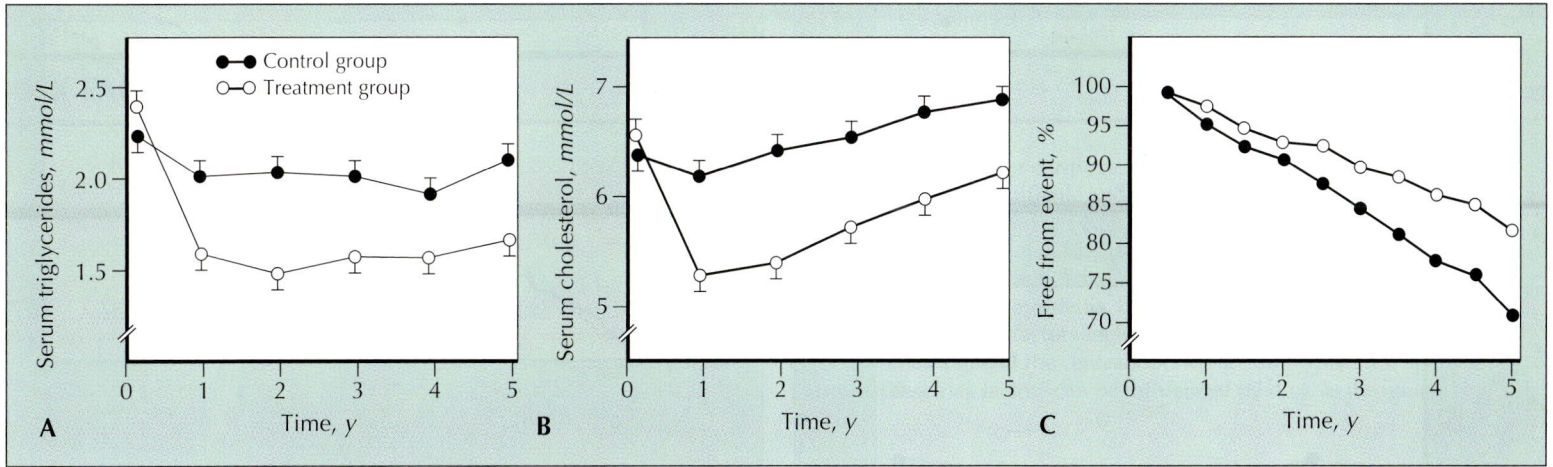

FIGURE 1-35. The Stockholm Ischemic Heart Disease Study was designed to assess plasma lipid reduction as a means of preventing recurrent coronary heart disease (CHD) in those patients who had experienced a myocardial infarction. Five hundred fifty-five men and women age under 79 years of age were assigned randomly to either niacin plus clofibrate or to placebo.

A, The total triglyceride level fell from 2.4 mmol/L (211 mg/dL) to 1.6 mmol/L (140 mg/dL) in the active treatment group. The control group experienced a decline from 2.2 mmol/L (191 mg/dL) to 2.0 mmol/L (176 mg/dL). **B,** The total cholesterol level was reduced from 6.6 mmol/L (254 mg/dL) to 5.2 mmol/L (200 mg/dL) initially; by the end of the study, however, the mean plasma cholesterol had risen to 6.1 mmol/L (235 mg/dL). The control group had a steady rise in cholesterol over the 5 years. **C,** The number of persons suffering a recurrent infarction or cardiovascular death was significantly reduced. At the end of the study, only 71% of the control group had not suffered an event whereas 83% of the treated group were event-free. The total mortality was also significantly reduced because of the marked decline in cardiovascular mortality (36%).

The reduction in CHD events was directly related to triglyceride reduction but had no correlation with the decline in cholesterol. However, LDL cholesterol and HDL cholesterol were not measured. Both the drugs used elevated HDL cholesterol significantly, and this probably minimized the change in total plasma cholesterol. (*Adapted from* Carlson and Rosenhamer [48].)

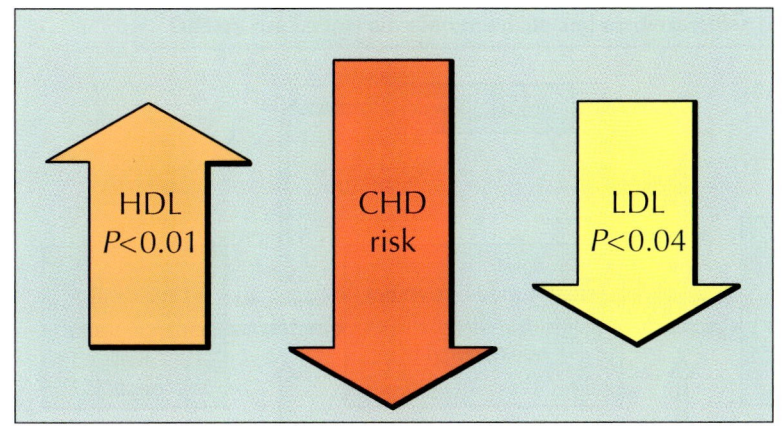

FIGURE 1-36. In the Helsinki Heart Study, significant correlations with reduced coronary heart disease (CHD) events were associated with an increase in HDL cholesterol (*P*<0.01) and a decrease in LDL cholesterol (*P*<0.04) during 5 years of treatment with gemfibrozil. A large reduction in triglycerides (35%) did not have a significant independent relationship to the observed reduction in cardiac endpoints [49].

EFFECTS OF VARYING CHOLESTEROL INTAKE

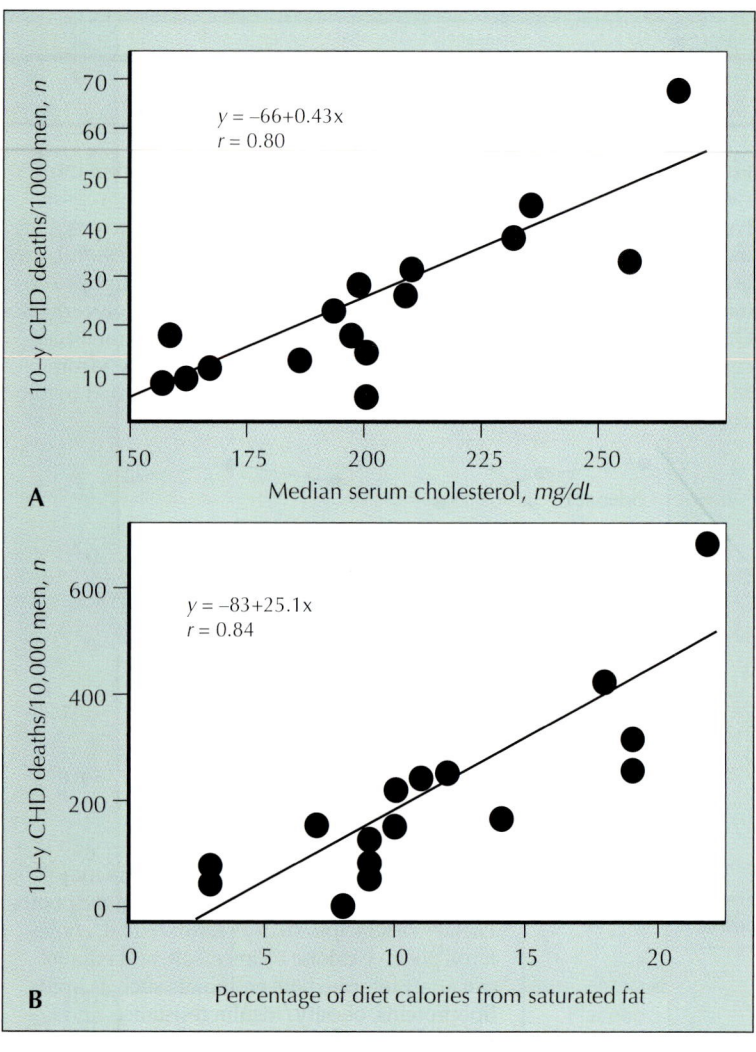

A

B

FIGURE 1-40. Comparison of the rates of coronary heart disease (CHD) mortality and serum cholesterol levels in countries consuming different average amounts of dietary fat and cholesterol. In 16 population groups from seven countries (The Seven Countries Study), there was a linear relationship between 10-year CHD mortality rates and median serum cholesterol levels (**A**). A similar relationship was demonstrated between CHD mortality rates and percentage of calories from fat (**B**). For example, in those countries where the consumption of fat constituted about 40% of calories and saturated fat accounted for about 20% of calories such as in Finland, the United States, and the Netherlands, there were higher average serum cholesterol levels and increased mortality from CHD as compared with countries such as Japan and Greece, where saturated fat consumption was less than 10% of calories and serum cholesterol levels were lower. (Part A *adapted from* Keys [51]; part B *adapted from* Keys *et al.* [52].)

PREVENTION TRIALS

DIETARY SECONDARY PREVENTION TRIALS

STUDY	SUBJECT AGE, y	CHOLESTEROL REDUCTION, %	RESULTS
Morrison [53]	40–78	29	Reduced CHD mortality
Rose *et al.* [54]	<70	No change	No effect on mortality or morbidity
Leren [55]	30–64	18	Mortality from MI reduced; overall mortality unchanged
MRC [56]	<65	17	No effect on mortality or morbidity
MRC [57]	<60	17	CHD relapse rate reduced; cardiovascular mortality unchanged
Bierenbaum *et al.* [58]	30–50	10	Reduction in fatal MI and total mortality
Woodhill *et al.* [59]	30–59	7	No dietary factors related to survival

FIGURE 1-41. Dietary secondary prevention trials performed between 1955 and 1980. In general, most studies in which there was a reasonable reduction in serum cholesterol (10% or greater) were associated with beneficial effects. CHD—coronary heart disease; MI—myocardial infarction. (*Adapted from* Pyorala [60].)

STRATEGIES TO IMPROVE COMPLIANCE

Explain reasons for requiring dietary change

Evaluate baseline (habitual) diet

Set specific dietary goals
 Select nutritious, tasty foods that are low in fat and cholesterol
 Develop diet that matches patient's lifestyle

Offer specific recommendations about dietary change

Provide educational materials

Follow-up regularly
 Reinforcement
 Answer questions
 Address problem areas

FIGURE 1-42. Strategies to improve compliance with a cholesterol-lowering diet. To aid compliance, the patient must understand the reason for recommending dietary change. The patient's baseline (habitual) diet should be assessed to determine what high-fat foods are usually consumed and whether to start with a Step I or Step II diet. It is important to set specific dietary goals for the patient. This includes selection of nutritious and tasty foods that are low in fat and cholesterol and provision of sufficient variety to prevent boredom. It is important to develop a diet that matches the patient's lifestyle, from the standpoints of ethnicity, practicality, and taste preferences. Specific recommendations about dietary change need to be made rather than generalizations. This is best done with the help of a qualified dietitian or nutritionist. Provision of educational materials can be helpful in allowing the patient to study aspects of the diet at leisure. Regular follow-up will enhance compliance. Follow-up will allow a reinforcement of the diet, the opportunity for the patient to ask questions related to specific foods, and to address difficulties with compliance.

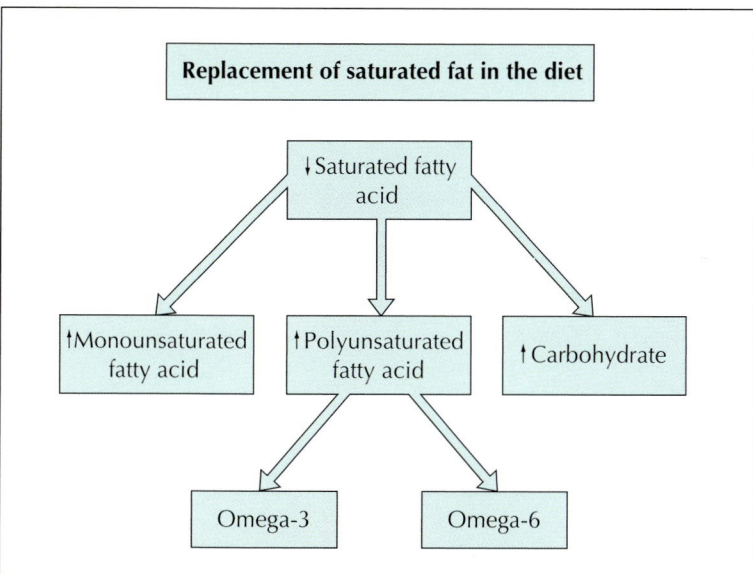

Replacement of saturated fat in the diet

↓Saturated fatty acid → ↑Monounsaturated fatty acid / ↑Polyunsaturated fatty acid / ↑Carbohydrate → Omega-3 / Omega-6

FIGURE 1-43. Replacement of saturated fatty acids in the diet. A decrease in the amount of saturated fatty acids, without replacement, will result in reduced caloric intake. A reduction in the saturated fat content of the diet also can be achieved isocalorically by replacing the saturated fatty acids with either carbohydrates, polyunsaturated fatty acids (either omega-6 or omega-3), or monounsaturated fatty acids. Because saturated fat and cholesterol often are found in the same foods, a reduction in the saturated fatty acid content of the diet is also accompanied by a reduction in dietary cholesterol.

FOODS RICH IN MONOUNSATURATED FATTY ACIDS

Olive oil

Canola (rape seed) oil

Peanut oil

Nuts

Avocados

FIGURE 1-44. Sources of monounsaturated fatty acids (oleic acid). The major oils that contain monounsaturated fatty acids are olive oil, rape seed oil (canola oil), and peanut oil. All these oils also contain small amounts of saturated and unsaturated fatty acids. Nuts and avocados are also rich dietary sources of monounsaturated fatty acids.

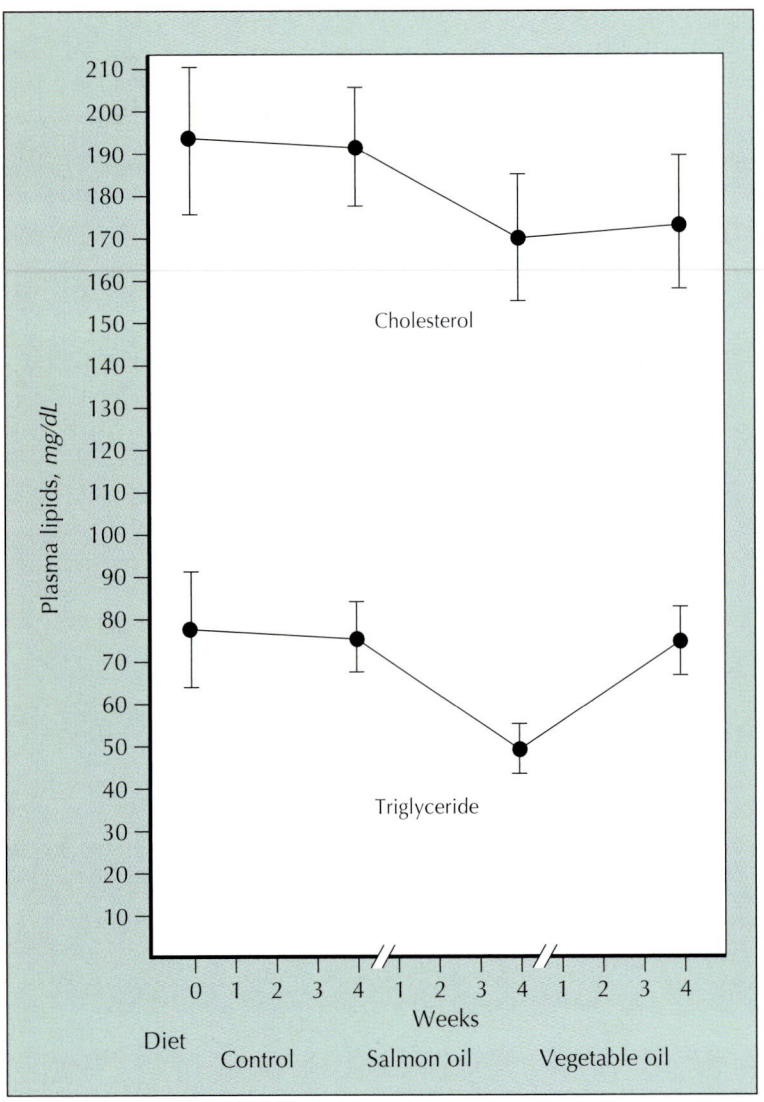

FIGURE 1-45. Effect of fish oils (omega-3 fatty acids) on plasma lipids. In normal subjects, supplements of omega-3 fatty acids primarily lower very low-density lipoprotein (VLDL) levels, which leads to a reduction in both triglycerides and cholesterol. However, LDL cholesterol levels do not change (not shown). HDL levels tend to increase, as is commonly seen, when triglyceride levels fall. Several studies in both humans and experimental animals have suggested that omega-3 fatty acids may reduce atherosclerotic artery disease. Several mechanisms may be responsible for this response. Diets rich in fish oils tend to be low in saturated fatty acids. Omega-3 fatty acids may have an antithrombotic effect, both by interfering with platelet aggregation and by modulating prostaglandin and leukotriene metabolism, which in turn may also impact on vascular tone. These fatty acids may thus be antithrombotic, with consequent effects on atherogenesis and thrombosis.

OBESITY

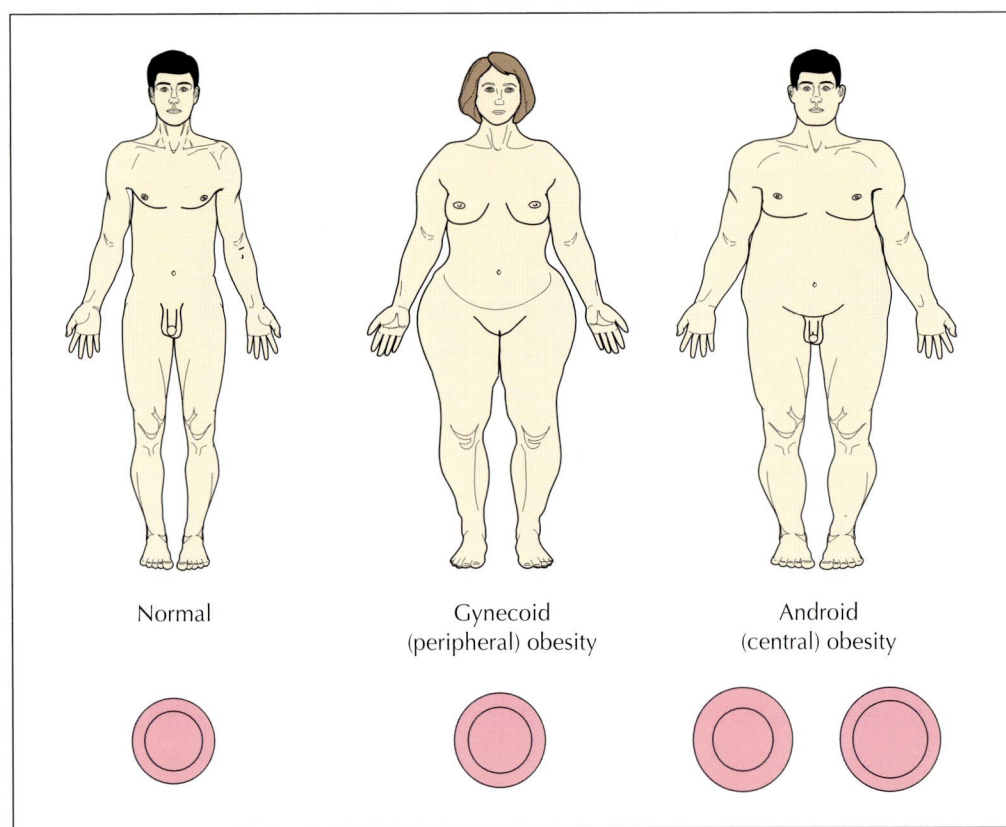

Normal

Gynecoid
(peripheral) obesity

Android
(central) obesity

FIGURE 1-46. There are two major forms of obesity. In gynecoid obesity, which occurs more frequently in females than males, the distribution of excess fat is predominantly around the buttocks and thighs, whereas the upper body fat distribution tends to be normal. Android obesity occurs more commonly in males than females; although the limbs tend to be normal, most of the fat is deposited around the abdomen and chest. Fat deposition in central obesity can either be predominantly subcutaneous, in which most of the excess fat occurs outside the abdominal cavity (central, subcutaneous obesity) or there can be an increased deposition of adipose tissue around the abdominal viscera (central visceral obesity). Central obesity tends to be associated with several atherogenic disorders (*see* Fig. 1–48). There is a hierarchy of association of obesity with atherosclerotic complication such that central visceral obesity is more commonly associated than central subcutaneous obesity, which occurs with greater frequency than gynecoid obesity. Although central obesity is more common in males, when it occurs in females it has the same metabolic and atherogenic consequences as in males.

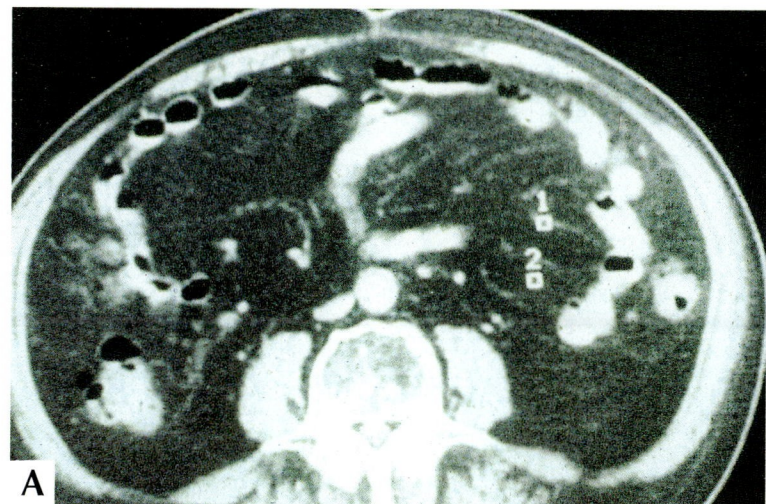
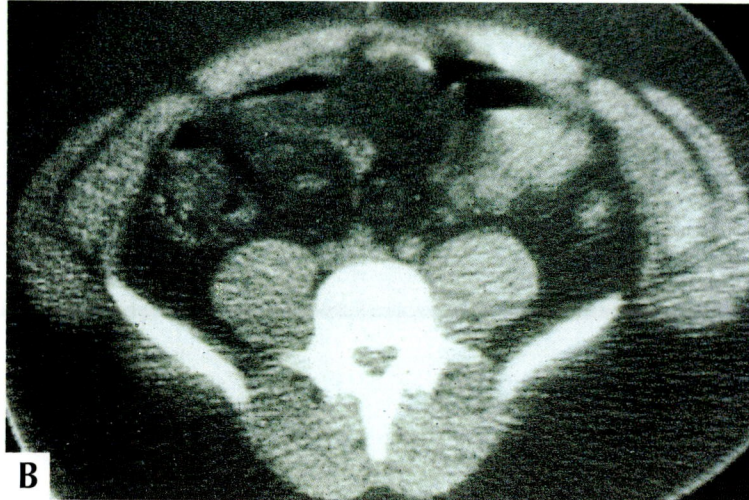

FIGURE 1-47. Computed tomography (CT) to demonstrate distribution of abdominal fat. CT across the central abdomen aorta is the best method of distinguishing visceral from subcutaneous fat deposition. The *black areas* represent fat.

A, This subject can clearly be shown to have an intra-abdominal (visceral) distribution of his adipose tissue that surrounds the viscera.

The amount of subcutaneous fat is normal. **B**, Although having a similar abdominal circumference as the subject in *A*, this subject demonstrates a clearly different distribution of abdominal fat. There is little fat surrounding the viscera, most of the excess fat being deposited subcutaneously and outside the abdominal cavity.

ATHEROGENIC ASSOCIATIONS WITH CENTRAL OBESITY

Insulin resistance

Glucose intolerance and NIDDM

Dyslipidemia

  Hypertriglyceridemia

  Small VLDL and remnants

  Low HDL

  Small dense LDL

Hypertension

FIGURE 1-48. Atherogenic associations with central obesity. Central, particularly visceral, obesity is associated with several metabolic and other disturbances that may increase the risk of cardiovascular disease. These include 1) insulin resistance; 2) glucose intolerance, which sometimes manifests as non–insulin-dependent diabetes mellitus (NIDDM); 3) dyslipidemia; and 4) hypertension. The dyslipidemia reflects one or more of the following abnormalities: hypertriglyceridemia because of the presence of small very low-density lipoprotein (VLDL) particles and their remnants; low levels of HDL; and the presence of small, dense LDL particles. Often the hypertriglyceridemia and low HDL are not very well marked. However, this combination of risk factors is associated with a markedly increased risk of atherosclerotic complications. The constellation of central obesity and insulin resistance, glucose intolerance or NIDDM (or both), dyslipidemia, and hypertension has been termed the "deadly quartet." The relationship between obesity and atherosclerosis is therefore likely to be partly due to the clustering of cardiovascular risk factors that are associated with central obesity.

ANTIOXIDANTS

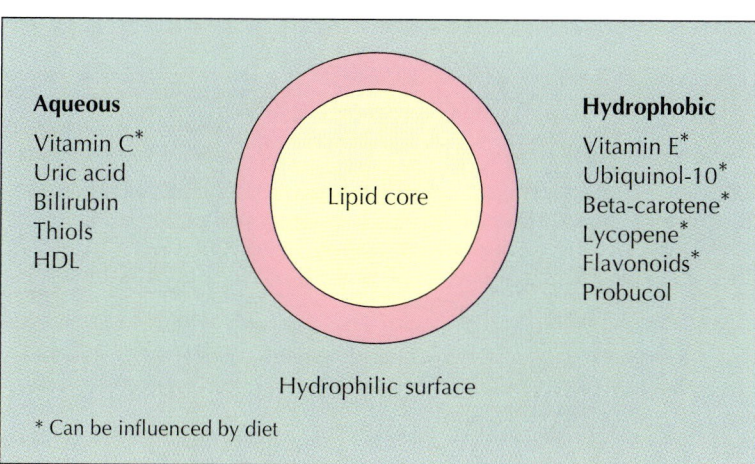

Aqueous

Vitamin C*
Uric acid
Bilirubin
Thiols
HDL

Lipid core

Hydrophobic

Vitamin E*
Ubiquinol-10*
Beta-carotene*
Lycopene*
Flavonoids*
Probucol

Hydrophilic surface

* Can be influenced by diet

FIGURE 1-49. Antioxidants and lipoprotein oxidation. Lipoprotein particles consist of a hydrophobic lipid core (containing cholesterol esters, triglycerides, and hydrophobic antioxidants) surrounded by a hydrophilic surface (comprised of unesterified cholesterol, phospholipids, and apolipoproteins). There are two major classes of antioxidants that can affect lipoprotein oxidation. The first includes antioxidants present in the aqueous milieu of the lipoproteins such as vitamin C, uric acid, bilirubin, thiols, and HDL. The second group of antioxidants, which are hydrophobic, includes vitamin E, ubiquinol-10, beta-carotene, lycopene, and flavonoids. These become incorporated into the central lipid core and are transported together with the lipoprotein particle. Antioxidant drugs such as probucol are very hydrophobic and become incorporated into the lipid core. Other antioxidant drugs can act in the aqueous milieu of the lipoprotein.

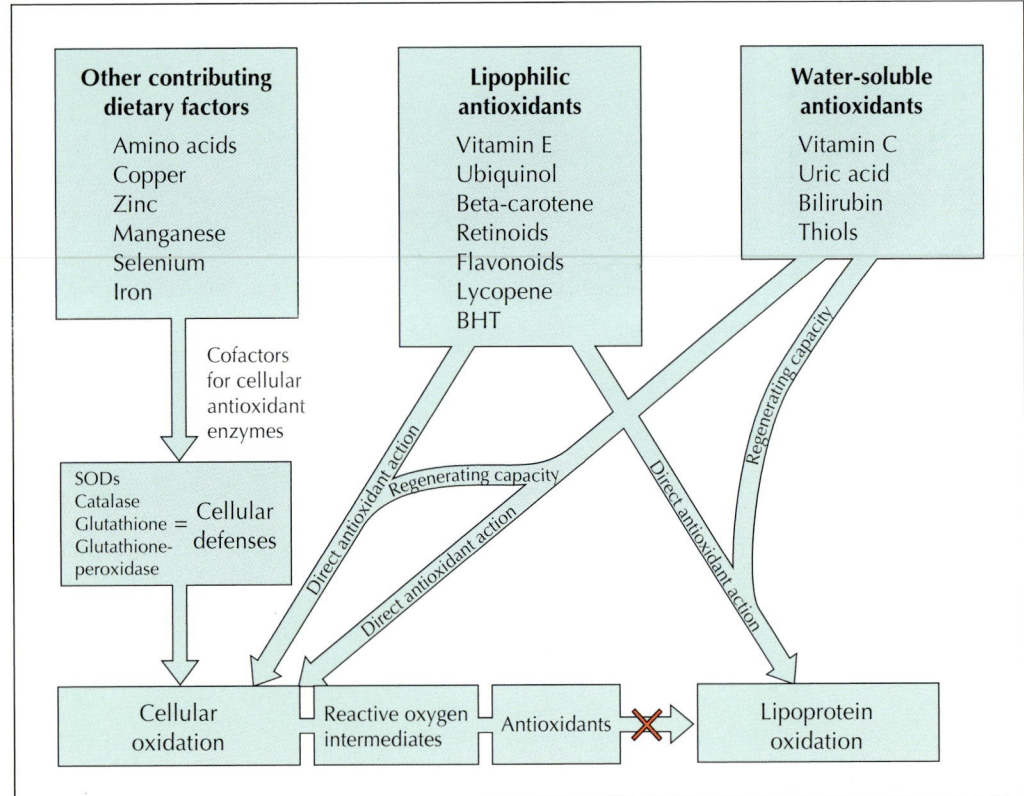

Figure 1-50. Potential roles of dietary factors in protection against destructive oxidative mechanisms. Normal cellular oxidative mechanisms occur in the mitochondria or plasma membranes of certain cells and contribute to the oxidative modification of lipoproteins by supplying reactive oxygen intermediates to initiate lipid peroxidation. This illustration demonstrates how dietary factors could contribute to regulating these processes by: 1) acting as chainbreaking antioxidants (*eg*, lipophilic dietary antioxidants such as vitamin E); 2) regenerating the antioxidant capacity of the lipophilic antioxidants (*eg*, water-soluble antioxidants such as vitamin C); or 3) stimulating the normal cellular antioxidant pathways (*eg*, other contributing dietary factors such as copper, zinc, manganese, and selenium, which are cofactors for antioxidant enzymes such as the superoxide dismutases [SODs] and glutathione peroxidase). BHT—butylated hydroxytoluene.

Drug Treatment

GUIDELINES FOR DRUG TREATMENT

GUIDELINES FOR DRUG TREATMENT OF LDL CHOLESTEROL		
	LEVEL FOR DRUG CONSIDERATION, *mg/dL (mmol/L)*	GOAL OF THERAPY, *mg/dL (mmol/L)*
Secondary prevention		
Clinical evidence of CHD or other atherosclerotic disease	≥130 (3.3)	≤100 (2.6)
Primary prevention		
With two (or more) other risk factors	≥160 (4.1)	<130 (3.3)
Without two (or more) other risk factors	≥190 (4.9)	<160 (4.1)

Figure 1-51. Guidelines for drug treatment of low-density lipo-protein (LDL) cholesterol. Secondary prevention includes all patients with clinical evidence of coronary heart disease (CHD), definite thrombotic stroke or transient ischemic attacks, abdominal aortic aneurysm, or evidence of peripheral arterial disease, including claudication or prior interventional procedures. For patients with CHD and LDL cholesterol levels between 100 and 129 mg/dL, clinical judgment is required to either initiate therapy or to add additional drug(s). In primary prevention, an LDL cholesterol level of 220 mg/dL or higher is suggested for initiating drug therapy in men younger than 35 years of age or premenopausal women in the absence of other risk factors.

FIGURE 1-52. *High risk,* defined as a net of two or more coronary heart disease (CHD) risk factors, leads to more vigorous intervention. Age (defined differently for men and women) is treated as a risk factor because rates of CHD are higher in the elderly than the young, and in men than women of the same age. Use of antihypertensive medication has not produced the expected reduction in CHD risk and, thus, treated hypertension continues as a risk factor. High-density lipoprotein (HDL) cholesterol levels decrease CHD risk and, thus, one risk factor is subtracted. Although obesity is not listed as a risk factor because it operates through other risk factors that are included (hypertension, hyperlipidemia, decreased HDL cholesterol, and diabetes mellitus), it should be considered a target for intervention. Physical inactivity is similarly not listed as a risk factor, but it too should be considered a target for intervention.

EFFECT OF DRUGS ON LIPOPROTEIN METABOLISM

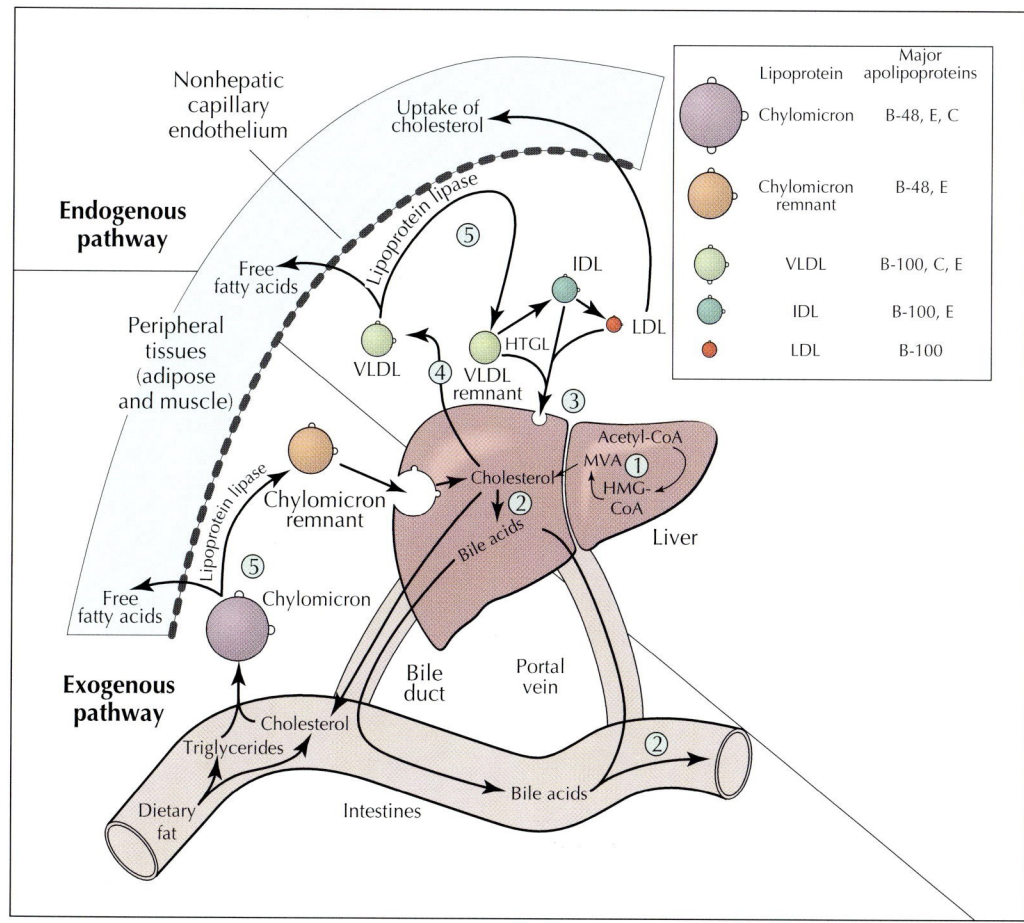

FIGURE 1-53. Overview of lipoprotein metabolism [61]. This illustration depicts the five major sites for drug action that are associated with LDL or triglyceride lowering. The major mechanism for lowering LDL involves an increase in LDL receptor numbers (3). Increases in the number of LDL receptors occur when there is a decrease in the cholesterol content of hepatic and other cells. This can occur either by decreasing the rate-limiting enzyme in cholesterol synthesis (hydroxymethyl glutaryl-coenzyme A [HMG-CoA] reductase) (1) or increasing the fecal excretion of bile acids with the resulting decrease in the bile acid pool (2). Enhanced receptor activity (3) increases the removal of LDL plus the precursors of LDL, very low-density lipoprotein (VLDL) remnants, and intermediate-density lipoprotein (IDL). Thus, the formation of LDL can also be decreased. VLDL remnants and IDL also contain triglycerides and thus a modest decrease in triglycerides may be observed. Inhibition of lipoprotein synthesis (4) decreases the synthesis or secretion of VLDL, the major triglyceride-carrying lipoprotein. Secondarily, the formation of VLDL remnants, IDL, and LDL are decreased and both LDL cholesterol and triglyceride levels are reduced. Increased lipoprotein lipase activity (5) facilitates the removal of triglycerides from both chylomicrons and VLDL. These smaller particles may then be removed from the circulation by the remnant receptor. Moreover, the VLDL remnants can proceed to the formation of IDL and LDL, which can be removed by the LDL receptor. Acetyl-CoA—acetyl coenzyme A; HTGL—hepatic triglyceride lipase; MVA—mevalonate.

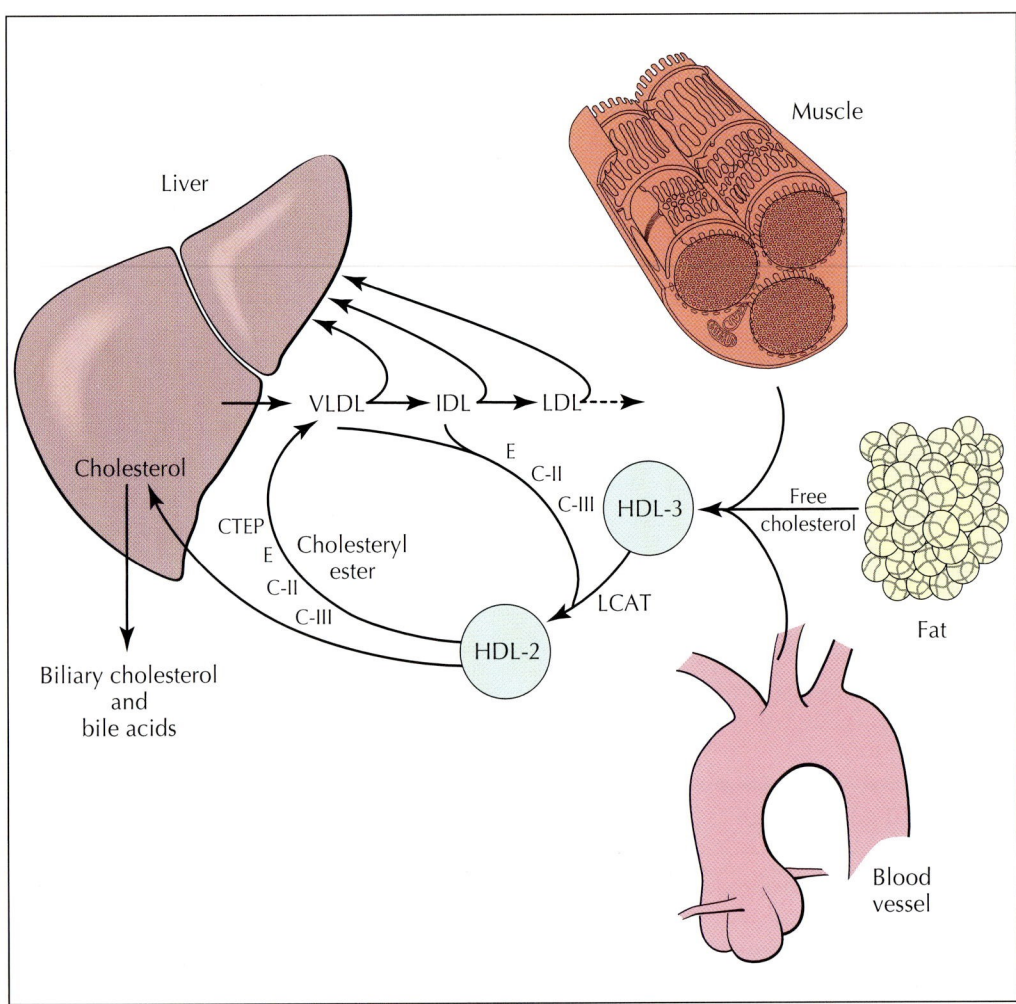

Figure 1-54. HDL metabolism. The formation and metabolism of HDL are very complex and the mechanism of action of drugs that either increase or decrease HDL have not been well established [62,63]. Apolipoprotein (apo) A-1 is the major protein in HDL, and apo A-1 levels appear to correlate best with changes in HDL levels. Thus, drugs that either increase the synthesis or decrease the catabolism of apo A-1 would be expected to increase HDL levels. However, the origins of the various components of HDL are diffuse and there is an extensive exchange of protein, phospholipid, cholesterol (free and esterified), and triglycerides between HDL and other lipoproteins. Drugs have the potential for influencing HDL levels and function by multiple mechanisms. Because of the complexity and poor understanding, no further discussion of the effects of individual drugs on HDL metabolism is included in this chapter. CETP—cholesteryl ester transfer protein; IDL—intermediate-density lipoprotein; LCAT—lecithin-cholesterol acyltransferase; VLDL—very low-density lipoprotein.

BILE ACID SEQUESTRANTS

OVERVIEW OF BILE ACID SEQUESTRANTS

Administered as a powder that must be hydrated in an aqueous vehicle

One sequestrant (colestipol) is available in tablet form

Not absorbed from the gastrointestinal tract

Evidence for reduction in risk of coronary heart disease

Evidence of long-term safety

Primary effect is to lower LDL cholesterol levels

Used as single-drug therapy or in combination with other lipid-lowering drugs

Recommended as initial therapy in young adults, women with childbearing potential, or low-risk patients

Acceptance by both patients and health professionals is frequently low because of inconvenience, poor palatability, gastrointestinal complaints, and interference with absorption of other drugs

For active drug in the powder form, efficacy of 5 g of colestipol is equal to 4 g of cholestyramine

Figure 1-55. Overview of bile acid sequestrants. Bile acid sequestrants are effective in lowering LDL cholesterol levels but patient acceptance, especially of higher doses, is frequently low. They are ideal drugs for initial therapy in low-risk patients with moderate elevations of LDL cholesterol or in patients in whom long-term safety considerations are of major importance.

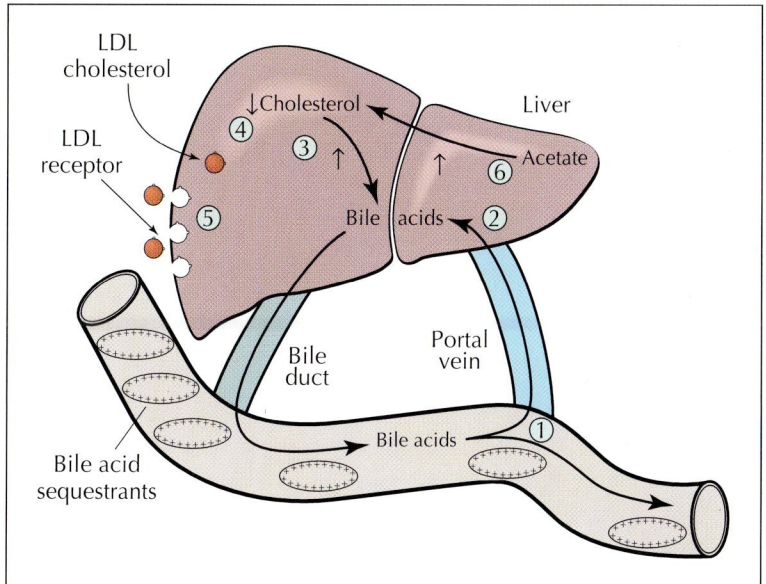

FIGURE 1-56. Mechanism of action of bile acid sequestrants [63,64]. The bile acid sequestrants are highly charged resins that are not absorbed. They form insoluble complexes with bile acids in the gut and increase their fecal excretion (1). There is a decrease in the recirculation and pool of bile acids (2) resulting in a compensatory increase in the conversion of cholesterol to bile acids (3). Hepatic cholesterol content is decreased (4) with an increase in LDL receptor numbers (5) and an increased rate of removal of LDL from the circulation. However, there is also a compensatory increase in cholesterol synthesis (6), which limits the increase in LDL receptors and the decrease in plasma LDL receptors that can be achieved.

STATINS

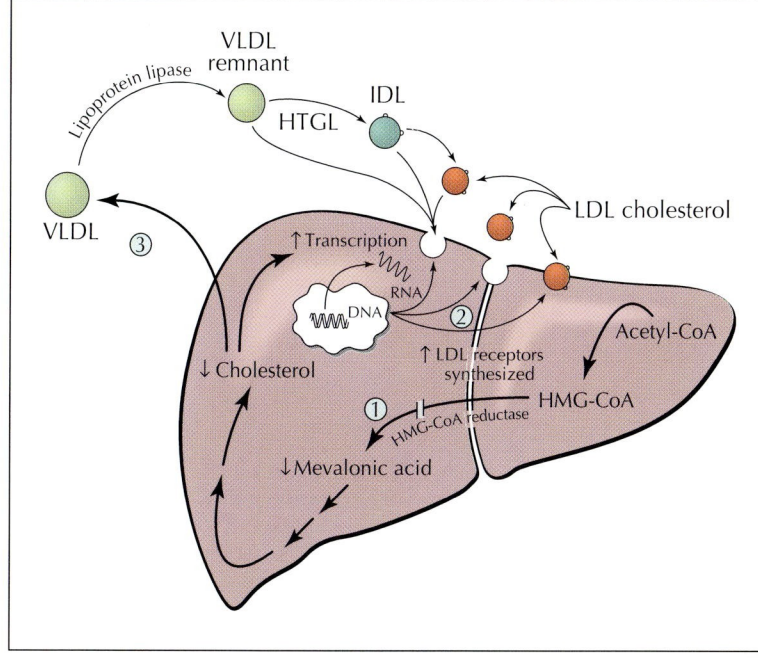

FIGURE 1-57. Mechanism of action of statins [65,66]. The statins inhibit the rate-limiting enzyme, hydroxymethyl glutaryl-coenzyme A (HMG-CoA) reductase, in cholesterol biosynthesis (1). The major organs for cholesterol biosynthesis are the small intestine and liver. The associated decrease in hepatic and cellular cholesterol concentration stimulates the production of LDL receptors, which increase the rate of removal of LDL from the plasma (2). There is also increased removal of very low-density lipoprotein (VLDL) remnants and intermediate-density lipoprotein (IDL), which are precursors to LDL formation. In some patients, there may also be a decrease in lipoprotein synthesis (3). The enhanced removal of VLDL remnants and IDL and the inhibition of lipoprotein synthesis may contribute to the modest triglyceride-lowering effect of the statins. Acetyl-CoA—acetyl coenzyme A; HTGL—hepatic triglyceride lipase.

CLINICAL TRIALS WITH STATINS

A. ANGIOGRAPHIC TRIALS

Clinical evidence of a beneficial effect on the atherosclerotic process:

Reduced rates of progression/increased regression in the coronary arteries

Preliminary evidence of reduced progression in the carotid and peripheral arteries (angiographic or ultrasound studies)

Some studies also show a reduced number of CHD events

Representative studies include:

Monitored Atherosclerosis Regression Study (MARS) [66]

Canadian Coronary Artery Intervention Trial (CCAIT) [67]

Pravastatin Limitation of Atherosclerosis in Coronary Arteries (PLAC–1) [68]

Pravastatin, Lipids, and Atherosclerosis in the Carotid Arteries (PLAC–2) [69]

Asymptomatic Carotid Artery Plaque Study (ACAPS) [70]

B. CLINICAL ENDPOINT TRIALS

Pravastatin Multinational Study [71]

Scandinavian Simvastatin Survival Study [72]

Most definitive trial to date involving 4444 participants with evidence of CHD who were followed for 5.4 y

Simvastatin administration associated with a 30%–44% reduction in total mortality and major CHD events

West of Scotland Study [73]

Pravastatin treatment reduced CHD events by 32% and mortality by 22%

Cholesterol and Recurrent Events (CARE) Trial (74)

Pravastatin treatment reduced coronary events by 24% in CHD patients with average total cholesterol (209 mg/dl)

Long-term Intervention with Pravastatin in Ischemic Disease (LIPID) Trial (75)

Pravastatin treatment reduced coronary events by 24% in CHD patients

Air Force/Texas Coronary Atherosclerosis Study (AFCAPS/TexCAPS) (76)

Lovastatin reduced fatal and nonfatal MI by 40% in normal middle-aged subjects

FIGURE 1-58. Clinical trials with statins [66–72]. **A,** Angiographic trials. **B,** Clinical endpoint trials. The Scandinavian Simvastatin Survival Study [72] conclusively demonstrated the benefits of LDL cholesterol lowering in patients with coronary heart disease (CHD). The recent West of Scotland Study has given very similar results in patients who did not have CHD at entry [72]. The smaller angiographic trials demonstrated reduced rates of progression in the coronary arteries. A reduction in clinical events has also been demonstrated in meta-analyses of these trials and also in some individual trials.

SIDE EFFECTS OF STATINS

INCREASED TRANSAMINASE LEVELS

1%–2% of treated patients develop increases of > 3 × upper-normal limit, especially at higher doses

Rapidly reversible, no evidence of chronic liver disease

MYOPATHY

Diffuse muscle pain and CPK > 10 × upper-normal limit

Primarily seen when higher doses of statins are used in combination with cyclosporine, gemfibrozil, and occasionally erythromycin and niacin

CATARACTS, LENS OPACITIES

No clinical evidence for increased risk

FIGURE 1-59. Side effects of statins [77,78]. The side effect profile of the statins is very favorable, considering their efficacy in lowering LDL cholesterol levels. Initial monitoring of transaminase levels is indicated, but abnormalities are rapidly reversible with a reduction in dosage; discontinuance of drug is rarely required. Myopathy is a clinical diagnosis that is confirmed by marked elevations of creatine phosphokinase (CPK) levels. Early diagnosis and reduction of dose or discontinuance of drug is required to prevent rhabdomyolysis and renal failure. The incidence of all side effects is low. If side effects do occur, use of another statin may be attempted.

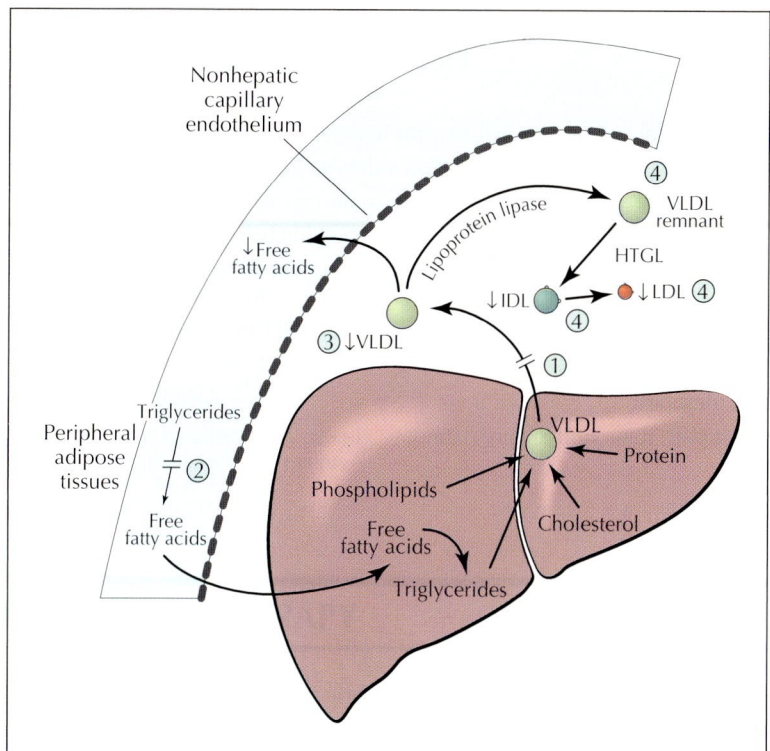

FIGURE 1-60. Mechanism of action of nicotinic acid. Inhibition of lipoprotein synthesis is generally considered to be the major effect of nicotinic acid (1). Inhibition of lipolysis of the stored fat in adipose tissue (2) with the resultant decrease in free fatty acids delivered to the liver could also indirectly decrease lipoprotein synthesis. The clinical significance of this mechanism has not been well documented in humans. Inhibition of lipoprotein synthesis decreases very low-density lipoprotein (VLDL) secretion or synthesis (3), and all subsequent lipoproteins in this pathway (VLDL remnants, intermediate-density lipoprotein [IDL] and LDL) are also decreased (4). Nicotinic acid may also modestly lower lipoprotein (a) levels by unknown mechanism(s). HTGL—hepatic triglyceride lipase.

NICOTINIC ACID PREPARATIONS

NICOTINAMIDE

No lipid-altering effects

NICOTINIC ACID

Crystalline- or immediate-release preparation

  Most effective drug for increasing HDL cholesterol

  Large doses are required to achieve significant decreases in LDL cholesterol

Sustained or slow-release preparation

  Used primarily for lowering LDL cholesterol or if crystalline-release preparation is not tolerated

  More effective than crystalline-release preparations for lowering LDL cholesterol, but less effective for raising HDL cholesterol

  Risk of severe hepatotoxicity is greater than for crystalline-release preparations

FIGURE 1-61. Nicotinic acid preparations [64,79,80]. Because these preparations are available without a prescription, patients must be instructed to take nicotinic acid or niacin only. The use of slow-release preparations is still controversial and some investigators and clinicians do not recommend their use.

44. Janus CK, Nicoll AM, Turner PR, *et al.*: Kinetic basis of the primary hyperlipidemias: studies of apolipoprotein B turnover in genetically defined subjects. *Eur J Clin Invest* 1980, 10:161–172.

45. Kissebah AH, Alfarsi S, Evans DJ: Low density lipoprotein metabolism in familial combined hyperlipidemia. Mechanisms of the multiple lipoprotein phenotypic expression. *Arteriosclerosis* 1984, 4:614–624.

46. Kesaniemi YA, Vega GL, Grundy SM: Kinetics of apolipoprotein B in normal and hyperlipidemic man: review of current data. In *Lipoprotein in Kinetics and Modeling*. Edited by Berman M, Grundy SM, Howard BV. New York: Academic Press; 1982:181–205.

47. Chait A, Robertson HT, Brunzell JD: Chylomicronemia syndrome in diabetes mellitus. *Diabetes Care* 1981, 4:343–348.

48. Carlson LA, Rosenhamer G: Reduction of mortality in the Stockholm Ischaemic Heart Disease Secondary Prevention Study by combined treatment with clofibrate and nicotinic acid. *Acta Med Scand* 1988, 223:405–418.

49. Manninen V, Elo O, Frick MH, *et al.*: Lipid alterations and decline in the incidence of coronary heart disease in the Helsinki Heart Study. *JAMA* 1988, 260:641–651.

50. Rubins HB, Robins SJ, Collins D, *et al.*: Gemfibrozil for the secondary prevention of coronary heart disease in men with low levels of high-density lipoprotein cholesterol. *N Engl J Med* 1999, 341:410–418.

51. Keys A: Coronary heart disease in seven countries. *Circulation* 1970, 41(suppl I):I-1–I-211.

52. Keys A, Menotti A, Karvonen MJ, *et al.*: The diet and 15-year death rate in the seven countries study. *Am J Epidemiol* 1986, 124:903–915.

53. Morrison LM: A nutritional program for prolongation of life in coronary atherosclerosis. *JAMA* 1955, 159:1425–1430.

54. Rose G, Thompson WB, Williams RT: Corn oil in treatment of ischaemic heart disease. *BMJ* 1965, 1:1531–1533.

55. Leren P: The Oslo Diet-Heart Study: eleven-year report. *Circulation* 1970, 62:935–942.

56. Research Committee to the Medical Research Council: Low fat diet in myocardial infarction: a controlled trial. *Lancet* 1965, 2:500–504.

57. Research Committee to the Medical Research Council: Controlled trial of soya bean oil in myocardial infarction. *Lancet* 1968, 2:693–699.

58. Bierenbaum MI, Fleischman AI, Raichelson RI, *et al.*: Ten year experience of modified-fat diets on younger men with coronary heart disease. *Lancet* 1973, 1:1404–1407.

59. Woodhill JM, Palmer AJ, Leelarthaepin B, *et al.*: Low fat, low cholesterol diet in secondary prevention of coronary heart disease. *Adv Exp Med Biol* 1978, 109:317–331.

60. Pyorala K: Clinical perspectives on blood lipids: clinical trials of lipid lowering. London: Current Medical Literature; 1988.

61. Ginsberg HN: Lipoprotein metabolism and its relationship to atherosclerosis. *Med Clin North Am* 1994, 78:1–20.

62. Shepherd J, Packard CJ: High density lipoprotein metabolism. *Atheroscler Rev* 1993, 24:17–43.

63. Sirtori CR, Manzoni C, Lovati MR: Mechanisms of lipid-lowering agents. *Cardiology* 1991, 78:226–235.

64. Hunninghake DB: Drug treatment of dyslipoproteinemia. *Endocrinol Metab Clin North Am* 1990, 19:345–360.

65. Bilheimer DW, Grundy SM, Brown MS, *et al.*: Mevinolin and colestipol stimulate receptor-mediated clearance of low density lipoprotein from plasma in familiar hypercholesterolemia heterozygoses. *Proc Natl Acad Sci USA* 1983, 80:4124–4128.

66. Blankenhorn DH, Azen SP, Kramsch DM, *et al.*: Coronary angiographic changes with lovastatin therapy. The Monitored Atherosclerosis Regression Study (MARS). *Ann Intern Med* 1993, 19:969–976.

67. Waters D, Higginson L, Gladstone P, *et al.*: Effects of monotherapy with an HMG-CoA reductase inhibitor on the progression of coronary atherosclerosis as assessed by serial quantitative arteriography. The Canadian Coronary Atherosclerosis Intervention Trial. *Circulation* 1994, 89:959–968.

68. Pitt B, Mancini GBJ, Ellis SG, *et al.*: Pravastatin limitation of atherosclerosis in the coronary arteries (PLAC I): reduction in atherosclerosis progression and clinical events. *J Am Coll Cardiol* 1995, 26:1133–1139.

69. Crouse JR, Byington RP, Bond MG, *et al.*: Pravastatin, lipids and atherosclerosis in the carotid arteries (PLAC-II). *Am J Cardiol* 1995, 75:455–459.

70. Furberg CD, Adams HP, Applegate WB, *et al.*: Effect of lovastatin on early carotid atherosclerosis and cardiovascular events. *Circulation* 1994, 90:1679–1687.

71. Pravastatin Multinational Study Group for Cardiac Risk Patients: Effects of pravastatin in patients with serum total cholesterol levels from 5.2 to 7.8 mmol/liter (200 to 300 mg/dl) plus two additional atherosclerotic risk factors. *Am J Cardiol* 1993, 72:1031–1037.

72. Scandinavian Simvastatin Survival Group: Randomized trial of cholesterol lowering 4,444 patients with coronary heart disease: the Scandinavian Simvastatin Survival Study (4S). *Lancet* 1994, 344:1383–1389.

73. Shepherd J, Cobbe SM, Ford I, *et al.*: Prevention of coronary heart disease with pravastatin in men with hypercholesterolemia. *N Engl J Med* 1995, 333:1301–1307.

74. Sacks FM, Pfeffer MA, Moye LA, *et al.*, for the Cholesterol and Recurrent Events Trial Investigators: The effect of pravastatin on coronary events after myocardial infarction in patients with average cholesterol levels. *N Engl J Med* 1996, 335(14):1001–1009.

75. The Long-Term Intervention with Pravastatin in Ischaemic Disease (LIPID) Study Group: Prevention of cardiovascular events and death with pravastatin in patients with coronary heart disease and a broad range of initial cholesterol levels. *N Engl J Med* 1998, 339(19):1349–57.

76. Downs JR, Clearfield M, Weis S, *et al.*, for the Air Force/Texas Coronary Atherosclerosis Research Group: Primary prevention of acute coronary events with lovastatin in men and women with average cholesterol levels: results of AFCAPS/TexCAPS. *JAMA* 1998, 279(20):1615–1622.

77. Bradford R, Sher CL, Chermos AN, *et al.*: Expanded Clinical Evaluation of Lovastatin (EXCEL) Study results: I. Efficacy in modifying plasma lipoproteins and adverse event profile in 8245 patients with moderate hypercholesterolemia. *Arch Intern Med* 1991, 51:43–49.

78. Blum CB: Comparison of properties of four inhibitors of 3-hydroxy-3-methylglutarylcoenzyme A reductase. *Am J Cardiol* 1994, 73(suppl):3D–11D.

79. Illingworth DR, Stein EA, Mitchel YB, *et al.*: Comparative effects of lovastatin and niacin in primary hypercholesterolemia: a prospective trial. *Arch Intern Med* 1994, 154:1586–1595.

80. McKenney JM, Proctor JD, Harris S, *et al.*: A comparison of the efficacy and toxic effects of sustained- vs immediate-release niacin in hypercholesterolemic patients. *JAMA* 1994, 271:672–677.

81. Coronary Drug Project Research Group: Clofibrate and niacin in coronary heart disease. *JAMA* 1975, 231:360–381.

82. Canner PL, Berge KG, Wenger NK, *et al.*: Fifteen-year mortality in coronary drug project patients: long-term benefit with niacin. *J Am Coll Cardiol* 1986, 8:1245–1255.

83. Stewart JM, Packard CJ, Lorimer AR, *et al.*: Effects of bezafibrate on receptor-mediated and receptor-independent low density lipoprotein catabolism in type II hyperlipoproteinaemic subjects. *Atherosclerosis* 1982, 44:355–365.

84. Blankenhorn DH, Nessim SA, Johnson RL, *et al.*: Beneficial effects of combined colestipol-niacin therapy on coronary atherosclerosis and coronary venous bypass grafts. *JAMA* 1987, 257:3233–3240.

85. Brown G, Albers JJ, Fisher LD, *et al.*: Regression of coronary artery disease as a result of intensive lipid-lowering therapy in men with high levels of apolipoprotein B. *N Engl J Med* 1990, 323:1289–1298.

86. Yuan J, Tsai M, Hunninghake DB: Changes in composition and distribution of LDL subspecies in hypertriglyceridemic and hypercholesterolemic patients during gemfibrozil therapy. *Atherosclerosis* 1994, 110:1–11.

87. WHO Monica Project: A co-operative trial in the primary prevention of ischemic heart disease using clofibrate. *Br Heart J* 1978, 40:1069–1118.

88. Committee of Principal Investigators: WHO cooperative trial on primary prevention of ischemic heart disease with clofibrate to lower serum cholesterol: final mortality follow-up. *Lancet* 1984, 2:600–604.

89. Frick MH, Elo O, Haapa K, *et al.*: Helsinki Heart Study: primary-prevention trial with gemfibrozil in middle-aged men with dyslipidemia: safety of treatment, changes in risk factors, and incidence of coronary heart disease. *N Engl J Med* 1987, 317:1237–1245.

90. Huttunen JK, Heinonen OP, Manninen V, *et al.*: The Helsinki Heart Study: an 8.5 year safety and mortality follow-up. *J Intern Med* 1994, 235:31–39.

91. Colditz GA, Willett WC, Stampfer MJ, *et al.*: Menopause and the risk of coronary heart disease in women. *N Engl J Med* 1987, 316:1105–1110.

92. Stampfer MJ, Colditz GA: Estrogen replacement therapy and coronary heart disease: a quantitative assessment of the epidemiologic evidence. *Prev Med* 1991, 20:47–63.

93. Sullivan JM, Vander Zwaag R, *et al.*: Estrogen replacement and coronary artery disease: effect on survival in postmenopausal women. *Ann Intern Med* 1990, 150:2557–2562.

94. Grady D, Rubin SM, Petitti DB, *et al.*: Hormone therapy to prevent disease and prolong life in postmenopausal women. *Ann Intern Med* 1992, 117:1016–1037.

95. Granfone A, Campos H, McNamara JR, *et al.*: Effects of estrogen replacement on plasma lipoproteins and apolipoproteins in postmenopausal, dyslipidemic women. *Metabolism* 1992, 41:1193–1198.

96. National Cholesterol Education Program: Second report of the National Cholesterol Education Program (NCEP) expert panel on detection, evaluation, and treatment of high blood cholesterol in adults (adult treatment panel II). *Circulation* 1994, 89:1329–1445.

97. Ridker PM: Novel risk factors and markers for coronary disease. *Adv Intern Med* 2000, 45:391–418.

98. Ridker PM, Genest J, Libby P: In *Heart Disease: A Textbook of Cardiovascular Medicine*, edn 6. Edited by Braunwald E, Zipes DP, Libby P. Philadelphia: WB Saunders; 2001:1010–1039.

99. Libby P, Ridker PM: Novel inflammatory markers of coronary risk: theory versus practice. *Circulation* 1999, 100(11):1148–1150.

100. Ridker PM, Glynn RJ, Hennekens CH: C-reactive protein adds to the predictive value of total and HDL cholesterol in determining risk of first myocardial infarction. *Circulation* 1998, 97(20):2007–2011.

101. Prevention of coronary heart disease in clinical practice. Recommendations of the Second Joint Task Force of European and other Societies on coronary prevention. *Eur Heart J* 1998, 19(10):1434–1503.

102. Ansell BJ, Watson KE, Fogelman AM: An evidence-based assessment of the NCEP Adult Treatment Panel II guidelines. National Cholesterol Education Program. *JAMA* 1999, 282(21):2051–2057.

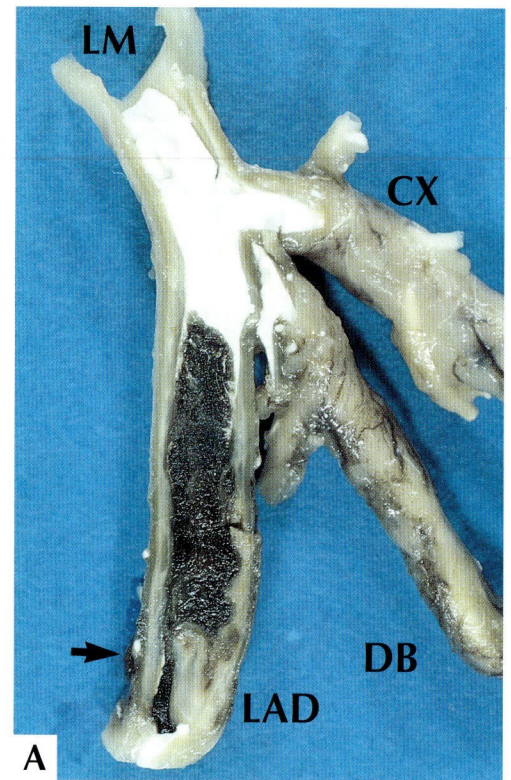

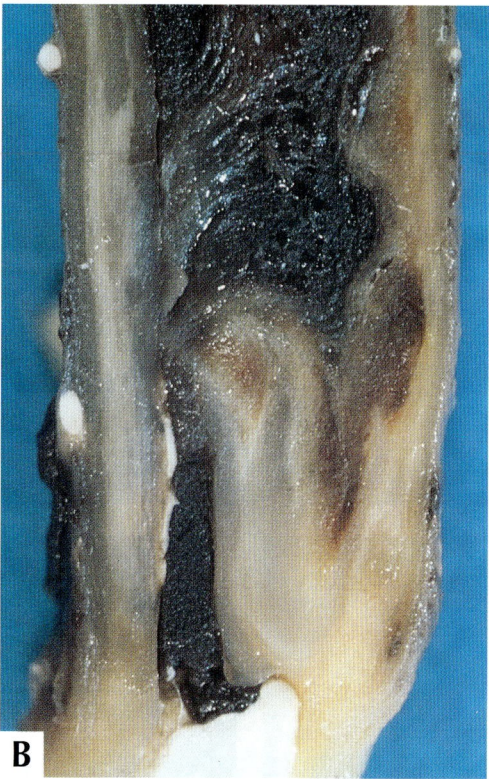

FIGURE 2-8. Secondary to flow reduction, a red stagnation thrombus may propagate upstream. **A** and **B,** The proximal left anterior descending coronary artery (LAD) has been cut open longitudinally. A ruptured plaque with a gray-white occluding thrombus (platelet-rich) can be seen at the *arrow* in *A* (magnified in *B*), and a red thrombus (erythrocyte-rich) is seen propagating upstream up to the first diagonal branch (DB). **C** and **D,** A thrombosed right coronary artery, showing a red thrombus propagating upstream and passing a side branch (SB) without occluding it. The platelet-rich thrombus causing the initial flow reduction is marked (*arrow*). **E** and **F,** Specimen of partly opened, thrombosed right coronary artery and corresponding angiogram showing total occlusion at and just proximal to the acute branch (AB) as well as an extensive filling defect propagating upstream without occluding any major side branches. CX—circumflex branch; LM—left main stem. (Panel A *from* Falk [10]; with permission; panel D *from* Falk [11]; with permission.)

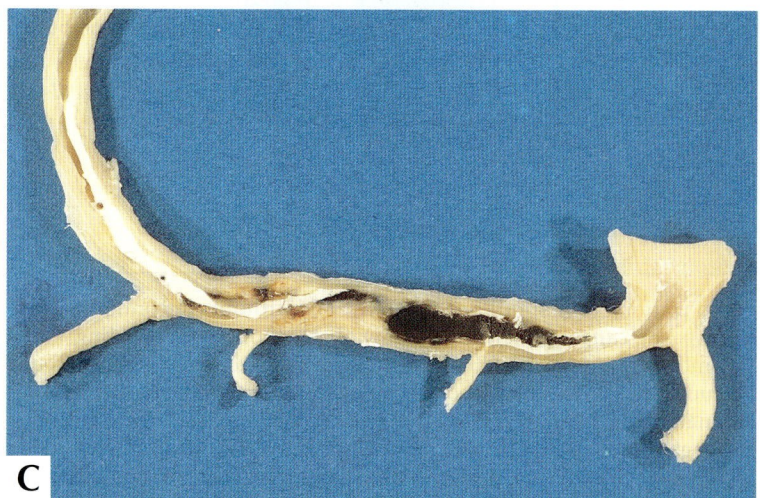

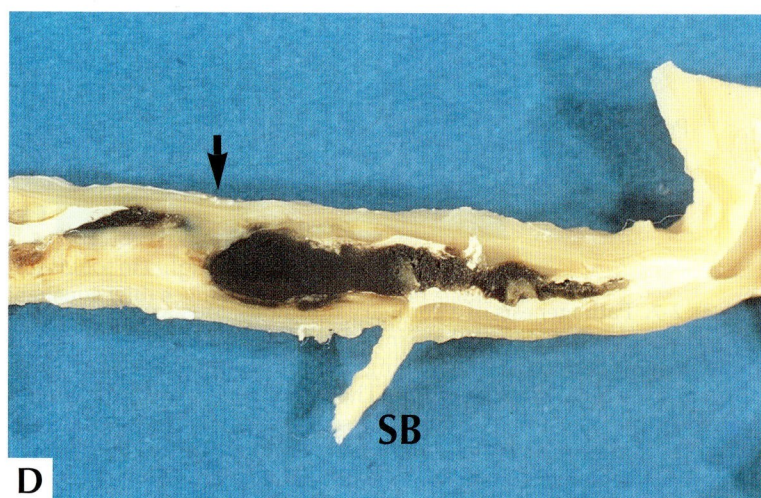

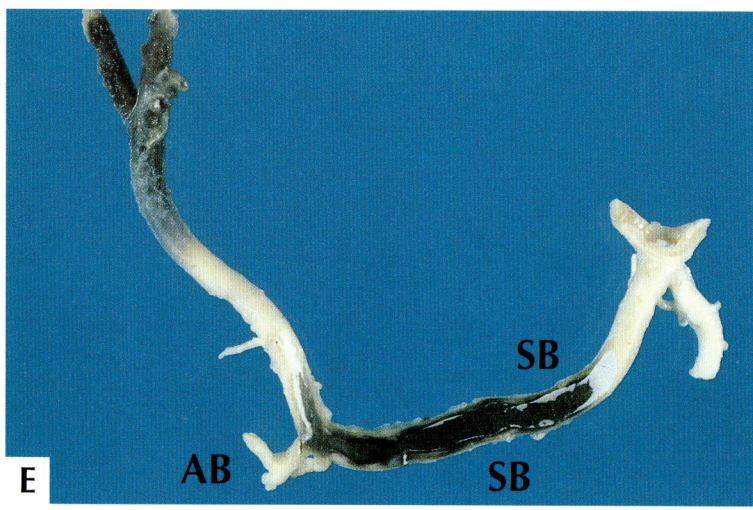

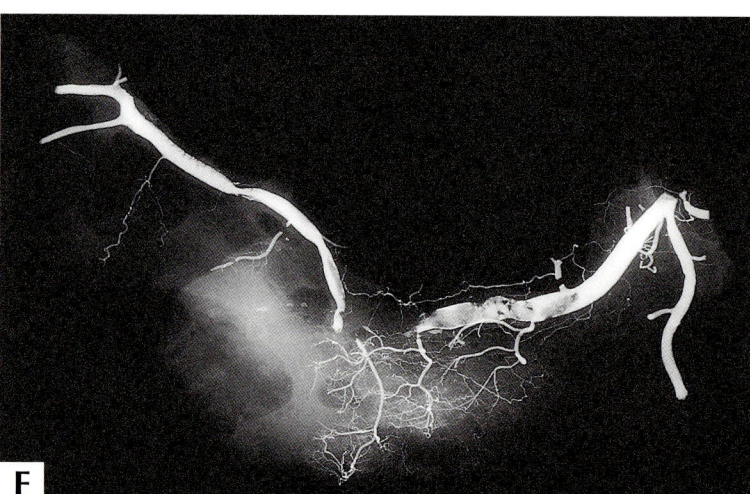

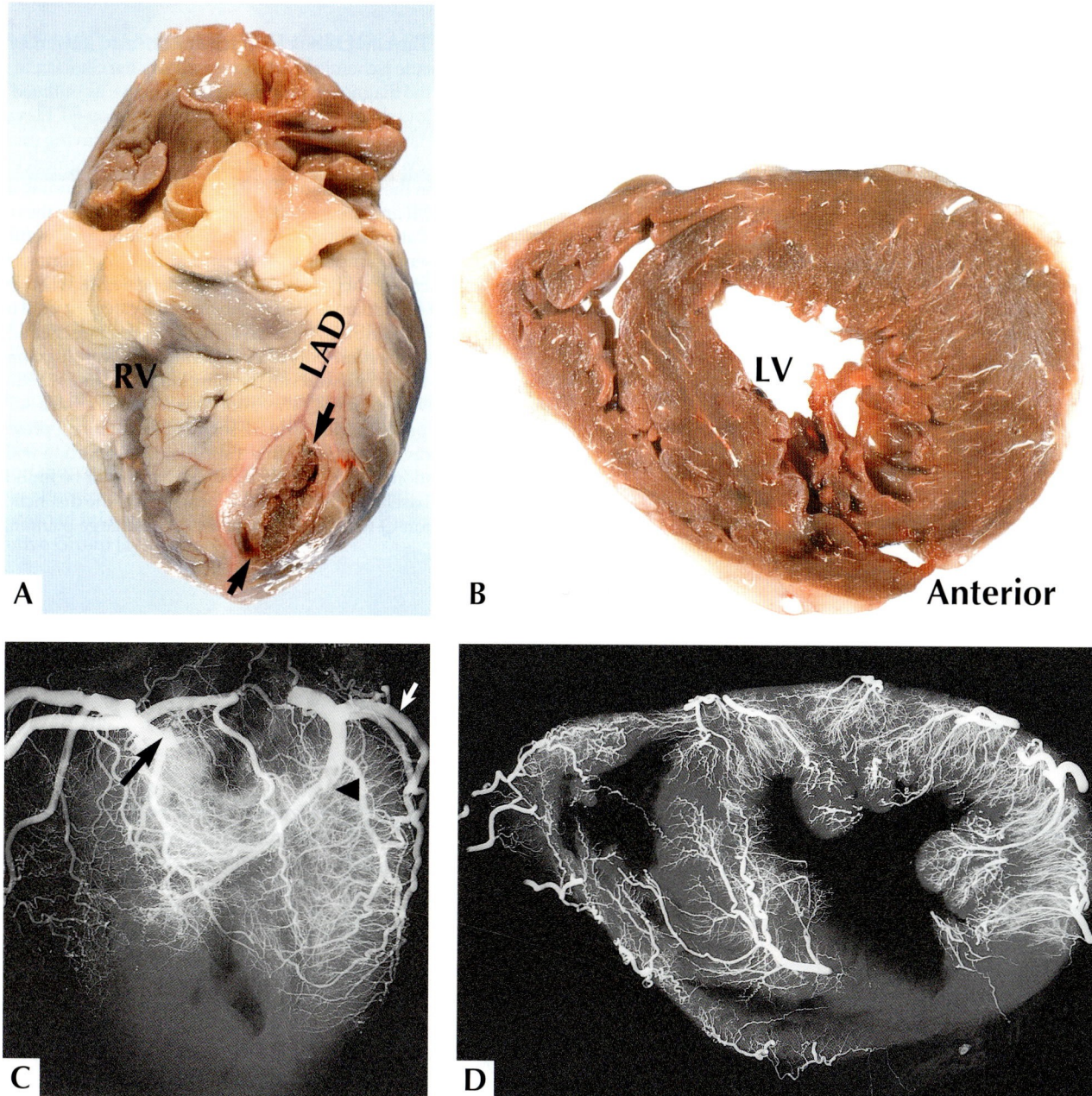

FIGURE 2-9. Rupture of the heart complicates acute myocardial infarction in about 10% of autopsied cases. Typically, it occurs during the first week after a first infarct and is more common in elderly women. The pathoanatomic substrate for postinfarction rupture of the left ventricular free wall or the interventricular septum includes total occlusion of a functional end artery (poor collateral circulation) causing transmural infarction in a perfusion area that was previously healthy (*ie*, no myocardial fibrosis). Usually, heart weight is normal. **A,** Rupture of the anterior wall of the left ventricle (LV; *between arrows*), parallel to the left anterior descending artery (LAD). **B,** Perforation of the free wall in this 11-hour-old infarct can be seen clearly on the transventricular myocardial slice (short-axis view). Thrombolytic therapy was not given. **C,** Postmortem angiogram of a similar case (28-hour-old infarct) showing LAD occlusion (*arrowhead*). The right coronary (*black arrow*) and left circumflex (*white arrow*) arteries appear almost normal (single-vessel disease). The LAD is occluded just distal to the first septal branch, with no distal collateral filling.

D, Angiographic short-axis view of transventricular myocardial slice reveals no vascular filling in the area normally perfused by the LAD. Note the treelike coronary branching pattern with well-defined perfusion areas, in contrast to the enlarged anastomotic network frequently seen with subendocardial infarction and, in particular, with diffuse subendocardial necrosis. RV—right ventricle.

CALCIUM ANTAGONISTS

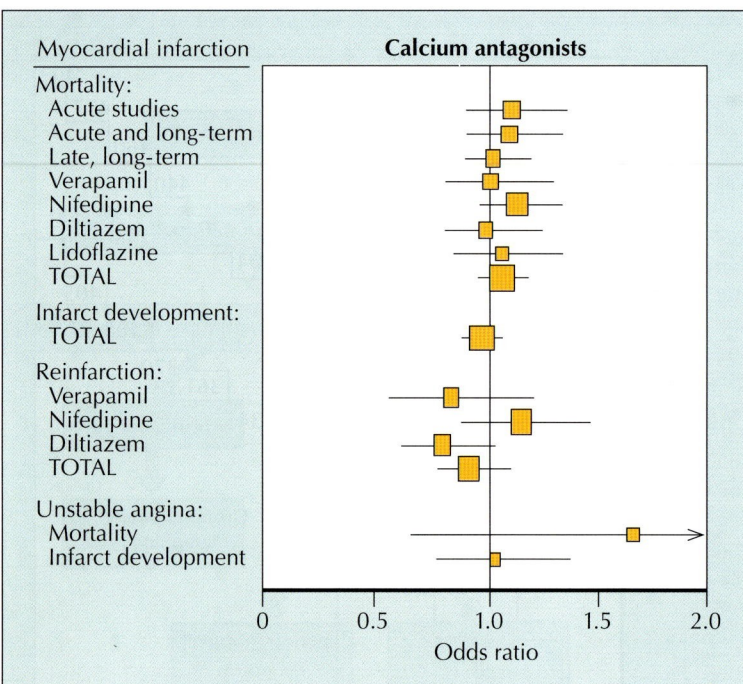

FIGURE 2-13. Results of therapy with calcium antagonists in acute coronary syndromes. This meta-analysis indicates that calcium antagonists have no significant beneficial effect on mortality in patients with acute MI and may even be associated with a trend toward an *increase* in mortality; no evidence of a beneficial effect was detected in patients with unstable angina either. Reinfarction rates tended to be lower in the patients treated with verapamil or diltiazem, but this value did not achieve statistical significance (confidence intervals overlap vertical line). Based on these observations, calcium antagonists cannot be recommended as primary therapy for unstable angina or acute MI. (*Adapted from* Held *et al.* [15].)

NITRATE THERAPY

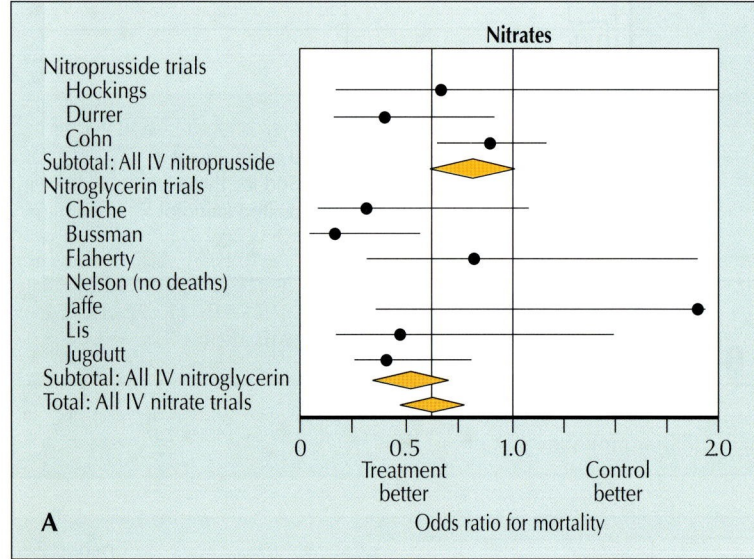

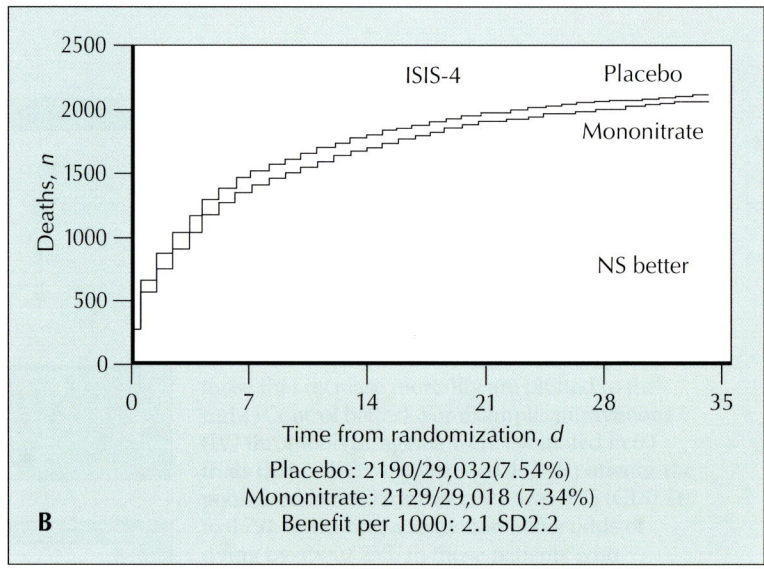

FIGURE 2-14. A, A meta-analysis of 10 trials from the prethrombolytic era indicated a favorable effect of nitrate-like compounds in the acute phase of MI [16]. **B,** In the current thrombolytic era, when important reductions in mortality can be achieved with reperfusion therapy and aspirin, the rela-tive benefit of nitrates is considerably smaller, although some evidence of a slight reduction in short-term mortality can still be seen in the ISIS-4 [17] and GISSI-3 [18] Trials. IV—intravenous. (Part A *adapted from* Yusuf *et al.* [16]; part B *adapted from* ISIS-4 Collaborative Group [17].)

ANGIOTENSIN-CONVERTING ENZYME INHIBITION

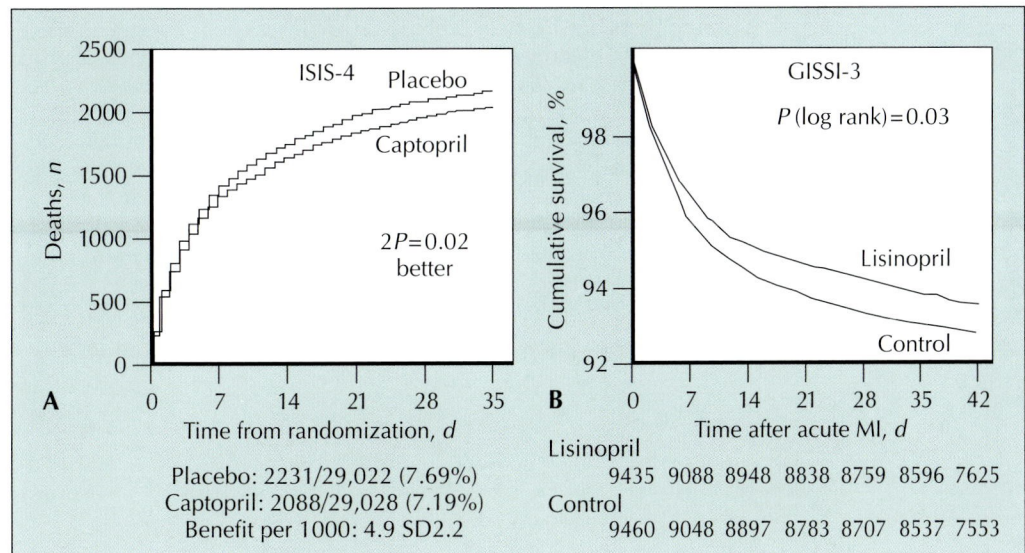

Placebo: 2231/29,022 (7.69%)
Captopril: 2088/29,028 (7.19%)
Benefit per 1000: 4.9 SD2.2

| Lisinopril | 9435 | 9088 | 8948 | 8838 | 8759 | 8596 | 7625 |
| Control | 9460 | 9048 | 8897 | 8783 | 8707 | 8537 | 7553 |

FIGURE 2-15. Results of treatment with angiotensin-converting enzyme (ACE) inhibitors after acute MI. Two trials of acute therapy in unselected patients (*ie*, both with and without evidence of left ventricular dysfunction) have shown that ACE inhibitors reduce mortality at 4 to 6 weeks [17,18]. This effect was seen in two different patient populations and with two different ACE inhibitors, captopril (A) and lisinopril (B), attesting to the consistency and generalizability of the observations. (Part A *adapted from* ISIS-4 Collaborative Group [17]; part B *adapted from* Gruppo Italiano per lo Studio della Sopravvivenza nell'Infarto Miocardico [18].)

PROPHYLACTIC ANTIARRHYTHMIC DRUG THERAPY

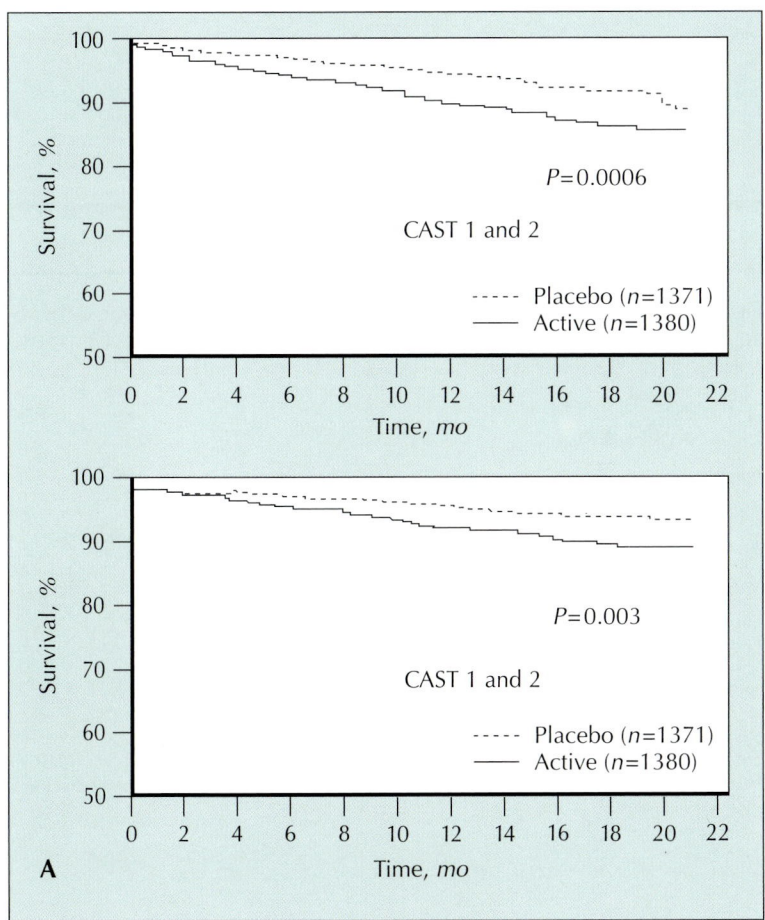

FIGURE 2-16. A, Results of CAST (Cardiac Arrhythmia Suppression Trial) [19]. This trial tested the hypothesis that the use of encainide, flecainide, or moricizine to suppress ventricular arrhythmias detected on Holter monitoring after MI would reduce the long-term risk for cardiac arrest and death. The first phase of the trial (CAST-1), which involved encainide and flecainide (class IC antiarrhythmic agents), was stopped prematurely because these drugs increased mortality; the second phase of the trial (CAST-2), in which moricizine (a class IA agent) was compared with placebo, was also discontinued prematurely due to both an increase in mortality during the titration phase of moricizine dosing and the fact that beneficial effects of moricizine in those patients who survived the titration phase were highly unlikely. Data from both CAST-1 and CAST-2 are combined here and clearly depict the adverse impact on long-term total mortality (*top panel*) and sudden cardiac death (*bottom panel*) with these antiarrhythmic agents versus placebo. (*continued*)

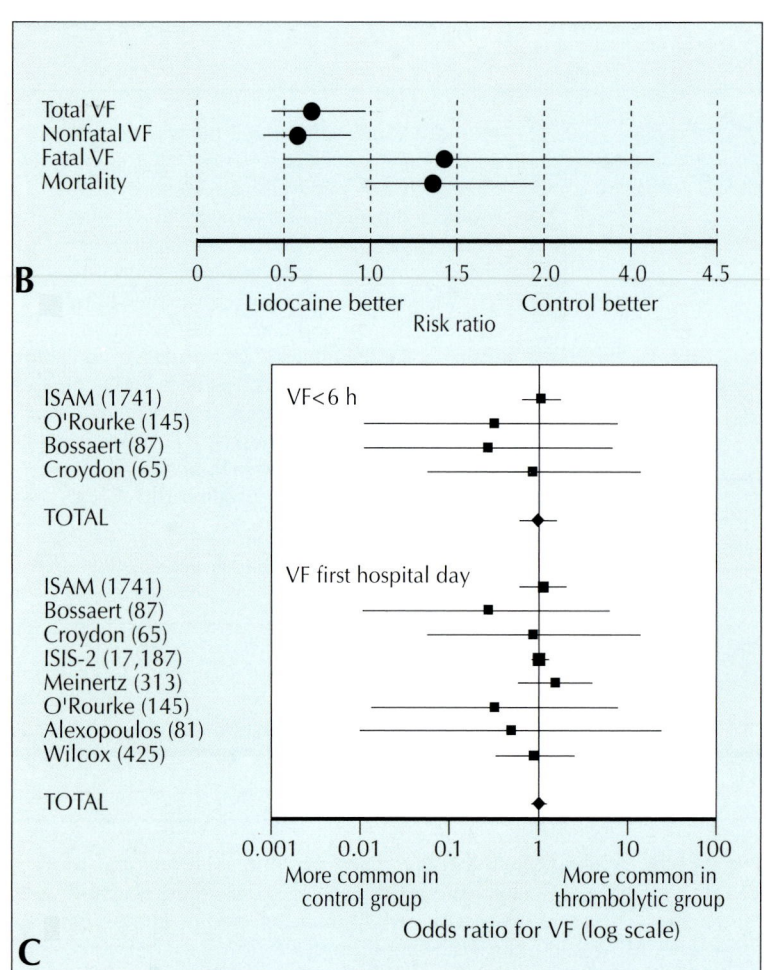

B

Lidocaine better | Control better
Risk ratio

C

ISAM (1741)
O'Rourke (145)
Bossaert (87)
Croydon (65)

TOTAL

ISAM (1741)
Bossaert (87)
Croydon (65)
ISIS-2 (17,187)
Meinertz (313)
O'Rourke (145)
Alexopoulos (81)
Wilcox (425)

TOTAL

VF<6 h

VF first hospital day

More common in control group | More common in thrombolytic group
Odds ratio for VF (log scale)

FIGURE 2-16. (*continued*) **B,** Although prophylactic lidocaine was clearly beneficial in reducing the risk for primary ventricular fibrillation (VF) in the absence of congestive heart failure or cardiogenic shock in the prethrombolytic era, its use was associated with a trend toward increased mortality, probably due to fatal bradycardia and asystolic arrest. **C,** Impact of thrombolytic therapy on the development of VF. Despite initial concerns about an increase in VF with reperfusion, the results of this meta-analysis show no difference in the incidence of VF in the first 6 hours or at any time during the first 24 hours in patients treated with a variety of thrombolytic agents compared with those given placebo. Based on this observation, the decision to administer a thrombolytic agent to patients treated in the hospital for acute MI does not appear to increase their risk for VF during the first day of treatment. (Part B *adapted from* MacMahon *et al.* [20]; part C *adapted from* Solomon *et al.* [21].)

WARFARIN THERAPY

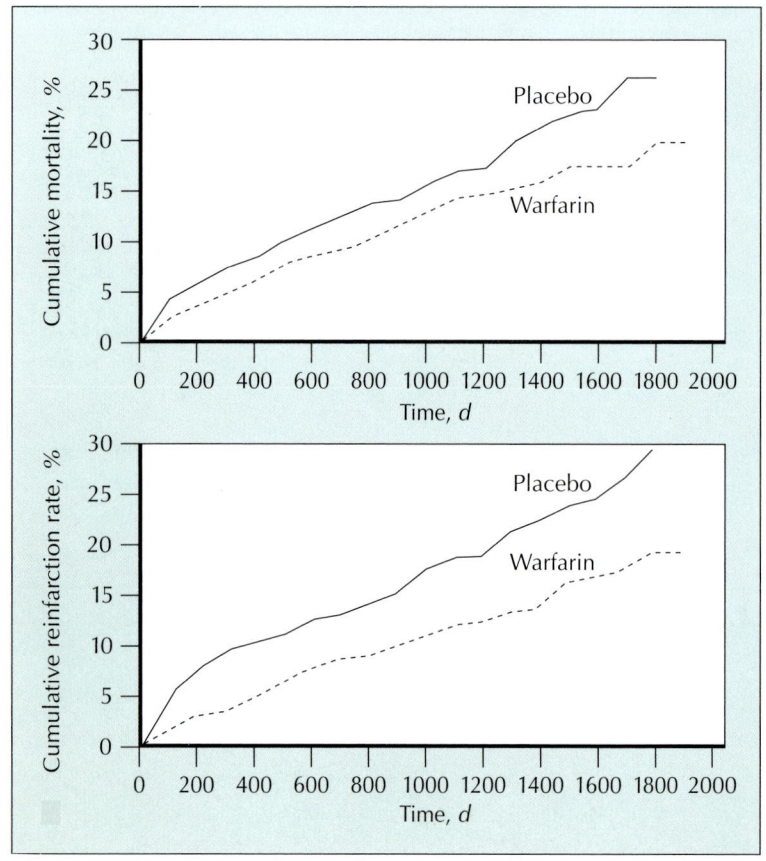

FIGURE 2-17. The Warfarin Reinfarction Study (WARIS) demonstrated reductions in mortality and the rate of reinfarction in patients given active therapy with warfarin compared with placebo (*Adapted from* Smith *et al.* [22].)

CLINICAL USE OF ANTITHROMBOTIC THERAPY

ORAL ANTIPLATELET THERAPY

Aspirin	Initial dose of 162–325 mg nonenteric formulation followed by 75–160 mg/d of an enteric or nonenteric formulation
Clopidogrel	75 mg/d, a loading dose of 4 to 8 tablets (300–600 mg) can be used when rapid onset of action is required
Ticlopidine	250 mg twice daily, a loading dose of 500 mg can be used when rapid onset of inhibition is required; monitoring of platelet and white cell counts during treatment is required

Heparins

Dalteparin	120 IU/kg subcutaneously every 12 hours (maximum 10,000 IU twice daily)
Enoxaparin	1 mg/kg subcutaneously every 12 hours; the first dase may be preceded by a 30 mg IV bolus
Heparin (UFH)	Bolus 60–70 units/kg (maximum 5000 units) IV followed by infusion of 12–15 units/kg/h (maximum 1000 u/h) titrated to aPTTT 1.5–2.5 times control

Intravenous antiplatelet therapy

Abciximab	0.25 mg/kg bolus followed by infusion of 0.125 μg/kg/min (maximum 10 μg/min) for 12 to 24 hours
Eptifibatide	180 μg/kg bolus followed by infusion of 2.0 μg/kg/min for 72 to 96 hours*
Tirofiban	0.4 μg/kg/min for 30 minutes followed by infusion of 0.1 μg/kg/min for 48 to 96 hours*

*Different dose regimens were tested in recent clinical trials before percutaneous interventions.
UFH—unfractionated heparin.

FIGURE 2-18. Clinical use of antithrombotic therapy. Antithrombotic therapy recommended in the guidelines for unstable angina in non-ST elevation myocardial infarction [23]. The change in heparin dosing is important to note; underdosing of heparin will lead to an increase in thrombotic events while overdosing will lead to an increase in both thrombotic and hemorrhagic events. Care must also be exhibited in combining the glycoprotein (GP) IIb/IIIa inhibitors with heparin or low molecular weight heparin. There is a pharmocodynamic interaction mandating an even lower dose of heparin when a GP IIb/IIIa inhibitor is used; the proper dose of a LVMW when a GP IIb/IIIa inhibitor is under study.

CLASS I RECOMMENDATIONS FOR ANTITHROMBOTIC THERAPY

POSSIBLE ACS	LIKELY/DEFINITE ACS	DEFINITE ACS WITH CONTINUE ISCHEMIA OR OTHER HIGH-RISK FEATURES* OR PLANNED INTERVENTION
Aspirin	Aspirin	Aspirin
	+	+
	SC LMWH	IV heparin
	or	+
	IV heparin	IV GP IIb/IIIa antagonist

Clinical data on the combination of low molecular weight heparin (LMWH) and GP IIb/IIIa antagonist are lacking. Their combined use is not currently recommended.

*High-risk features include diabetes, recent myocardial infarction, and elevated troponin T or I.

FIGURE 2-19. Class I recommendations for antithrombotic therapy. Patients with possible acute coronary syndrome (ACS) should be treated with aspirin. Patients with definite ACS should be treated with aspirin and either low molecular weight heparin or unfractionated heparin. Patients with high-risk features should be treated with aspirin, IV heparin, and an IV glycoprotein (GP) IIb/IIIa antagonist. Aspirin is recommended for possible ACS because of its demonstrated benefit and very low risk of bleeding complications. The addition of the antithrombin regimen is based on less conclusive data, but the global community is convinced of the benefit and the empirical support is substantial. The addition of GP IIb/IIIa inhibitor in high-risk situations is based upon definitive clinical trial results [23].

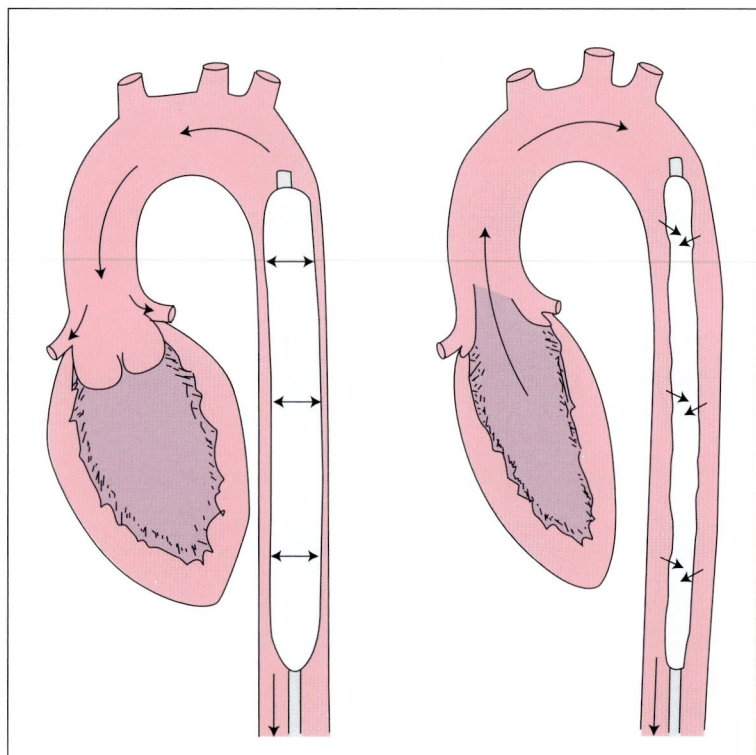

FIGURE 2-20. The major mode of action of the intra-aortic balloon pump (IABP) in unstable angina is improvement of diastolic coronary blood flow. In addition, the mechanical effect of the balloon inflation and deflation decreases afterload substantially, therefore reducing myocardial wall stress. Functioning IABP. During diastole (*left panel*), the balloon is inflated, which increases volume in the aorta, raises diastolic pressure, and increases perfusion of coronary arteries. Just before and during systole (*right panel*), the balloon is deflated, which decreases the volume in the aorta, decreases aortic pressure (afterload), and facilitates ejection by the left ventricle.

OVERVIEW OF MEDICAL MANAGEMENT OF ACUTE CORONARY SYNDROMES

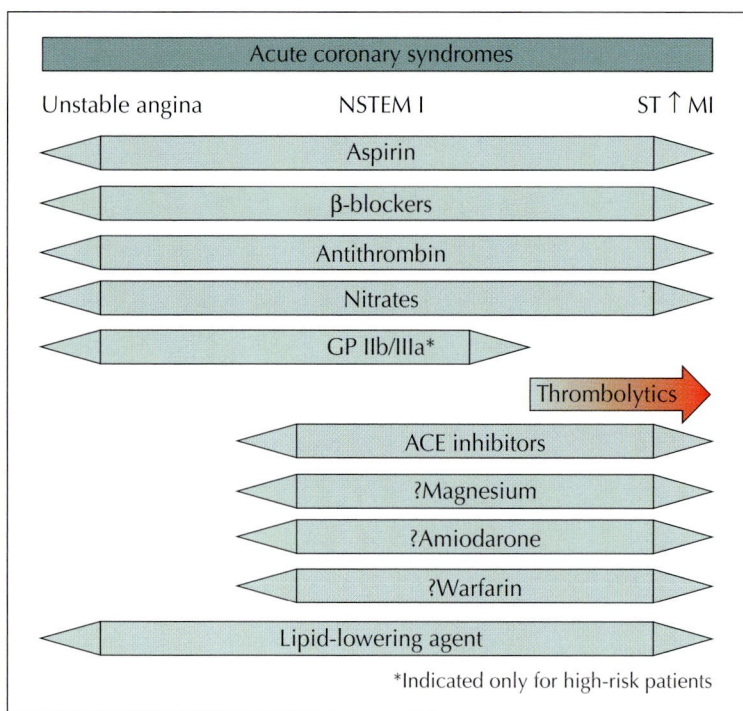

FIGURE 2-21. Summary of results of medical therapy for acute coronary syndromes. Aspirin, beta blockers, and an antithrombin (*eg*, heparin or the new direct antithrombins), alone and in combination, have been shown to

reduce morbidity and mortality across the entire spectrum of acute coronary syndromes. Although nitrates are useful for relieving recurrent episodes of ischemic-type discomfort, these agents probably provide only a small short-term benefit with regard to reducing mortality in patients with acute MI who receive the other therapies noted above. Of the various forms of medical therapy, intravenous thrombolytic agents offer the most dramatic reductions in mortality for patients with Q-wave MI. Based on available data, the thrombolytic agents and regimens now available do not appear to benefit patients with unstable angina/NQMI. Angiotensin-converting enzyme (ACE) inhibitors have clearly been shown to reduce long-term mortality in patients with left ventricular (LV) dysfunction following MI, and recent data suggest that they reduce short-term mortality (4 to 6 weeks) even when patients are not selected for the presence of LV dysfunction. However, before ACE inhibitors can be recommended on a broad basis for patients with either NQMI or Q-wave MI, even in the absence of LV dysfunction, additional analyses and more long-term follow-up are needed. The benefits of magnesium remain controversial, and decisions regarding the use of class III antiarrhythmic agents such as amiodarone or low-dose warfarin in combination with aspirin should await the findings of ongoing clinical trials.

Lipid-lowering therapy is clearly helpful in reducing risk for recurrent ischemic events and probably will lead to a reduction in mortality, although the latter outcome has not been rigorously established in the current therapeutic era. Recent recommendations from the National Cholesterol Education Program Adult Treatment Panel-2 have proposed a much more aggressive approach to lipid lowering than clinicians have used in the past. A target goal for low-density lipoprotein cholesterol below 100 mg/dL has been recommended for patients with a history of coronary heart disease. NSTE MI—non-ST elevation myocardial infarction.

CONSEQUENCES OF CORONARY OCCLUSION AND REPERFUSION

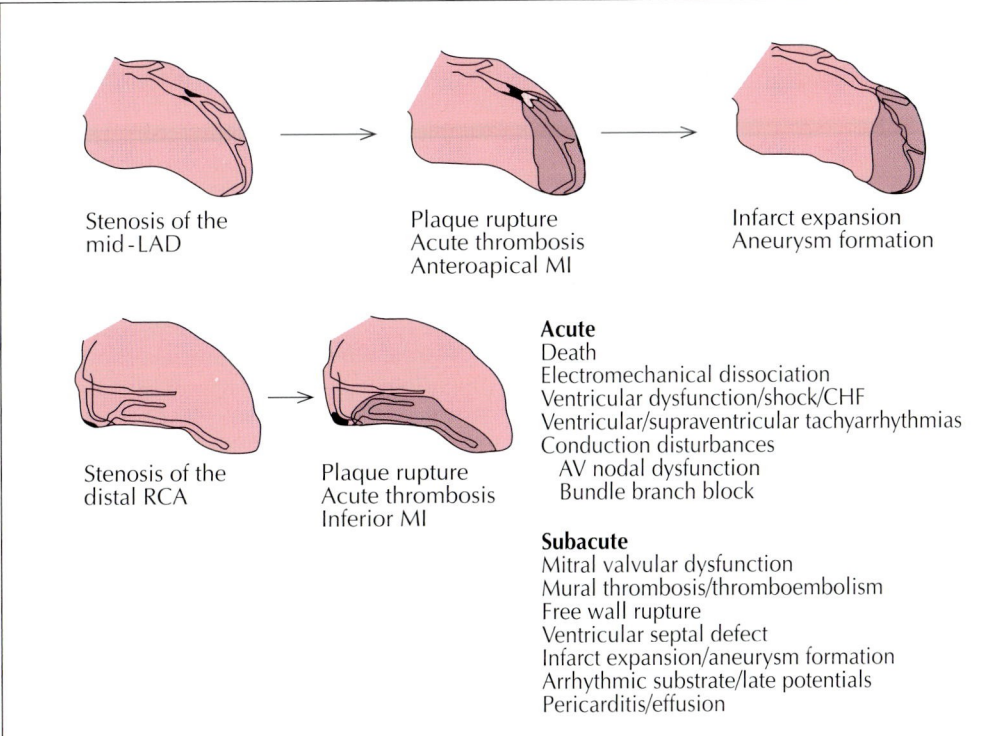

Stenosis of the mid-LAD

Plaque rupture
Acute thrombosis
Anteroapical MI

Infarct expansion
Aneurysm formation

Stenosis of the distal RCA

Plaque rupture
Acute thrombosis
Inferior MI

Acute
Death
Electromechanical dissociation
Ventricular dysfunction/shock/CHF
Ventricular/supraventricular tachyarrhythmias
Conduction disturbances
  AV nodal dysfunction
  Bundle branch block

Subacute
Mitral valvular dysfunction
Mural thrombosis/thromboembolism
Free wall rupture
Ventricular septal defect
Infarct expansion/aneurysm formation
Arrhythmic substrate/late potentials
Pericarditis/effusion

FIGURE 2-22. Myocardial consequences of acute coronary occlusion. Complications of MI are direct consequences of the loss of ventricular myocardium. Acutely, ventricular dysfunction may result in congestive heart failure (CHF) or shock, severely compromising survival. In the subacute period, compromised integrity of infarcted myocardium may lead to rupture of the free wall (usually leading to pericardial tamponade), rupture of the septum (leading to a large intracardiac shunt), or disruption of the mitral apparatus (leading to acute valvular regurgitation). In the convalescent phase, infarct expansion and/or aneurysm formation may lead to unfavorable ventricular mechanics and may exacerbate CHF. Acutely and chronically, noncontractile or dyskinetic myocardial regions predispose to mural thrombosis and thromboembolic complications. Electrical instability predisposing to potentially fatal ventricular arrhythmias may occur in the acute or chronic phase, with the infarct scar servingas arrhythmic substrate. AV—atrioventricular; LAD—left anterior descending artery; RCA—right coronary artery.

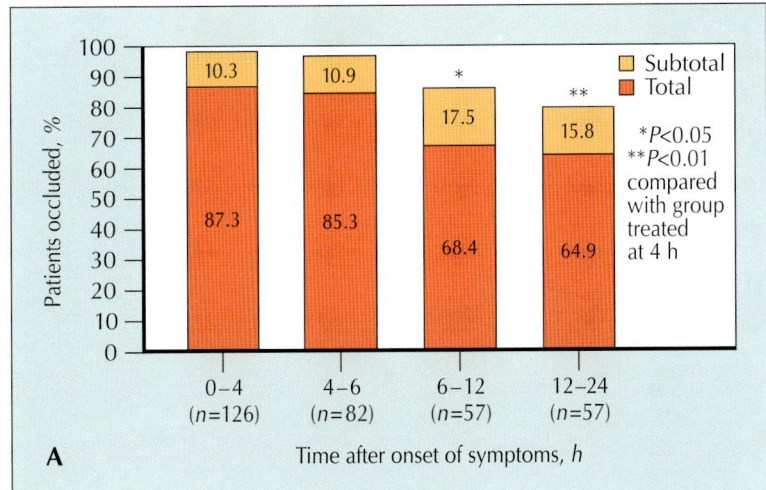

$*P<0.05$
$**P<0.01$ compared with group treated at 4 h

A Time after onset of symptoms, h

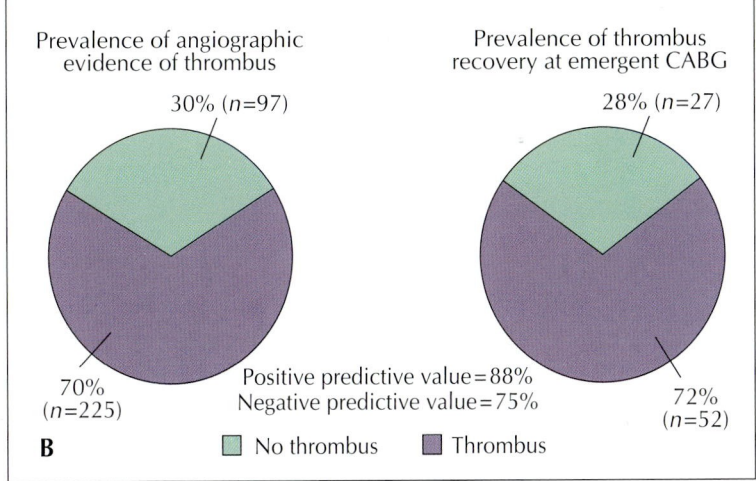

Prevalence of angiographic evidence of thrombus

30% (n=97)

70% (n=225)

Positive predictive value=88%
Negative predictive value=75%

Prevalence of thrombus recovery at emergent CABG

28% (n=27)

72% (n=52)

B □ No thrombus ■ Thrombus

FIGURE 2-23. Prevalence of total and subtotal occlusion in acute MI. The role of acute thrombotic occlusion in the pathogenesis of MI has guided therapeutic efforts since publication of the landmark study by DeWood *et al.* [24] in 1980. DeWood *et al.* performed coronary angiography on 322 patients (out of 1210 patients admitted with early transmural MI between March 1971 and December 1978) within 24 hours of onset of symptoms. **A,** The prevalence of total and subtotal coronary occlusions was found to be highest in the earliest hours following symptom onset, prompting ther-apeutic strategies aimed at restoration of coronary blood flow. The numbers inside each bar are percentages of total and subtotal occlusions.

B, The high prevalence of angiographic evidence of thrombus, corroborated by the recovery of thrombus at the time of emergent coronary artery bypass graft surgery (CABG), provides the rationale for the strategy of thrombolytic/antithrombotic approaches to the treatment of acute MI. (*Adapted from* DeWood *et al.* [24].)

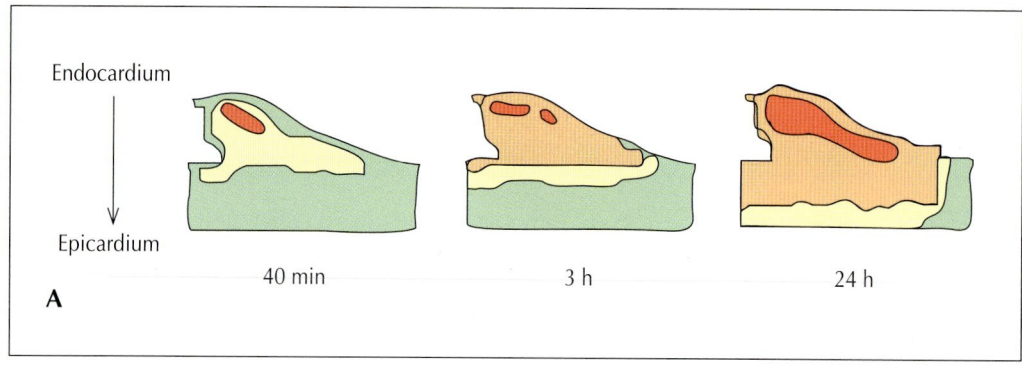

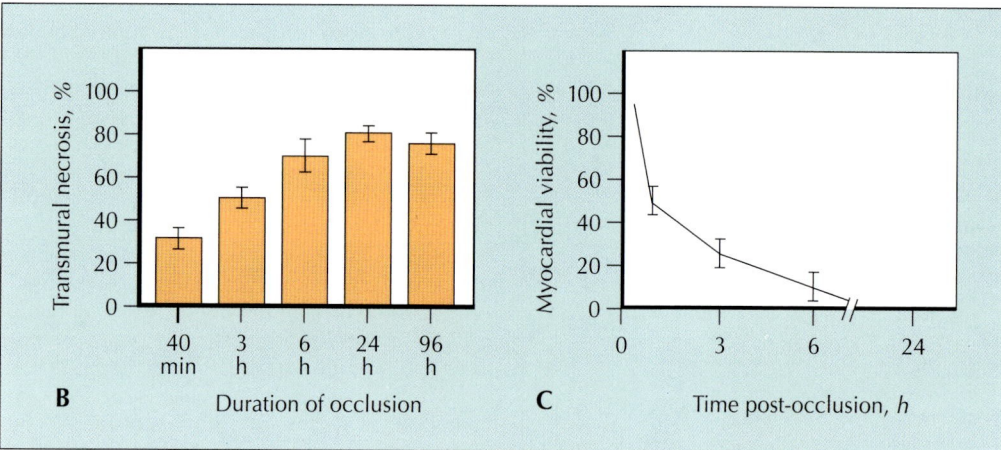

a dog papillary muscle preparation. Necrosis following coronary occlusion occurs in "wavefront" form, advancing from the endocardial surface outward to the subepicardial region over time. *Yellow area* indicates the anatomic boundary between ischemic circumflex and nonischemic left anterior descending coronary beds. *Orange area* indicates interstitial hemorrhage. *Red area* represents the central core of necrotic muscle devoid of either hemorrhage or inflammatory response, which results from complete cessation of microvascular perfusion.

B, In the dog papillary model, the percentage of sections exhibiting transmural infarction continues to rise over the first 6 hours following coronary occlusion. **C,** Conversely, the amount of viable myocardium diminishes rapidly over the first hour, and continues to decline to small amounts of salvageable myocardium beyond 6 hours (plot shows proportion of viable, potentially salvageable myocardium in a dog papillary model as a function of time after coronary occlusion, plotted as a percentage of 24-hour infarct size). Myocardial loss in acute MI in humans has been found to follow a similar time dependency, forming the basis of the quest for therapeutic strategies emphasizing earlier diagnosis and triage, and the earliest possible restoration of coronary blood flow. *T-bars* indicate ±SEM. (*Adapted from* Reimer *et al.* [25].)

FIGURE 2-24. Progression of myocardial necrosis in acute coronary occlusion. **A,** The extent of myocardial necrosis in acute MI is a time-dependent process, as elucidated by Reimer *et al.* [25] in

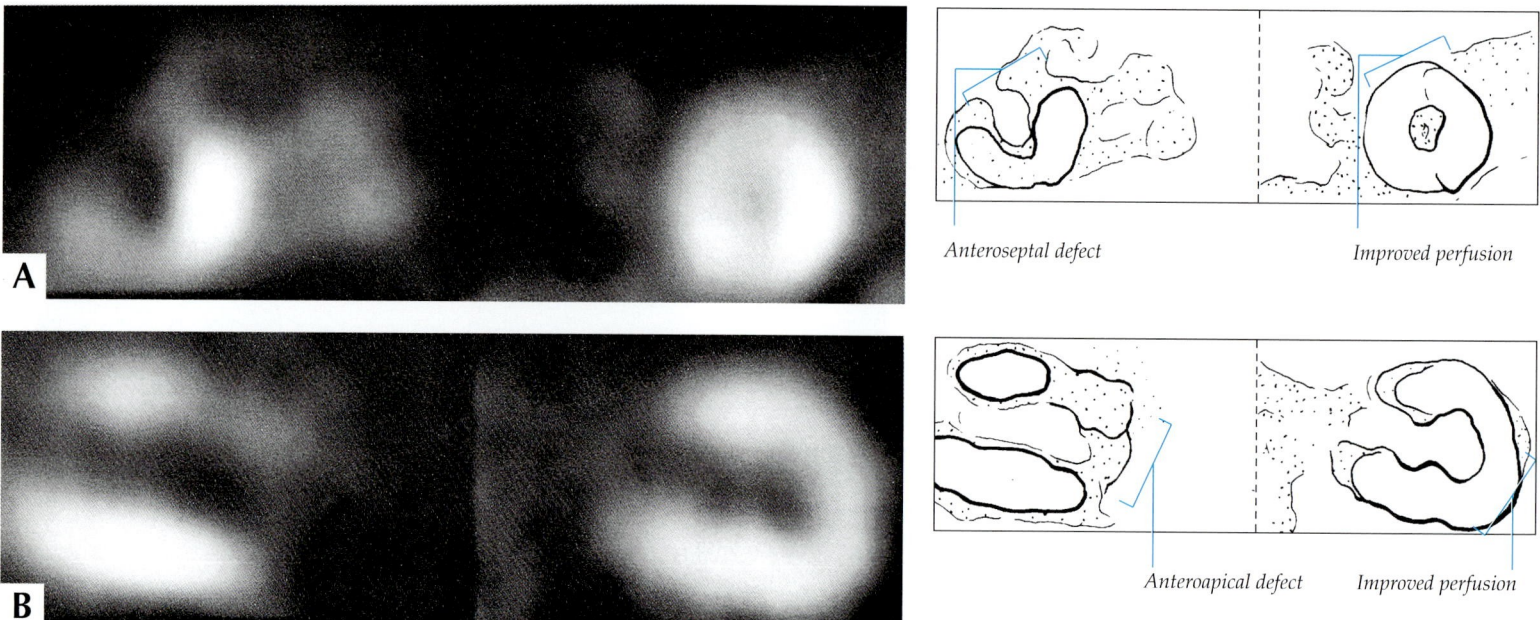

FIGURE 2-25. Radionuclide perfusion imaging: Assessment of myocardium at risk and myocardial salvage. Tomographic images of a patient with acute anterior MI. **A,** Midventricular short-axis slices. **B,** Vertical long-axis slices. The images in the *left panels* were acquired following acute MI prior to administration of thrombolytic therapy. Repeat imaging performed 1 week later (*right panels*) revealed resolution of the initial large anterior perfusion defects indicative of successful reperfusion. (*From* Gibbons [26]; with permission.)

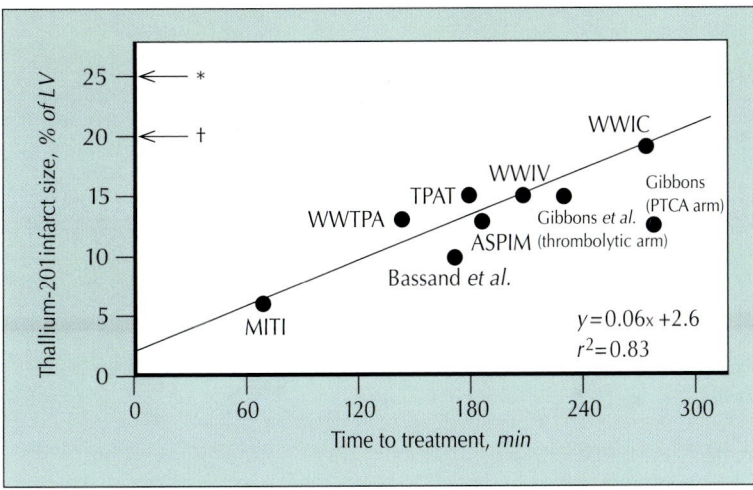

Figure 2-26. Effect of time to reperfusion therapy and infarct size. This graph shows infarct size, as determined by radionuclide tomographic perfusion imaging in trials of thrombolytic therapy and direct angioplasty,

plotted against the mean time to initiation of reperfusion therapy. Indicated are the approximate infarct sizes that might be expected in the presence of treated but persistently occluded vessels (*asterisk*), and in patients treated by conservative means (*dagger*) as suggested by the results of the TPAT (Tissue Plasminogen Activator: Toronto) [27,28] and Western Washington [29,30] trials. A remarkably consistent correlation exists between time to treatment and infarct size across these studies. At approximately 4 to 5 hours, the infarct size might be expected to be similar in treated and untreated groups, thus reperfusion beyond this time is not likely to result in significant myocardial salvage. Of interest, the farthest outlier (not included in regression) is the direct percutaneous transluminal coronary angioplasty (PTCA) group of the study by Gibbons [26]. While the thrombolytic arm of this study [31] appears consistent with other thrombolytic trials, the smaller infarcts experienced by the PTCA group, even at a later time to treatment, may reflect the greater likelihood of *complete reperfusion* with this strategy. The non-zero intersection of the regression line reflects the limitations of both symptom-based infarction diagnosis and reperfusion therapy [32–36]. APSIM—Anisoylated Plasminogen Streptokinase Activator Complex in Acute MI; LV—left ventricle; WWTPA—Western Washington Myocardial Infarction Registry and Tissue Plasminogen Activator trial. (*Adapted from* Martin and Kennedy [33].)

CORONARY PATENCY, VENTRICULAR FUNCTION, AND SURVIVAL

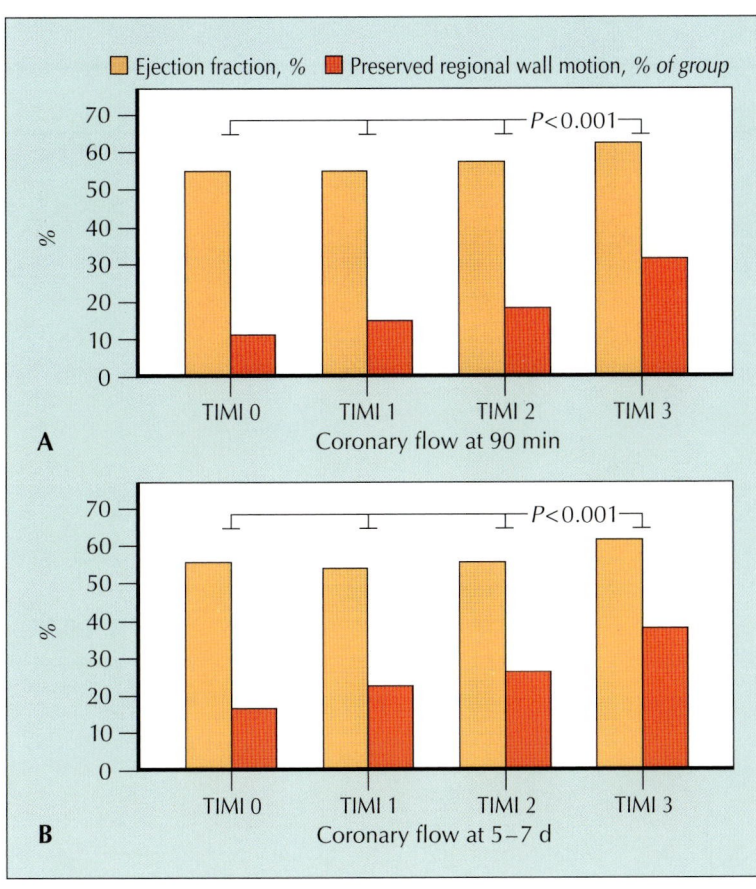

A
B

Figure 2-27. GUSTO: Coronary patency and ventricular function. The potential for myocardial salvage through restoration of coronary blood flow early in the course of acute MI has been demonstrated dramatically by the GUSTO angiographic substudy. In this group of patients treated with various thrombolytic regimens, significant relationships of flow to various measures of ventricular function were observed. In addition to global ejection fraction and the percentage of patients with completely preserved regional wall motion, measures of end-systolic volume index, wall motion (SD/chord, by left ventriculography), and number of abnormal chords all were significantly better in the group with normal flow (TIMI 3) when compared with no (TIMI 0 to 1) or only partial (TIMI 2) reperfusion. These relationships were observed both acutely (by angiography at 90 minutes post-thrombolytic administration; **A**) and in the convalescent period (5 to 7 days; **B**). (*Adapted from* the GUSTO Angiographic Investigators [37].)

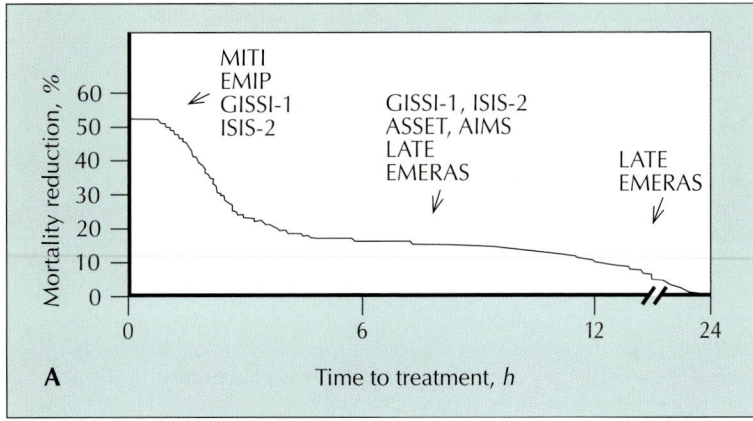

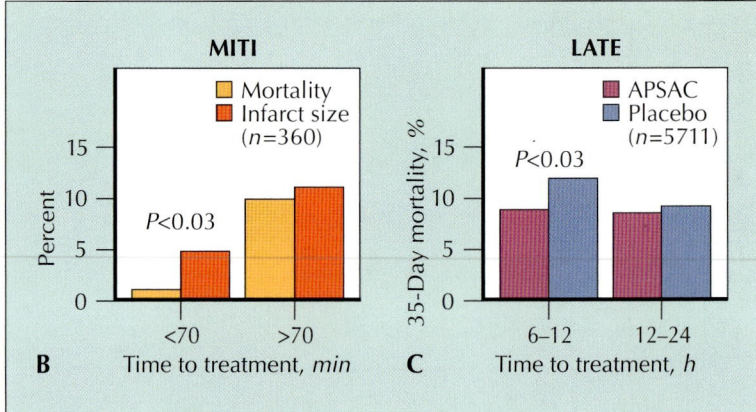

FIGURE 2-28. Mortality reduction and time to initiation of reperfusion therapy. **A,** Mortality reduction through thrombolytic therapy for acute MI is clearly a time-dependent phenomenon, reflecting the increased likelihood of successful reperfusion as well as the greater potential for myocardial salvage in the early hours following the onset of symptoms. **B,** The greatest benefit may be achieved in the first 1 to 2 hours. In the MITI trial [32], dramatic decreases in mortality and infarct size were noted in patients treated within 70 minutes (compared with patients treated after 70 minutes). **C,** As demonstrated by the LATE (Late Assessment of Thrombolytic Efficacy) trial [38], modest benefit may still be derived if

treatment is initiated as late as 12 hours after the onset of infarction. Therapy initiated between 12 and 24 hours is of uncertain merit; to date, no clinical trials have demonstrated mortality reduction in patients treated with therapy in this time frame. However, individuals with significant coronary collateralization or "stuttering" infarcts may possess significant amounts of viable, vulnerable myocardium, and may be at risk for infarct extension and/or recurrent ischemia during this later time frame. Such situations may warrant revascularization. APSAC—anisoylated plasminogen-streptokinase activator complex. (Part A *adapted from* Lincoff and Topol [39].)

SPECIFIC THROMBOLYTIC AGENTS

CHARACTERISTICS OF MAJOR FIBRINOLYTIC AGENTS

AGENT	STREPTOKINASE	ANISTREPLASE	ALTEPLASE	SARUPLASE	RETEPLASE	TENECTEPLASE	STAPHYLOKINASE
Source	Gp C streptococci	Gp C streptococci; plasminogen; anisoylated	Recombinant, human	Recombinant, human	Recombinant, human deletion mutation	Recombinant, triple substitution mutant	Recombinant *Staphylococcus aureus*
Fibrin specificity	No	No	++	+	+	+++	++++
Half-life, *min*	18–23	70–120	3–4	6–8	18	20	6
Mode of administration	infusion	Single bolus	90-min infusion	infusion	Double bolus	Single bolus	Double bolus
Mode of action	Activator complex	Direct	Direct	Direct	Direct	Direct	Activator complex
Antigenicity	Yes	No	No	No	No	No	Yes
Patency 90 min TIMI-3, %	32	50	54		60	54	68
Estimated hospital cost, in US dollars	280	1700	2200	Not determined	2200	Not determined	Not determined

FIGURE 2-29. Streptokinase remains a commonly used fibrinolytic agent in many parts of the world, especially where there are greater cost restraints. Anistreplase is not commonly used, and saruplase (pro-urokinase) is promising based on patency studies and a trial showing similar clinical outcomes as streptokinase, but it is not approved for acute myocardial infarction in the United States. Alteplase (t-PA) [40], reteplase (rPA) [41], and tenecteplase (TNK-t-PA) [42] all have similar 90-minute coronary

artery patency, with reteplase having the advantage of the ease of double-bolus administration, and tenecteplase the ease of single-bolus administration and lower risk of noncerebral bleeding. Staphylokinase, which is even more fibrin specific than tenecteplase, is in development [43]. Angiographic patency rates are derived from different trials and therefore are not directly comparable.

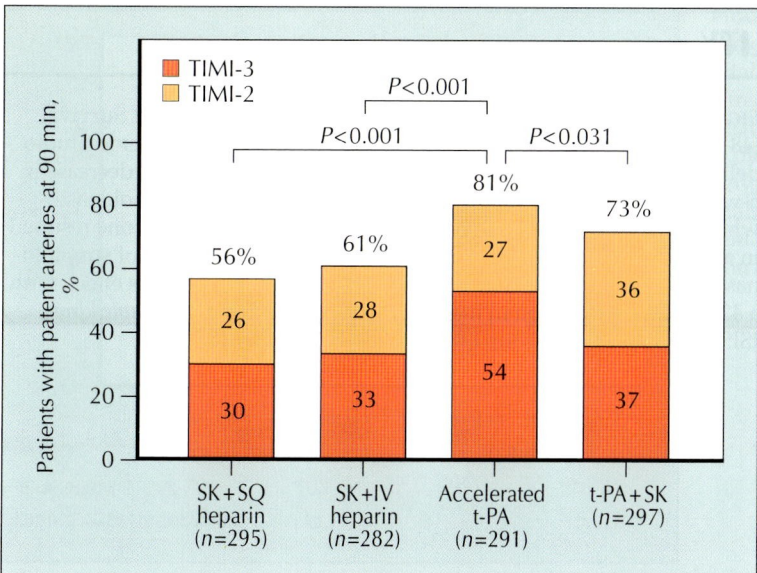

FIGURE 2-30. The GUSTO trial included an angiographic substudy of approximately 2400 patients enrolled at 75 North American, European, and Australian hospitals. Half were randomly assigned to have angiograms 90 minutes after enrollment [8]. Patients assigned to accelerated t-PA had significantly higher infarct-related artery patency (both TIMI-2 or -3 and TIMI-3 flow) at 90 minutes. IV—intravenous; SK—streptokinase; SQ—subcutaneous; TIMI—Thrombolysis in Myocardial Infarction.

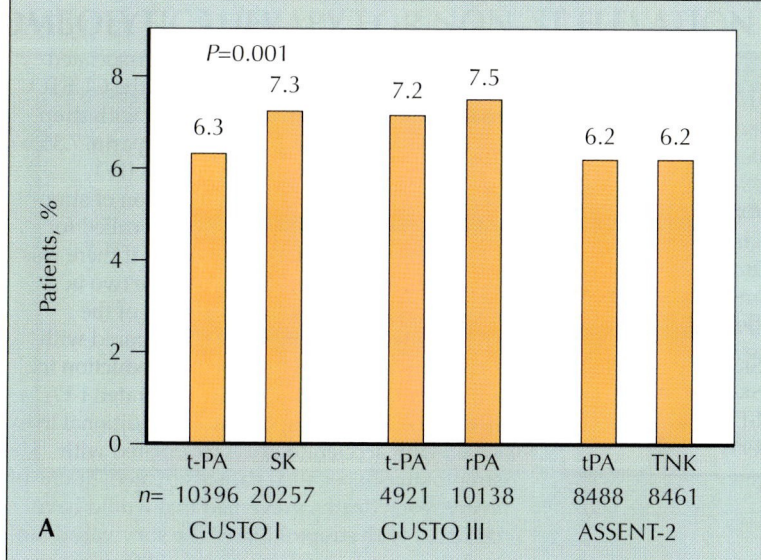

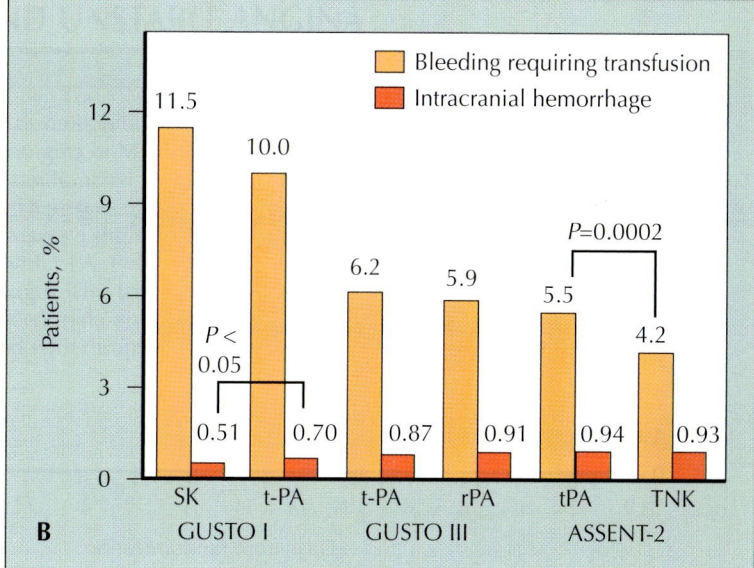

FIGURE 2-31. A and **B**, Selected clinical trials comparing fibrinolytic agents. Since the ISIS-3 trial [44] that showed that streptokinase (SK), 4-hour t-PA (dutelplase) infusion, and anistreplase resulted in similar mortality when administered with either delayed subcutaneous or no routine heparin, there have been three large trials comparing currently available fibrinolytic agents. All three included patients within 6 hours of symptom onset and with ST segment elevation or left bundle branch block on the qualifying electrocardiogram (ECG). All used 30-day mortality as the primary endpoint. GUSTO I [45] showed a 1.0% absolute survival advantage of accelerated t-PA over streptokinase (95% confidence interval 0.4 to 1.6%). GUSTO III [46] showed a 0.2% excess mortality with reteplase (rPA) compared with alteplase (95% confidence

interval -1.1 to 0.6%). ASSENT-2 [47] showed nearly identical mortality with tenecteplase versus alteplase (6.16 vs 6.18%, with the 95% confidence interval of the difference being -0.67 to 0.74). Intracranial hemorrhage was higher with alteplase than streptokinase and was similar for reteplase and tenecteplase vs alteplase. Of concern, the overall rate of intracranial hemorrhage with alteplase has tended to increase since the early 1990s (GUSTO-I) to the late 1990s (ASSENT-2), a finding that cannot be explained by changing patient characteristics such as age. Noncerebral bleeding was higher for those taking streptokinase than alteplase, and higher for those taking alteplase than tenecteplase. Bleeding and transfusion rates are dependent on definitions, country norms, and intervention rates; therefore, comparisons between trials are limited.

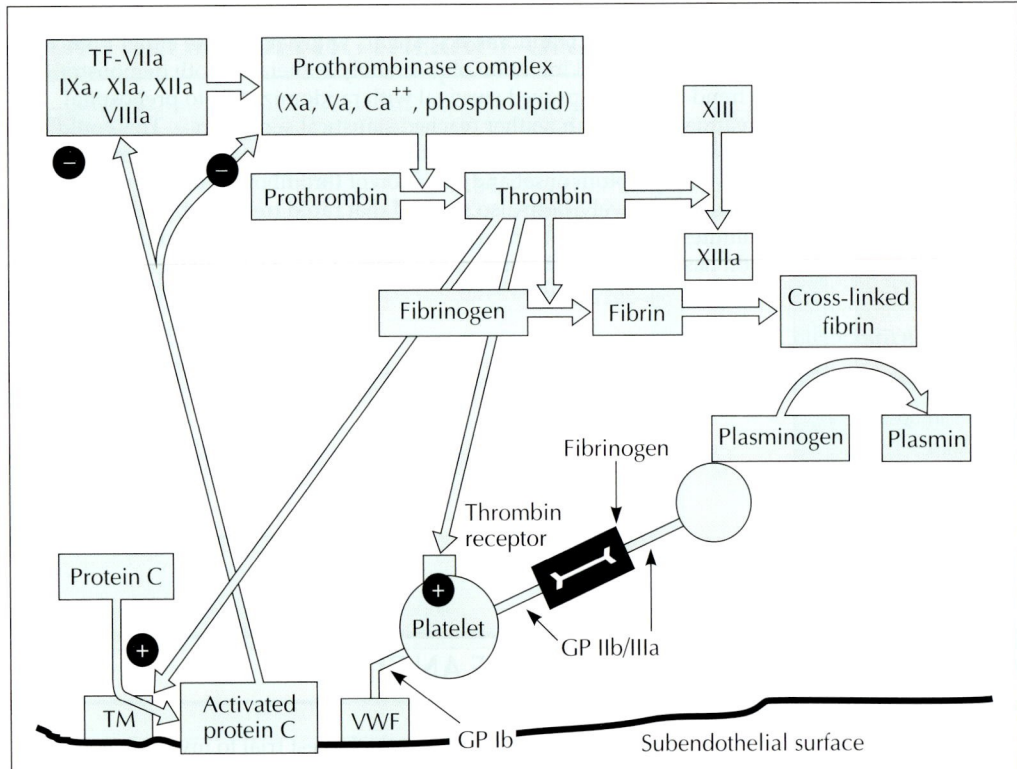

FIGURE 2-38. Investigations over the last decade have shown the interdependence of platelet hemostasis and the coagulation system. Thrombosis is a complex series of interactions between these two systems. The interplay between agonists and inhibitors of these systems maintains the balance between hemostasis and hemorrhage. A fascinating array of new approaches to altering the balance of the coagulation system is becoming available. Agonists and antagonists of each step of the coagulation cascade are now available for preclinical or clinical investigation. The search for the most appropriate balance of inhibition of thrombosis versus production of bleeding will demand substantial empiric evidence. GP—glycoprotein; TF—tissue factor; TM—thrombomodulin; VWF—von Willebrand factor.

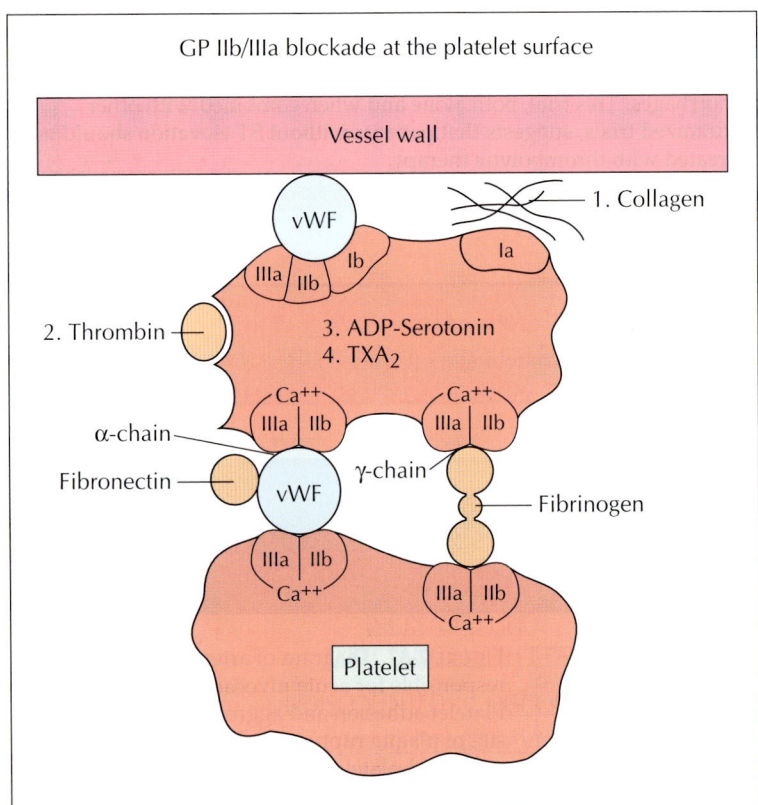

FIGURE 2-39. Despite its effectiveness, aspirin is a relatively weak platelet antagonist and does not effectively inhibit the platelet aggregation caused by many of the stimuli thought to be important in active ischemic heart disease (*eg*, thrombin). Recent studies have demonstrated that blockade of the glycoprotein (GP) IIb/IIIa receptor on the platelet surface (thought to be the final common pathway of platelet aggregation) leads to a beneficial clinical outcome, albeit posing an increased risk for bleeding, when given during the very acute phase of unstable angina, particularly when this syndrome is treated with percutaneous revascularization [55]. (*Adapted from* Fuster *et al.* [55].)

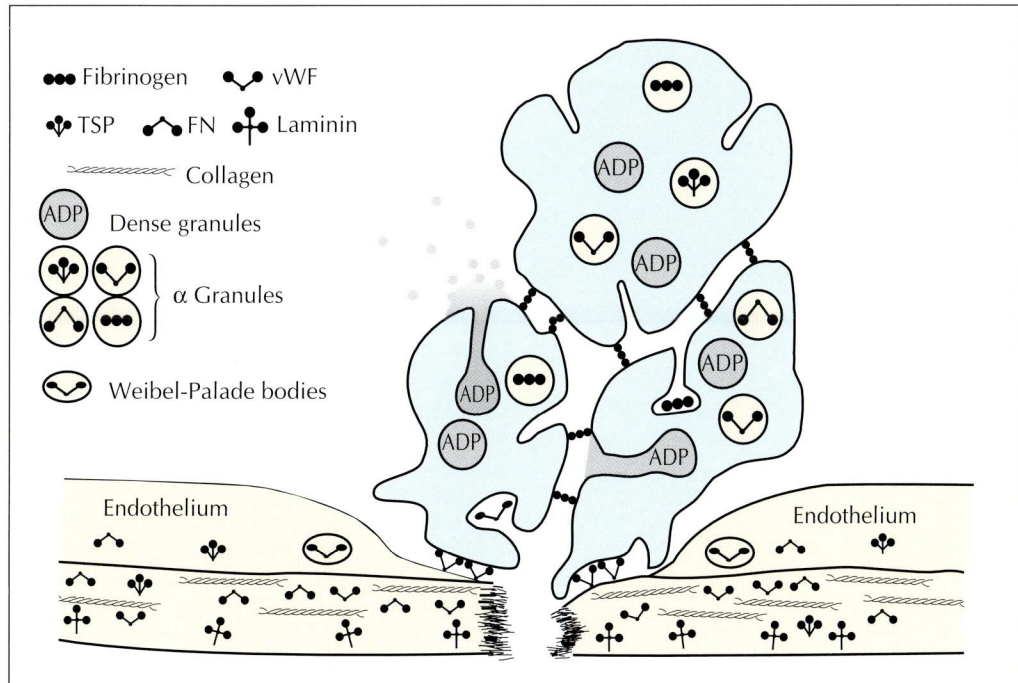

FIGURE 2-40. Platelet aggregation occurs primarily through platelet-platelet cross-linking by fibrinogen. Although the fibrinogen receptor glycoprotein IIb-IIIa is present on the platelet surface at all times, it is able to bind fibrinogen only after the platelet has undergone some level of "activation" and ADP has been provided, from either the platelet itself or other locations such as endothelial cells. Platelets may also be cross-linked through an ADP-dependent mechanism by von Willebrand factor (vWF). FN— fibronectin; TSP—thrombospondin. (*Adapted from* Hawiger [56].)

Legend:
- ●●● Fibrinogen
- vWF
- TSP
- FN
- Laminin
- Collagen
- ADP Dense granules
- α Granules
- Weibel-Palade bodies

Endothelium

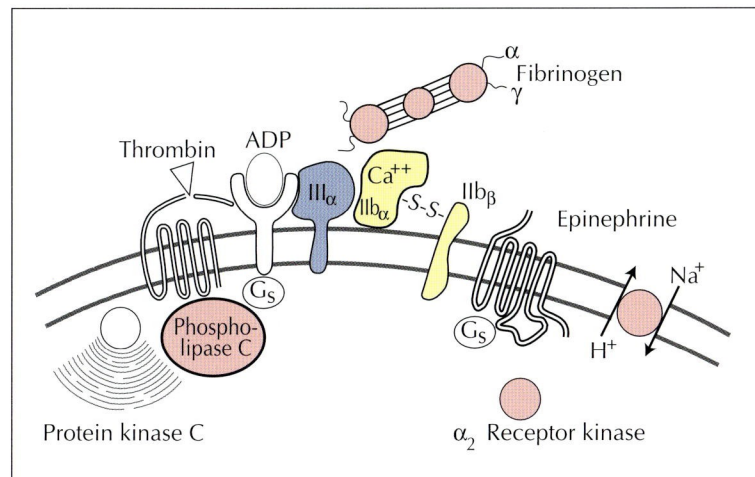

FIGURE 2-41. The three known agonist receptors on human platelets. Once the appropriate ligand has come into place, the role of these receptors is at least in part to activate the glycoprotein IIb-IIIa fibrinogen receptor so that platelet aggregation can take place. Thrombin "receptor" is actually a misnomer, since it is not a receptor at all but rather a substrate for thrombin [57]. This "receptor" and the epinephrine receptor (a true "receptor") are coupled to G proteins (G$_s$) and phospholipase C. Both receptors are members of a protein superfamily characterized by seven domains believed to be transmembranous. The ADP receptor is not well understood at this time; it is believed to be closely associated with the glycoprotein IIb-IIIa fibrinogen receptor, but the details await discovery. Binding of platelets to other extracellular matrix components such as collagen and fibronectin through specific receptors also results in activation, although less is known about these receptors. (*Adapted from* Hawiger [58].)

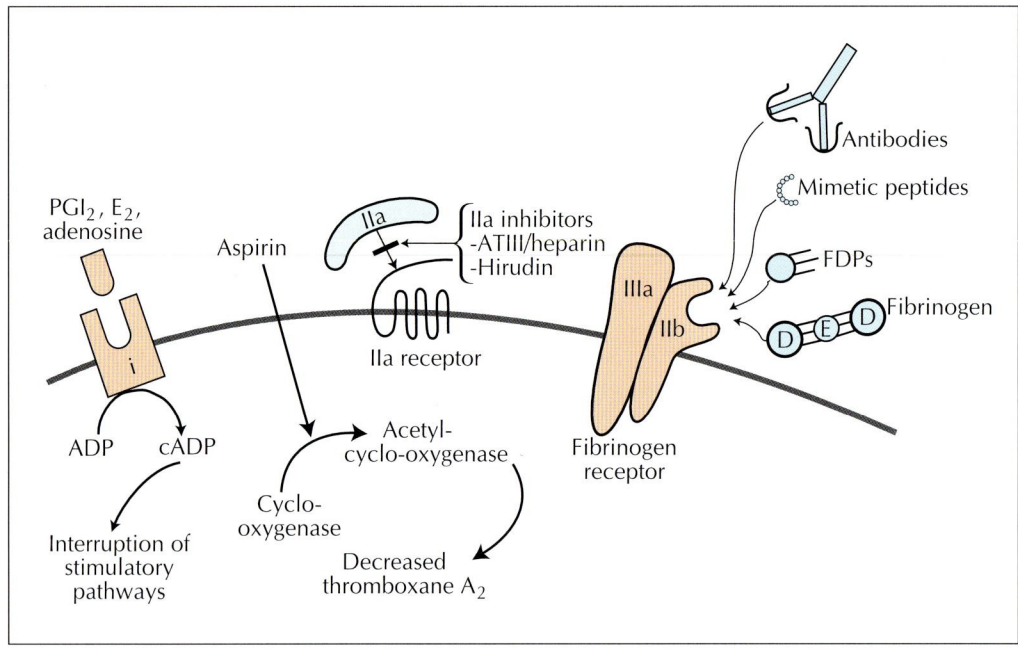

FIGURE 2-42. Four major classes of platelet inhibitors. Inhibitory prostaglandins (PGI_2, PGE_2), along with adenosine, act as inhibitors by binding to specific inhibitory receptors (i), thereby generating cADP, which interrupts the phospholipase A_2 and phospholipase C stimulatory pathways. Aspirin,

which is receiving increased attention as a means of preventing coronary heart disease, works by irreversibly acetylating the cyclo-oxygenase enzyme, thereby reducing the concentration of the stimulator thromboxane A_2 [59]. Thrombin (IIa) acts as a platelet agonist by cleaving the thrombin receptor and producing the "tethered ligand." Therefore, any effective thrombin inhibitor will act as a platelet inhibitor. Such inhibitors include heparin, the leech anticoagulant hirudin (and recent genetically engineered modifications of hirudin), and other inhibitors of the thrombin active site. Finally, platelet cross-linking during thrombus formation occurs via the interaction of fibrinogen (and in some cases von Willebrand factor) with the activated glycoprotein IIb-IIIa receptor. Therefore, any compound that can occupy this receptor will act as a platelet inhibitor in the sense that it will inhibit platelet aggregation by competition for the IIb-IIIa receptor. Such compounds include specific anti–IIb-IIIa antibodies; small synthetic peptides that mimic the part of fibrinogen which binds to the receptor; and fibrin(ogen) degradation products (FDPs), which contain the IIb-IIIa binding site from fibrinogen

ANTIPLATELET THERAPY

ASPIRIN

ANTIPLATELET TRIALISTS' COLLABORATION: REDUCTION IN VASCULAR EVENTS ACHIEVED BY ANTIPLATELET THERAPY FOLLOWING ACUTE MI			
EVENT	REDUCTION, %	STANDARD DEVIATION, %	P VALUE
All vascular events	25	4	<0.001
Nonfatal infarction	31	5	<0.001
Nonfatal stroke	42	11	<0.001
Vascular death	13	5	<0.005

FIGURE 2-43. In an analysis of 10 trials of antiplatelet agents (predominantly aspirin) for secondary prophylaxis of vascular events following acute MI, the Antiplatelet Trialists' Collaboration reported

striking reductions in nonfatal MI and nonfatal stroke in patients treated chronically with antiplatelet therapy (n=18,441). There was also a highly significant reduction in cardiovascular mortality. Interestingly, similar reductions were seen for patients receiving antiplatelet therapy following stroke. There were no differences in effect between varying doses of aspirin or aspirin with or without dipyridamole. Based on these data, it was estimated that if 100 patients underwent treatment with antiplatelet therapy for 2 years following acute MI, two deaths and three nonfatal events would be prevented. Based on a smaller number of patients with unstable angina, one death and two nonfatal events would be prevented [60].

TRIALS OF ANTITHROMBIN AND ANTIPLATELET THERAPY

TRIALS		PATIENTS WITH EVENT, % DEATH OR MI				P VALUE
	n	Active	Placebo			
ASA vs placebo				5-day to 2-year endpoint		
Lewis, et al. (VA)	1266	5.0	10.1			0.005
Cairns, et al.	555	10.5	14.7			0.137
Théroux, et al.	239	3.3	11.9			0.012
RISC Group	388	7.4	17.6			0.003
All ASA vs placebo	2448	6.4	12.5			0.0005
UFH +ASA vs ASA				1 week endpoint		
Théroux, et al.	243	1.6	3.3			0.40
RISC Group	399	1.4	3.7			0.140
ATACS Group	214	3.8	8.3			0.170
Gurfinkel, et al.	143	5.7	9.6			0.380
ALL UFH vs ASA	999	2.6	5.5			0.018
LMWH + ASA vs ASA				1 week endpoint		
Gurfinkel, et al.	141	0.0	9.6			n/a
FRISC Group	1498	1.8	4.8			0.001
All heparin or LMWH vs ASA	2629	2.0	5.3			0.0005
GP IIb/IIIa antagonist + UFH vs UFH				30-day endpoint		
CAPTURE	1265	4.8	9.0			0.003
PARAGON*	1516	10.6	11.7			0.410
PRISM-PLUS	1570	8.7	11.9			0.034
PRISM[†]	3232	5.8	7.1			0.110
PURSUIT	9461	3.5	3.7			0.042
All GP IIb/IIIa[‡]	170444	5.1	6.2			0.0022

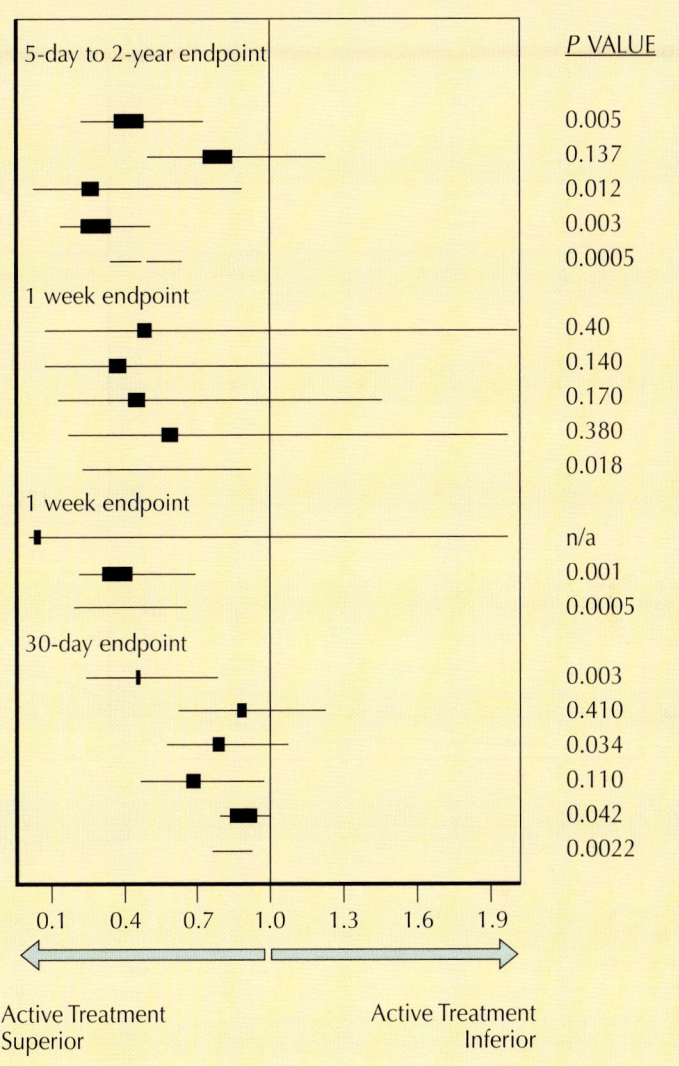

Axis values: 0.1 0.4 0.7 1.0 1.3 1.6 1.9

Active Treatment Superior — Active Treatment Inferior

*Best results group; [†]GP IIb/IIIa with no heparin; [‡]all trials except PRISM compared GP IIb/IIIa with UFH vs UFH.
ASA—acetylsalicylic acid; UFH—unfractionated heparin.

FIGURE 2-44. Trials of antithrombin and antiplatelet therapy. The aspirin trials in unstable angina all show a benefit; although the number of patients is relatively small, the magnitude of the benefit is great [23].

The trials of unfractionated heparin versus aspirin alone also show a benefit of UFH, but the magnitude of the benefit is difficult to estimate due to the fact that few than 1000 patients have been studied. The small number of patients has created difficulty in the development of new therapies attempting to show equivalence of noninferiority to unfractionated heparin. Definitive equivalence studies require substantial evidence that the active control, standard treatment (in this case, unfractionated heparin) is actually better than no treatment.

The trials of low molecular weight heparin plus aspirin versus aspirin have achieved mixed results. Trials with enoxaparin have shown benefit, while other trials have been neutral. These results have spawned a debate about whether there is heterogeneity in the clinical benefit of low molecular weight heparin or whether the apparent differences are due to random chance.

When combining all trials of either low molecular weight heparin or unfractionated heparin versus aspirin, the magnitude of the benefit is highly significant and very substantial. These results from the combined unfractionated and low molecular weight heparin trials provide the best support for the Class I recommendation for antithrombin therapy.

It is important to note that all the trials with antithrombin therapy had only a one week endpoint. The small amount of longer term follow-up for unfractionated heparin has shown an erosion of the benefit over time while the result with enoxaparin has been a sustenance of the benefit over time.

The final portion of the figure demonstrates the results of the 4P trials and CAPTURE, all of which used glycoprotein (GP) IIb/IIIa inhibitors in the setting of unstable angina or non-ST elevation myocardial infarction. The overall effect and the result in every trial favor using GP IIb/IIIa inhibitors.

ADVANTAGES AND DISADVANTAGES OF THROMBOLYTIC THERAPY

ADVANTAGES	DISADVANTAGES
Does not require access to catheterization laboratory facilities	Despite widespread availability, thrombolytic therapy is only given in approximately 30%–40% of patients with acute MI; absolute or relative contraindications frequent
Treats the underlying problem of a central occluding thrombus	Not effective for hemodynamic instability
Documented efficacy in large, well-controlled trials	Early reperfusion rates range from 55%–80% depending on agent used
	Achievement of TIMI-3 flow in <50%–60% of patients
	Reliable assessment of reperfusion often not possible
	Residual stenosis

FIGURE 2-47. Advantages and disadvantages of thrombolytic therapy. Proponents of thrombolytic therapy are equally vocal. One of the most important advantages is that thrombolytic therapy can be given in a variety of settings—primary, secondary, and tertiary hospitals, emergency rooms, and even in the field by trained paramedical personnel. It does not require access to a cardiac catheterization laboratory. This ability to administer the drug in a wider range of settings enhances the chance of giving it early and salvaging substantial myocardium. The other major advantage is that it has been documented to be effective in reducing morbidity and mortality in more than 150,000 patients in well-designed, scientifically controlled trials [24,48,61–65].

There are several disadvantages as well. Even though thrombolytic therapy is widely available, the most recent data indicate that it is given to only 30% to 40% of patients with acute MI in the United States. The frequency of administration in patients with acute MI may be higher in other countries, and it is increasing in this country. It remains the case that a large number of patients presenting with acute MI do not receive thrombolytic therapy either because of relative or absolute contraindications or concerns about risk-benefit issues. Despite the fact that early reperfusion is the goal of therapy, in contrast to direct PTCA, which is characterized by success rates of more than 90%, lytic therapy results in early reperfusion in only 55% to 80% of patients depending on the agent used [37]. In addition, achievement of TIMI-3 flow is even less frequent, although this may be the most important goal to optimize outcome. As previously mentioned, TIMI-3 flow is associated with substantially better improvement in left ventricular function and survival than TIMI-2 flow [37,66]. Other disadvantages include the fact that reliable assessment of reperfusion noninvasively is often not possible and, finally, that a significant residual stenosis often remains.

CHARACTERISTICS OF TRIALS COMPARING PTCA WITH INTRAVENOUS THROMBOLYSIS

				PTCA		
STUDY	PATIENT POPULATION	DURATION OF SYMPTOMS, h	PRIMARY FOLLOW-UP PERIOD	NO. OF PATIENTS (n=1290)	TIME TO TREATMENT, MIN	NO. OF PATIENTS (n=1316)
Zijlstra et al.	≤ 75 y; ST ↑	< 6	Discharge	152	62 †	142
Ribiero et al.	< 75 y; ST ↑	< 6	Discharge	50	238	50
Grinfeld et al.	ST ↑	< 12	30 d	54	63 ‡	58
Zijlstra et al.	ST ↑; low risk	< 6	30 d	45	68 †	50
DeWood	≤76 y; ST ↑	< 12	30 d	46	126 †	44
Grines et al.	ST ↑	< 12	Discharge	195	60 ‡	20
Gibbons et al.	< 80 y; ST ↑	< 12	Discharge	47	45 ‡	56
Ribichini et al.	< 80 y; inferior MI; anterior ST ↓	< 6	Discharge	41	40 ‡	42
Garcia et al.	Anterior MI	5	30 d	95	84 †	94
GUSTO IIb	ST ↑; LBBB	< 12	30 d	565	114 ‡	573

* All patients were treated with oral aspirin, except for those in the study by Zijlstra et al., who received intravenous angioplasty; ST ↑— ST-segment elevation; ST ↓—ST-segment depression; t-PA—tissue-type plasminogen activator thromboplastic time; MI—myocardial infarction; LBBB—left bundle branch block.
†From admission; ‡from randomization.

FIGURE 2-48. Meta-analysis of ten randomized clinical trials of thrombolytic therapy compared with direct angioplasty. A total of 2606 patients were included in this analysis. Overall, outcome was improved with direct angioplasty; mortality was 4.4% for patients undergoing direct PTCA and 6.5% in patients receiving thrombolytic therapy. The duration of follow-up reported for some of these trials was confined to the hospital stay and was 30 days for others. For this reason, as well as because of patient selection factors, the observed mortality is lower than that reported in broader epidemiologic studies. Overall, other secondary endpoints such as nonfatal reinfarction and recurrent ischemia were reduced in the primary PTCA groups compared with patients undergoing thrombolysis [67]. These trials were performed before the current era of stent placement and GP IIb/IIIa antagonist therapy, both of which have been associated with improved outcome in PCI patients. (*Adapted from* Weaver *et al.* [67].)

CARDIOGENIC SHOCK

PATHOPHYSIOLOGY OF LEFT VENTRICULAR SHOCK

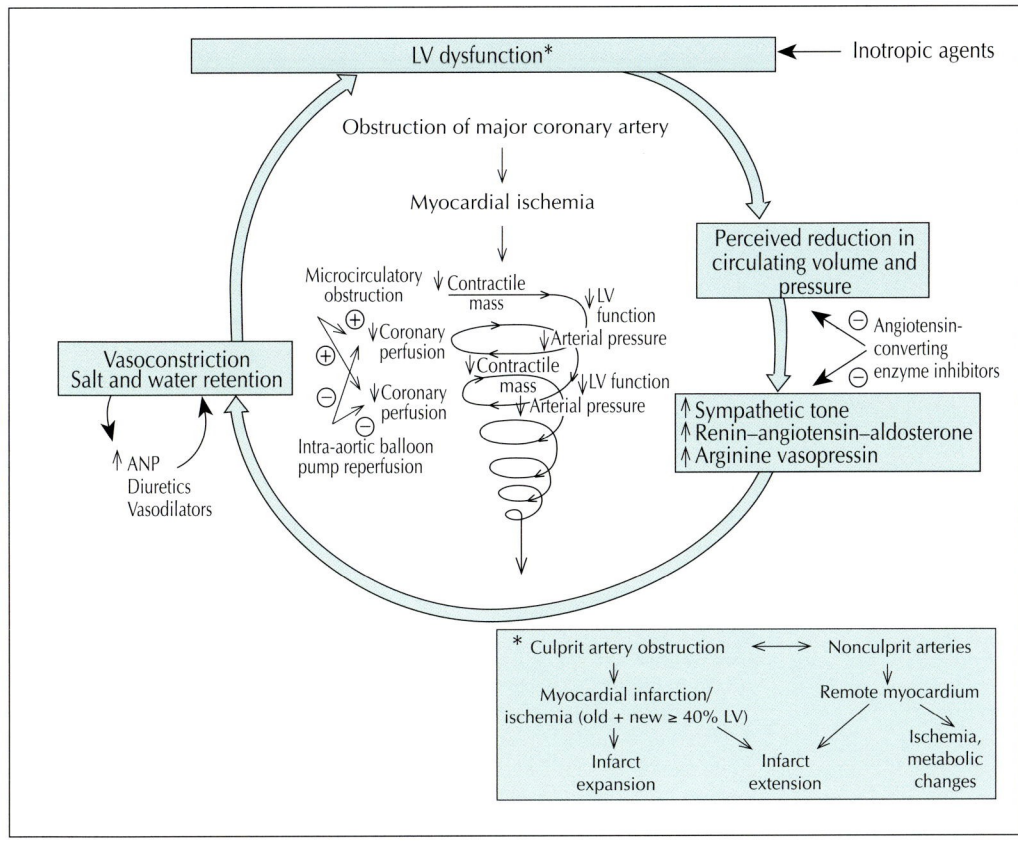

FIGURE 2-49. Cardiogenic shock can develop either early or late after the onset of MI. Early cardiogenic shock may be secondary to massive necrosis of the left ventricle (LV), but the combi-

nation of more modest necrosis plus widespread ischemia may also be responsible. Cardiogenic shock that develops later reflects more complex pathophysiology. The infarct can extend to areas of myocardium at risk as a result of re-occlusion of a recanalized artery or propagation of the existing thrombus into previously patent branches. In addition, LV dysfunction leads to hypotension and increases in LV end-diastolic pressure (LVEDP), further exacerbating coronary hypoperfusion. This low coronary blood flow compromises not only the jeopardized region but also distant myocardium. This "ischemia at a distance" is particularly profound when multivessel disease is present.

The development of LV dilatation and tachycardia associated with cardiogenic shock markedly increases the metabolic demands of the myocardium at a time when coronary flow reserve is too low to compensate, leading to more global ischemia and further dysfunction. This vicious circle is then perpetuated, as shown in the classic downward spiral of cardiogenic shock presented by Califf and Bengtson [68]. Infarct expansion characterized by thinning and dilatation of the infarct zone as well as acute LV "functional" aneurysm formation can further compromise cardiac output and increase wall stress and metabolic demands. ANP—atrial natriuretic peptide. (*Adapted from* Califf and Bengtson [68].)

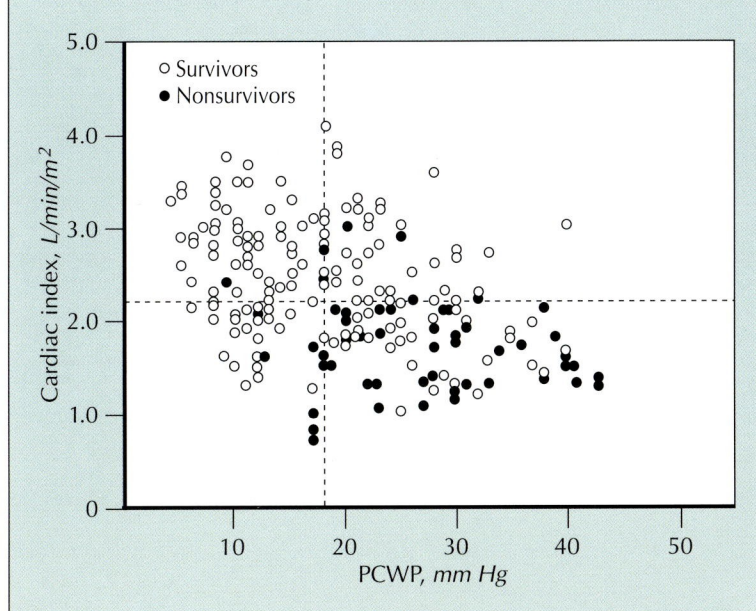

FIGURE 2-50. Cardiac index versus pulmonary capillary wedge pressure (PCWP) in 200 patients after acute myocardial infarction (MI), demonstrating an inverse relationship between mortality and cardiac performance [69]. A PCWP exceeding 18 mm Hg and a cardiac index less than 2.2 L/min/m^2 represent severe left ventricular (LV) failure (with or without

hypotension) and were associated with the highest mortality. This subset includes patients with classic LV cardiogenic shock. The results of this study by Forrester *et al.* [69] illustrate the importance of optimizing the PCWP to maximize cardiac index.

Based on the American College of Cardiology/American Heart Association (ACC/AHA) Task Force guidelines for the early management of patients with acute MI [70], patients with LV pump failure can be divided into two subsets. Subset 1 includes those with an LV filling pressure above 15 mm Hg, systolic arterial blood pressure above 100 mm Hg, and a cardiac index below 2.5 L/min/m^2, representing LV failure without classic shock. Subset 2 is defined as an LV filling pressure above 15 mm Hg, arterial pressure below 90 mm Hg, and a cardiac index below 2.5 L/min/m^2, representing more classic shock. Typically, the cardiac index is lower (*ie*, <2.0 L/min/m^2) and PCWP higher (*ie*, >20 mm Hg) when classic cardiogenic shock is the result of LV failure (without hypovolemia). This distinction has important clinical implications in terms of therapeutic intervention. When systolic arterial blood pressure exceeds 100 mm Hg, treatment options would include afterload reduction with nitroglycerin or nitroprusside, drugs that are usually employed in conjunction with inotropic agents. Agents that combine inotropy and vasodilation, such as dobutamine or milrinone (or amrinone), can be used either alone or in combination.

Subset 2 constitutes the classic cardiogenic shock population. Frank hypotension and hypoperfusion are present. In addition to inotropic and vasopressor support, intra-aortic balloon counterpulsation for afterload reduction, increased coronary blood flow, and augmented systemic diastolic pressure are frequently needed. (*Adapted from* Forrester *et al.* [69].)

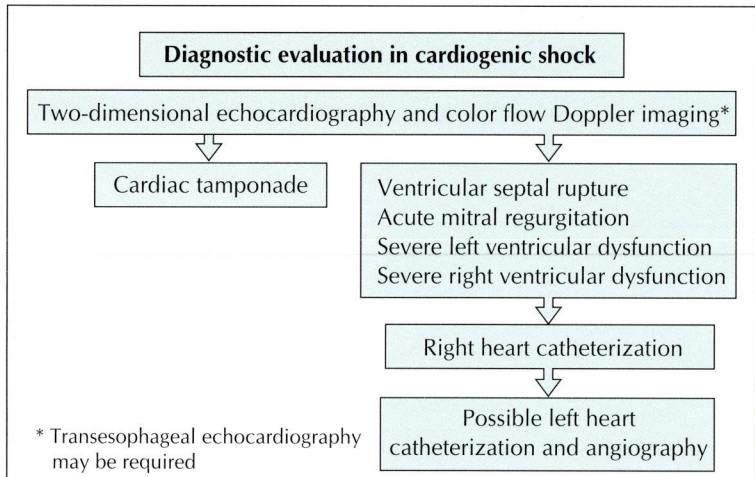

FIGURE 2-51. The diagnostic investigation for patients with cardiogenic shock should include an evaluation of volume status and an assessment of both RV and LV function. Swan-Ganz catheterization is used to measure right heart pressures, pulmonary artery pressure, and pulmonary capillary wedge pressure. Oxygen saturation should be measured routinely in the right-sided chambers in all patients with cardiogenic shock to assess whether a left-to-right shunt (*ie*, ventricular septal rupture) is present. Two-dimensional echocardiography and color flow Doppler imaging should be performed in all patients with cardiogenic shock. These tests are invaluable for the bedside assessment of ventricular function and the detection of valvular heart disease, shunts, and tamponade. Left heart catheterization with coronary angiography is indicated when an intervention such as PTCA or cardiac surgery is contemplated. At times the urgency of the situation (*eg*, acute cardiac tamponade) may preclude such testing prior to the intervention.

TREATMENT OF LEFT VENTRICULAR SHOCK

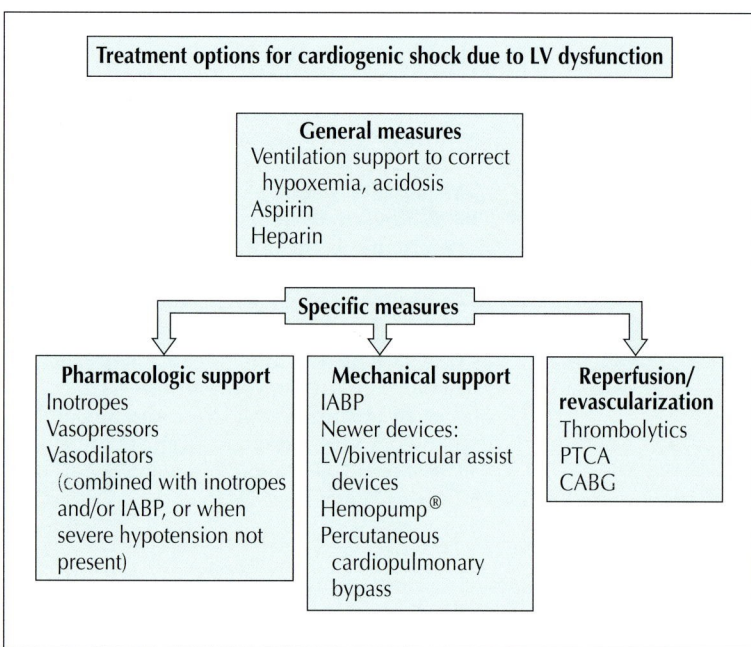

FIGURE 2-52. Specific treatment of cardiogenic shock secondary to left ventricular (LV) pump failure may include one or more of the three major modalities, including pharmacologic circulatory support, mechanical circulatory support, and reperfusion or revascularization. General measures such as maintaining adequate ventilation and correcting acidosis are extremely important. Aspirin is of documented efficacy in acute MI, and heparin is particularly important in the setting of low flow and high filling pressures to prevent LV thrombus, deep vein thrombosis, and coronary thrombus formation and propagation.

The use of vasopressors such as norepinephrine or dopamine may be necessary to support systemic perfusion pressure in the event of profound hypotension and hypoperfusion [71]. However, this may be at the expense of increasing systemic vascular resistance at a time when it is typically already elevated, increasing cardiac work. Borderline cases of cardiogenic shock, defined as systolic pressures greater than 80 to 90 mm Hg in the presence of increased pulmonary capillary wedge pressure, decreased cardiac output, and increased systemic vascular resistance, may be approached differently. In these instances, treatment with inotropic agents plus vasodilators may be useful for improving LV function and decreasing systemic vascular resistance. β-adrenergic agonists, such as dobutamine, and phosphodiesterase inhibitors, such as milrinone, are used frequently for this purpose. The latter are potent vasodilators and should be used with caution only when systolic blood pressure is greater than 100 mm Hg.

The use of mechanical circulatory support devices in combination with pharmacologic support has distinct advantages in classic cardiogenic shock when there is hypotension or hypoperfusion. These devices help support systemic circulation while concomitantly increasing coronary perfusion, decreasing cardiac work, and reducing ischemia. The most commonly used device is the intra-aortic balloon pump (IABP), which increases diastolic flow to the ischemic coronary bed and reduces aortic impedance and afterload, thus improving the cardiac index. Newer devices such as LV and biventricular assist devices, the Hemopump (Medtronics), and percutaneous cardiopulmonary bypass with extracorporeal membrane oxygenators have been used to provide circulatory support [72–78]. Although more invasive and difficult to implement, these newer devices offer more circulatory support than the IABP, serving as bridges for patients who will eventually undergo myocardial revascularization or cardiac transplantation.

Reperfusion with thrombolytic agents or revascularization by percutaneous transluminal coronary angioplasty (PTCA) or coronary artery bypass graft (CABG) surgery can re-establish flow to the infarct zone and potentially benefit patients in cardiogenic shock associated with acute MI. Potential mechanisms of benefit include reduction of infarct size and reversal of ischemia in the peri-infarct area, acute reduction in infarct expansion, and improved infarct healing, resulting in beneficial effects on chronic LV remodeling.

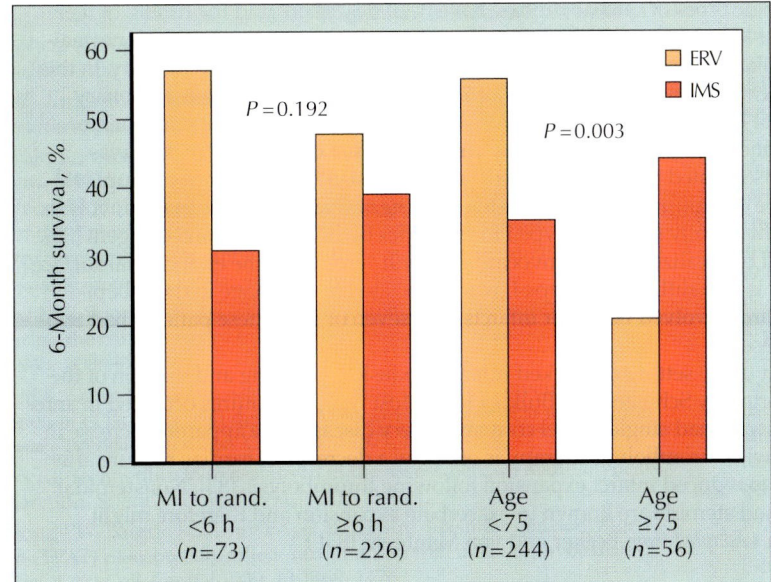

21.
22.
23.
24.
25.
26.
27.
28.
29.
30.
31.
32.
33.
34.
35.
36.
37.
38.
39.
40.
41.
42.

FIGURE 2-53. Six-month survival data from the SHOCK trial [79]. These prospective subgroups were tested for differential treatment effects. The subgroup variable of age (<75 years vs ≥ 75 years) interacted significantly with treatment effect at 30 days, 6 months, and 12 months (P=0.01, P=0.003, and P=0.029, respectively). There was no significant difference in the treatment effect for those with anterior myocardial infarction (MI) versus those without anterior MI. There was a trend toward survival in the early intervention group with prior MI.

MITRAL REGURGITATION, VENTRICULAR SEPTAL DEFECT AND CARDIAC RUPTURE

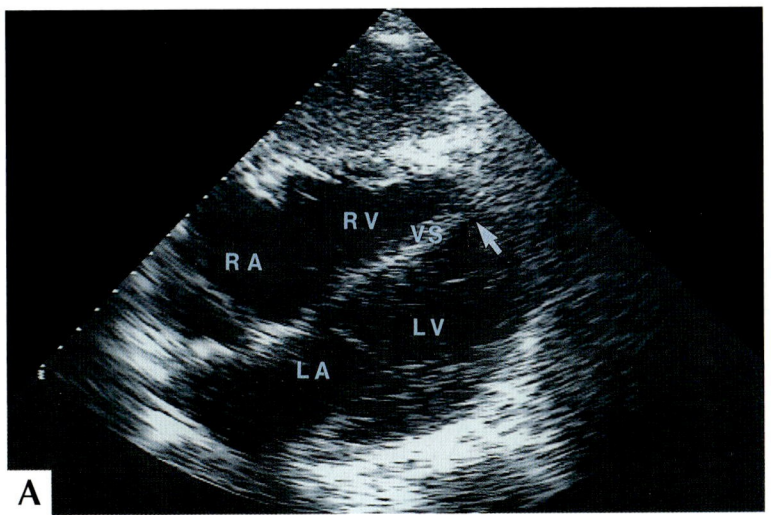

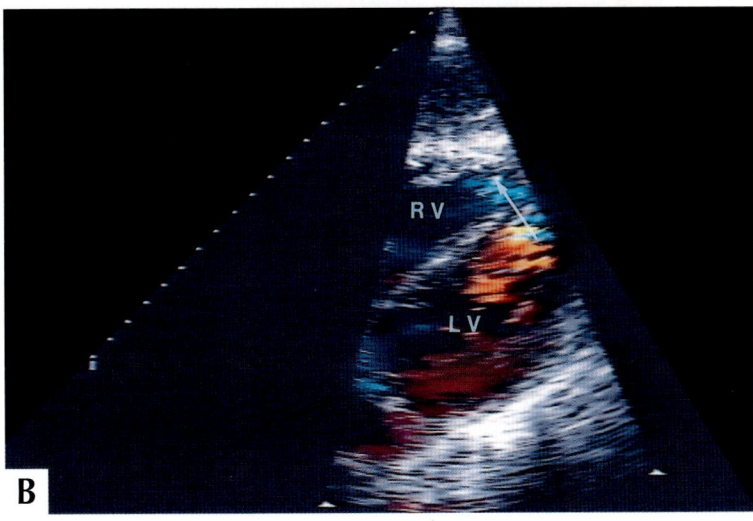

FIGURE 2-54. A, Two-dimensional echocardiogram demonstrating ventricular septal (VS) rupture (VSR). The *arrow* indicates the defect in the apical portion of the VS. **B,** Color Doppler flow through the VSR. The *arrow* shows systolic flow from the left ventricle (LV) to the right ventricle (RV) across the VSR. LA—left atrium; RA—right atrium. (*Courtesy of* Alan Mogtader, MD, St. Luke's-Roosevelt Hospital Center and Columbia University, New York, NY.)

67. Weaver WD, Simes RJ, Betriu A, *et al.*: Comparison of primary coronary angioplasty and intravenous thrombolytic therapy for acute myocardial infarction: a quantitative review. *JAMA* 1997, 278:2093–2098.

68. Califf RA, Bengston JR: Cardiogenic shock. *N Engl J Med* 1994, 330:1724–1730.

69. Forrester JS, Diamond G, Chatterjee K, *et al.*: Medical therapy of acute myocardial infarction by application of hemodynamic subsets. *N Engl J Med* 1976, 295:1356–1362.

70. Gunnar RM (Chairman), on behalf of the ACC/AHA Task Force: ACC/AHA Task Force Report: Guidelines for the early management of patients with acute myocardial infarction. *J Am Coll Cardiol* 1990, 16:249–292.

71. Mueller H, Aynessem, Gianellis, *et al.*: Effect of isoproterenol, I-norepinephrine and intraaortic counterpulsation on hemodynamics and myocardial metabolism in shock following acute myocardial infarction. *Circulation* 1971, 45:335–351.

72. Pennington DG, Kanter KR, McBride LR, *et al.*: Seven years' experience with the Pierce-Donachy ventricular assist device. *Thorac Cardiovasc Surg* 1988, 96:901–911.

73. Portner PM, Oyer PE, Pennington DG, *et al.*: Implantable electrical left ventricular assist system: bridge to transplantation and future. *Ann Thorac Sug* 1989, 47:142–150.

74. Joyce LD, Johnson KE, Toninato CJ, *et al.*: Results of the first 100 patients who received Symbion total artificial hearts as a bridge to cardiac transplantation. *Circulation* 1989, 80(suppl):III-192–III-201.

75. Gacioch GM, Ellis SG, Lee L, *et al.*: Cardiogenic shock complicating acute myocardial infarction: the use of coronary angioplasty and the integration of the new support devices into patient management. *J Am Coll Cardiol* 1992, 19:647–653.

76. Shawl FA, Domanski MJ, Hernandez TJ, *et al.*: Emergency percutaneous cardiopulmonary bypass support in cardiogenic shock from acute myocardial infarction. *Am J Cardiol* 1989, 64:967–970.

77. Pennington DG, Merjavy JP, Cood JE, *et al.*: Extracorporeal membrane oxygenation for patients with cardiogenic shock. *Circulation* 1984, 70(suppl):I-130–I-137.

78. Lincoff AM, Popma JJ, Bates ER, *et al.*: Successful coronary angioplasty in two patients with cardiogenic shock using the Nimbus Hemopump support device. *Am Heart J* 1990, 120:970–972.

79. Hochman JS, Sleeper L, Webb J, *et al.*: Effect of early revascularization for cardiogenic shock on one-year mortality: the SHOCK Trial Results [abstract]. *Circulation* 1999, 100:1939.

80. Becker AE, van Mantgem J-P: Cardiac tamponade: a study of 50 hearts. *Eur J Cardiol* 1975, 3/4:349–358.

81. Bloor CM: *Cardiac Pathology*. Philadelphia: JB Lippincott Co; 1978:176–221.

82. Schuster EH, Bulkley BH: Expansion of transmural myocardial infarction: a pathophysiologic factor in cardiac rupture. *Circulation* 1979, 60:1532–1538.

83. Becker R, Charlesworth A, Wilcox R, *et al.*: Cardiac rupture associated with thrombolytic therapy: impact of time to treatment in the Last Assessment of Thrombolytic Efficacy (LATE) Study. *J Am Coll Cardiol* 1995, 25:1063–1068.

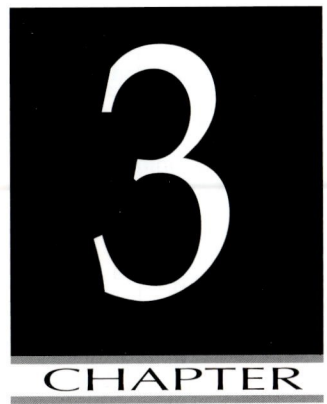

3

CHAPTER

CHRONIC ISCHEMIC HEART DISEASE

Edited by George A. Beller

*Jonathan Abrams, Barry D. Bertolet, Bernard R. Chaitman,
Delos M. Cosgrove III, David P. Faxor, Bernard J. Gersh,
Bruce W. Lytle, Carl J. Pepine, Michael H. Picard, Eric R. Powers,
Frans J. Th. Wackers, Arthur E. Weyman*

PATHOPHYSIOLOGY OF ANGINA

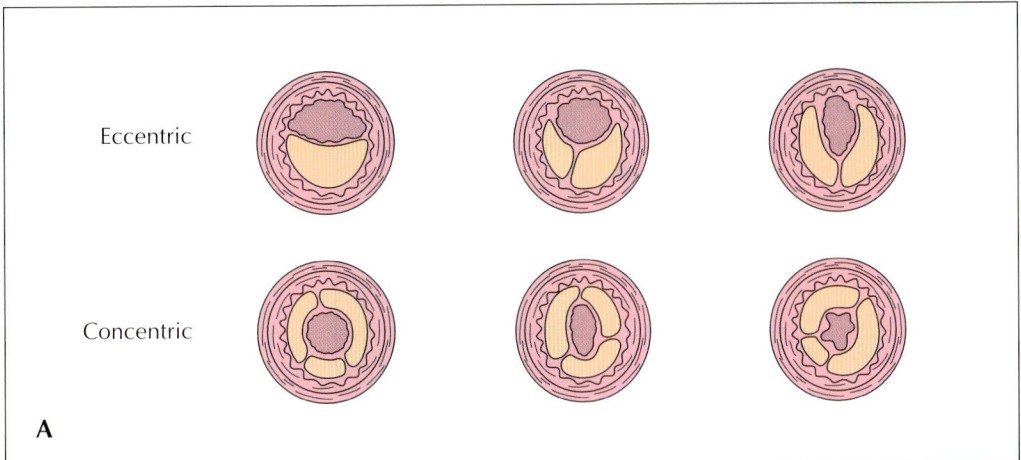

Eccentric

Concentric

A

FIGURE 3-1. Coronary stenosis as a cause of angina. It is now recognized that coronary artery obstructions are capable of changing caliber, and constriction or narrowing of a preexisting lesion can be a factor in precipitating angina and myocardial ischemia.

    A, If the coronary segment has sufficient smooth muscle (media) that is not involved in the atherosclerotic process, the vessel can dilate or constrict at the site of the stenosis. In general, vasoconstriction is most likely to occur with eccentric or asymmetric lesions, which consist of coronary atherosclerotic plaque in a segment of the vessel wall, with some relatively normal media intact. Concentric stenoses are less likely to constrict further or dilate. In concentric atherosclerosis, the atherosclerotic plaque circumferentially involves the entire area of the vessel. It is believed that at least 25% of an arc or rim of media in the coronary artery must be preserved to allow for stenosis vasomotion. (*continued*)

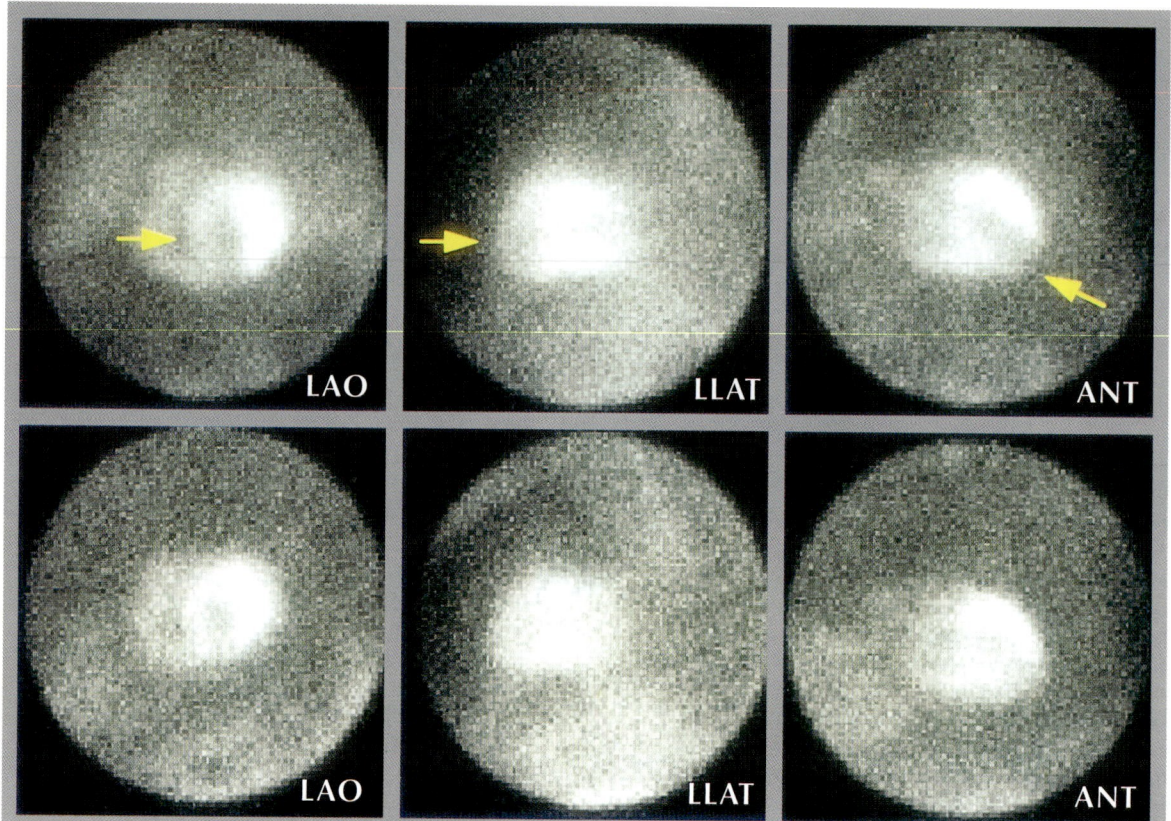

FIGURE 3-9. Abnormal planar exercise-redistribution Tl-201 images of myocardial perfusion showing reversible myocardial perfusion defects. On the exercise images (*top*), an anteroseptal myocardial perfusion defect is present (*arrows*). The defect is most apparent on the left anterior oblique (LAO) view and is almost completely reversed on redistribution imaging (bottom). These images are consistent with transient ischemia in the territory of the left anterior descending coronary artery. Ant—anterior; LLAT—left lateral.

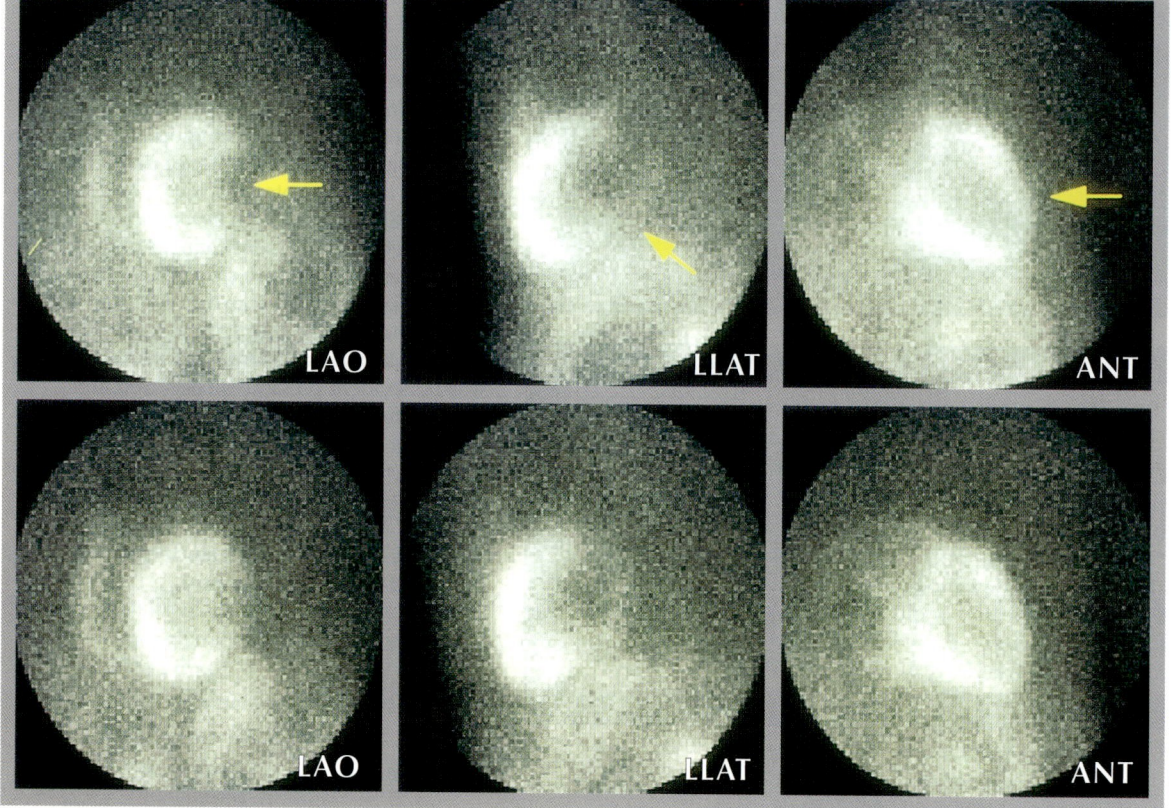

FIGURE 3-10. Abnormal planar exercise and redistribution Tl-201 myocardial perfusion images showing a fixed myocardial perfusion defect. On the exercise images (*top*), a large posterolateral and inferoposterior defect is present (*arrows*), and is unchanged at redistribution imaging (*bottom*). These images are consistent with infarction in the territory of the left circumflex coronary artery. ANT—anterior; LAO—left anterior oblique; LLAT—left lateral.

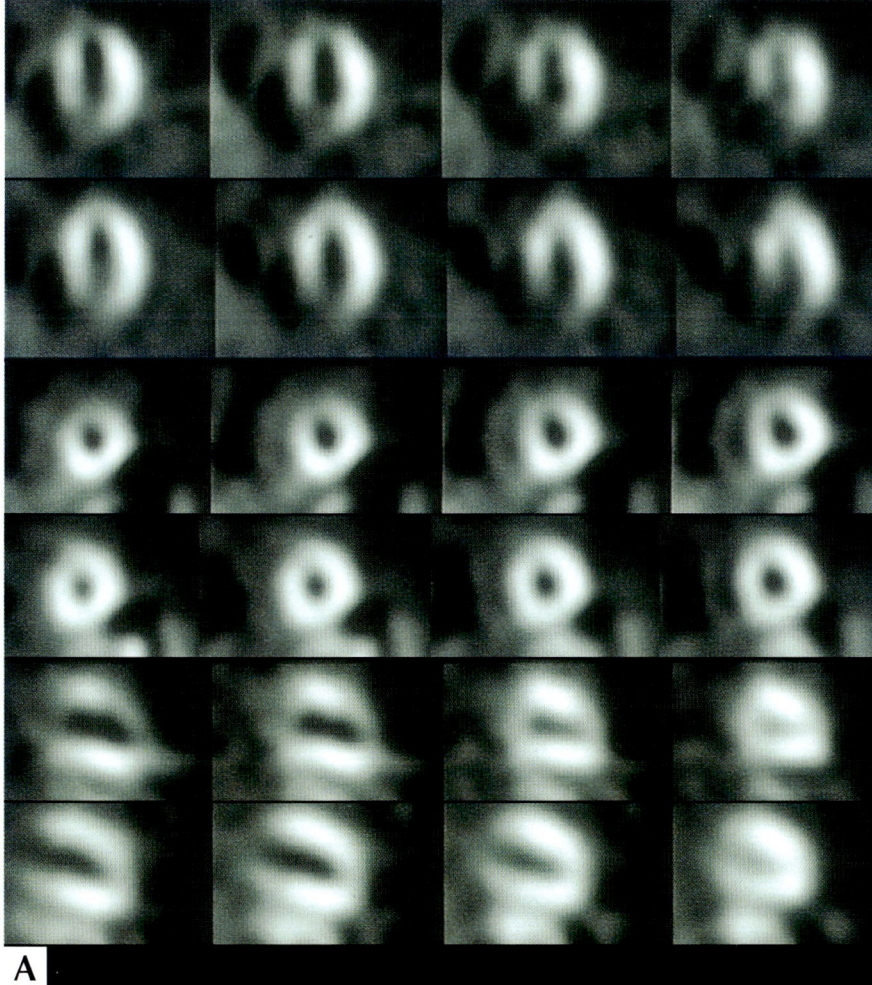
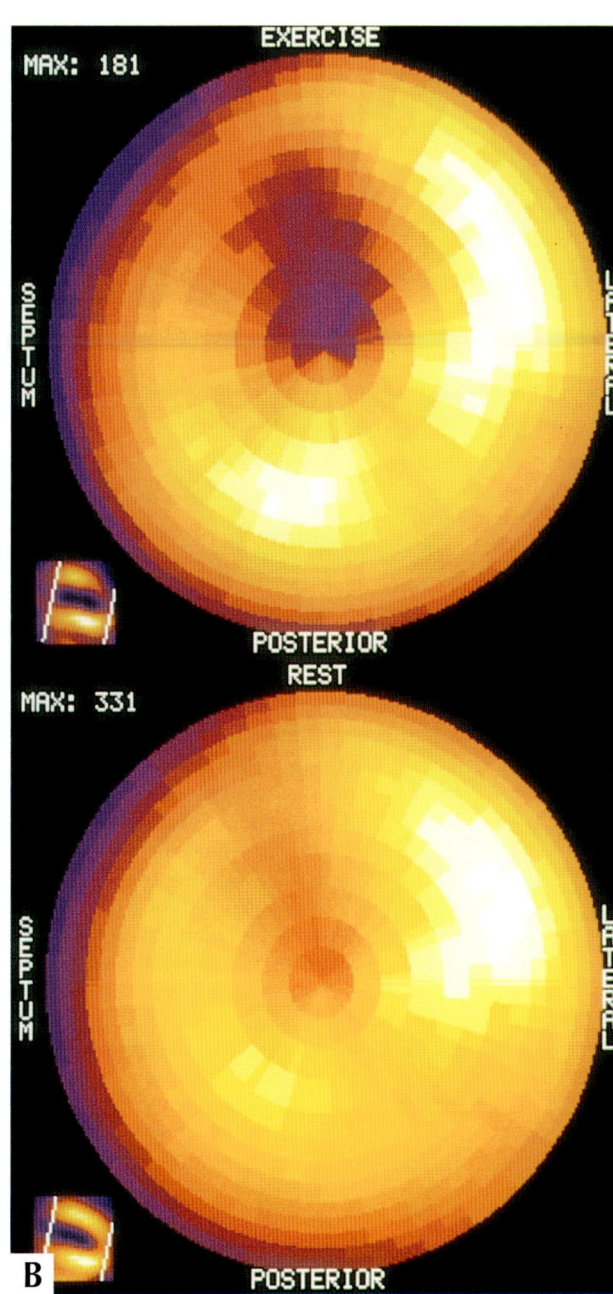

FIGURE 3-11. Myocardial perfusion imaging on single-photon emission computed tomography (SPECT) with Tc-99m tetrofosmin and polar map display. **A**, SPECT images. **B**, The exercise polar map (*top*) shows an anteroseptal defect (dark area), and the rest polar map (*bottom*) shows reversibility (homogeneous coloring). In display, the highest counts appear as white and yellow, and the lowest counts as purple and blue.

PROGNOSTIC VALUE OF MYOCARDIAL PERFUSION IMAGING

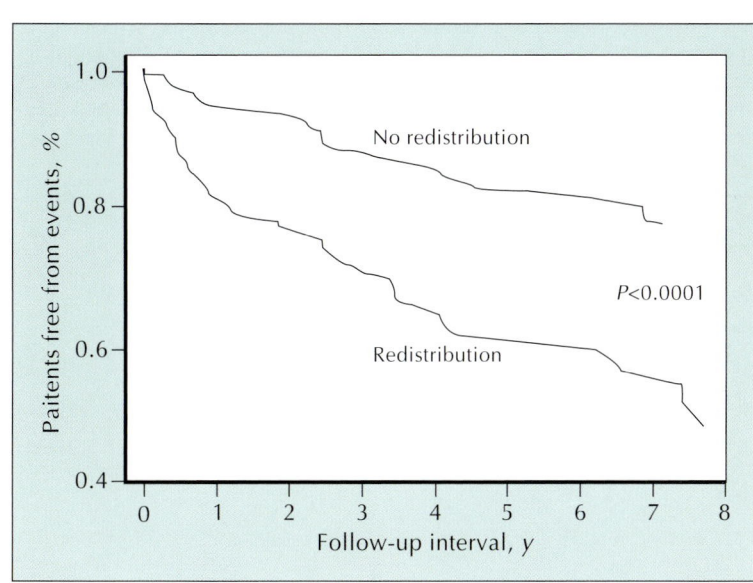

FIGURE 3-12. Event-free survival of patients with and without Tl-201 redistribution. Numerous investigators have shown that, in addition to detection of coronary artery disease, important prognostic and functional information can be obtained from exercise and rest myocardial perfusion images. This illustration demonstrates the significant difference in event-free survival in patients who had angiographic coronary artery disease with and without evidence of Tl-201 redistribution. "Event-free" indicates freedom from death, nonfatal myocardial infarction, coronary bypass surgery, or angioplasty for 3 months or longer after completion of the study. Five-year event-free survival was 82% for patients with no redistribution and 60% for patients with redistribution [8].

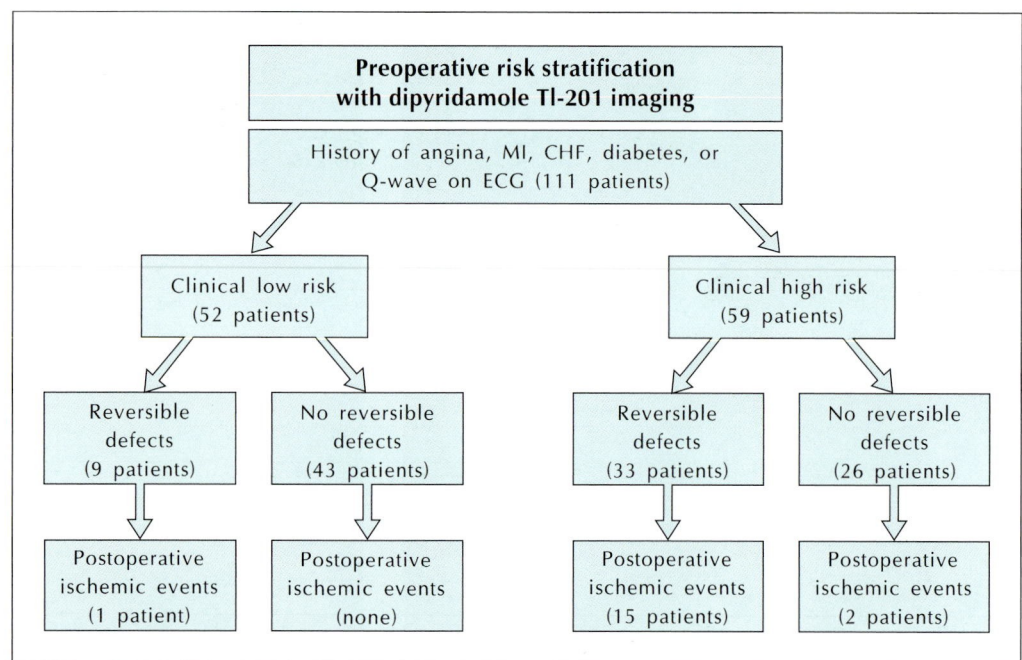

FIGURE 3-13. Preoperative risk stratification with dipyridamole Tl-201 myocardial perfusion imaging. Dipyridamole Tl-201 imaging has been used extensively for preoperative risk stratification of patients who are scheduled to undergo peripheral arterial surgery and for elderly patients who are scheduled for other types of major surgery. These patients have a high prevalence of associated coronary artery disease and are at risk for a perioperative cardiac event. Several investigators have demonstrated that the presence of reversible myocardial perfusion defects on dipyridamole Tl-201 imaging effectively predicts the occurrence of perioperative infarction and death [9]. Eagle *et al.* [10] showed that not all patients scheduled for surgery need to have dipyridamole myocardial perfusion imaging. Low-, intermediate-, and high-risk groups can be recognized by clinical criteria. Clinical variables that place a patient at increased risk are a history of angina, myocardial infarction (MI), congestive heart failure, diabetes, and Q wave on the electrocardiogram (ECG). If none of these variables is present, the patient is at relatively low risk and dipyridamole-myocardial perfusion imaging is unnecessary. If all clinical variables are present, the patient is at increased risk and dipyridamole-myocardial perfusion imaging is indicated. This diagram shows the result of myocardial perfusion imaging and the occurrence of cardiac events. Cardiac events occurred predominantly in patients with evidence of redistribution on perfusion imaging in the high-risk patient group. (*Adapted from* Eagle *et al.* [10].)

ASSESSMENT OF LEFT VENTRICULAR FUNCTION

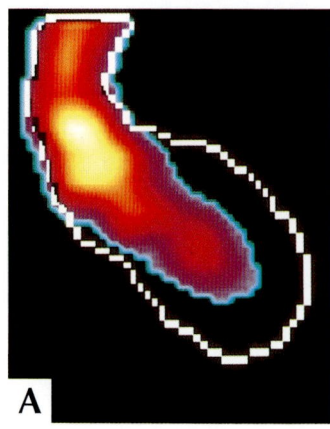
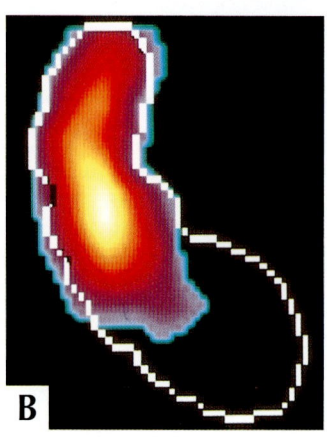

A **B**

FIGURE 3-14. Normal first-pass radionuclide angiography at rest and during exercise. In this illustration the left ventricular end-diastolic (ED) outline (white) in the anterior position is superimposed on the end-systolic (ES) image. This display allows assessment of regional wall motion from a static image; such images are best interpreted by dynamic display as an endless loop cine on a computer screen. Here, maximum count activity is yellow and the lowest activity is green. Resting left ventricular ejection fraction (LVEF) in this patient is 60% (**A**), and peak exercise LVEF is 80% (**B**). Regional wall motion shows uniformly increased contraction. In order to meet the increased demand during exercise, cardiac output must increase; this is achieved by increasing heart rate and LVEF (LVEF = ED volume - ES volume/ED volume). A normal LVEF response is defined as an increase in LVEF of 5% or greater compared with baseline LVEF and a uniform increase of regional wall motion [11].

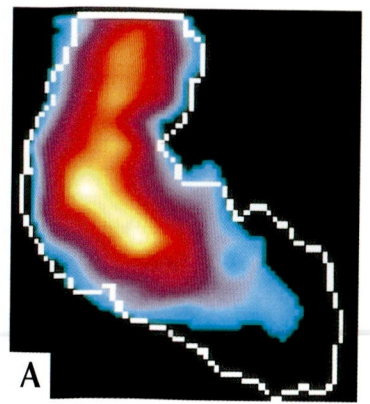
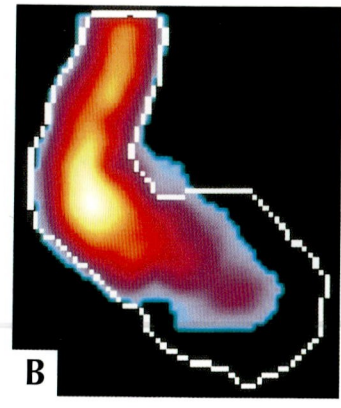

FIGURE 3-15. Abnormal first-pass radionuclide angiograms at rest and during exercise. In this patient, resting left ventricular ejection fraction (LVEF) is 60% (**A**), and peak exercise LVEF is 45% (**B**), with uniformly decreased regional wall motion. An abnormal response is defined as either a decrease greater than 5%, or no change in LVEF compared with baseline. In patients with a high baseline LVEF (*ie*, 70% or greater), only a decrease in LVEF is considered an abnormal response.

ECHOCARDIOGRAPHY

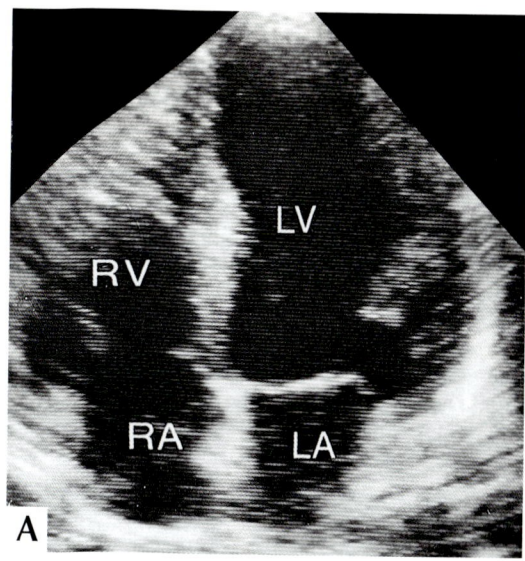
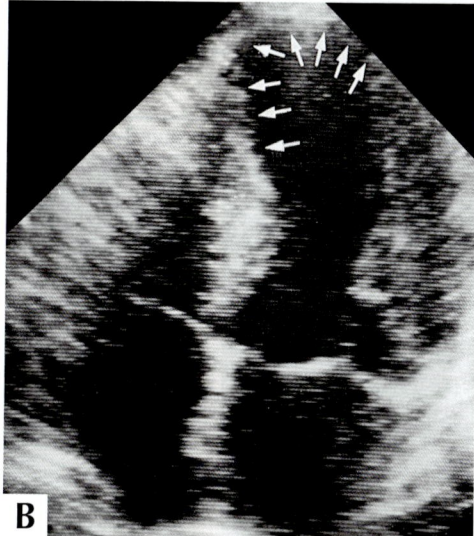

FIGURE 3-16. Wall motion abnormality is the hallmark of coronary artery disease on echocardiography. This abnormality is one of the earliest signs of myocardial ischemia or infarction. **A,** Two-dimensional echocardiographic apical four-chamber view at end-diastole. **B,** Two-dimensional echocardiographic apical four-chamber view at end-systole. The right ventricle (RV) and the septal and lateral walls at the base of the left ventricle (LV) demonstrate normal inward motion from diastole through systole; however, the distal septum and apex demonstrate akinesis (arrows in B). The wall motion abnormality demonstrated in this frame was caused by ischemia from a lesion in the mid-left anterior descending artery. LA—left atrium; RA—right atrium.

NATURAL HISTORY OF WALL MOTION ABNORMALITIES

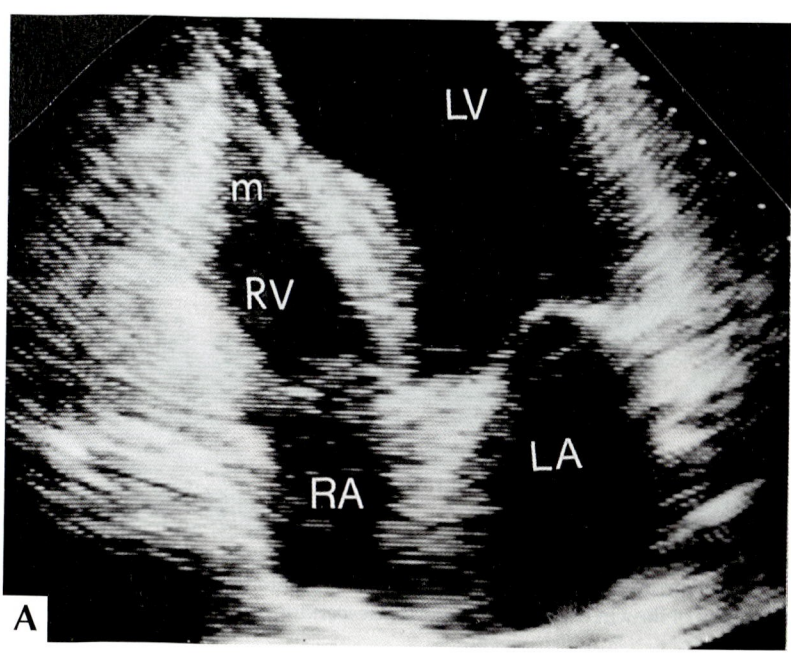

FIGURE 3-17. Infarct expansion, which is caused by thinning and stretching of infarcted myocardium without further myocyte necrosis, is observed to occur in up to 39% of patients after the first anterior Q-wave infarction. Such expansion is a substrate for aneurysm formation. Anteroapical location, rather than infarct size, has been reported as the most important predictor of infarct expansion [12]. Microscopically, slippage of myocytes and sarcomere stretching is observed [13]. Infarct expansion is detected by two-dimensional echocardiography as increased endocardial surface area within the region of abnormal wall motion. In clinical studies, infarct expansion has been observed as early as 2 hours after onset of myocardial infarction, with continued expansion observed over the months after infarction. **A,** Apical four-chamber echocardiogram from a patient 6 weeks after anteroapical myocardial infarction. (*continued*)

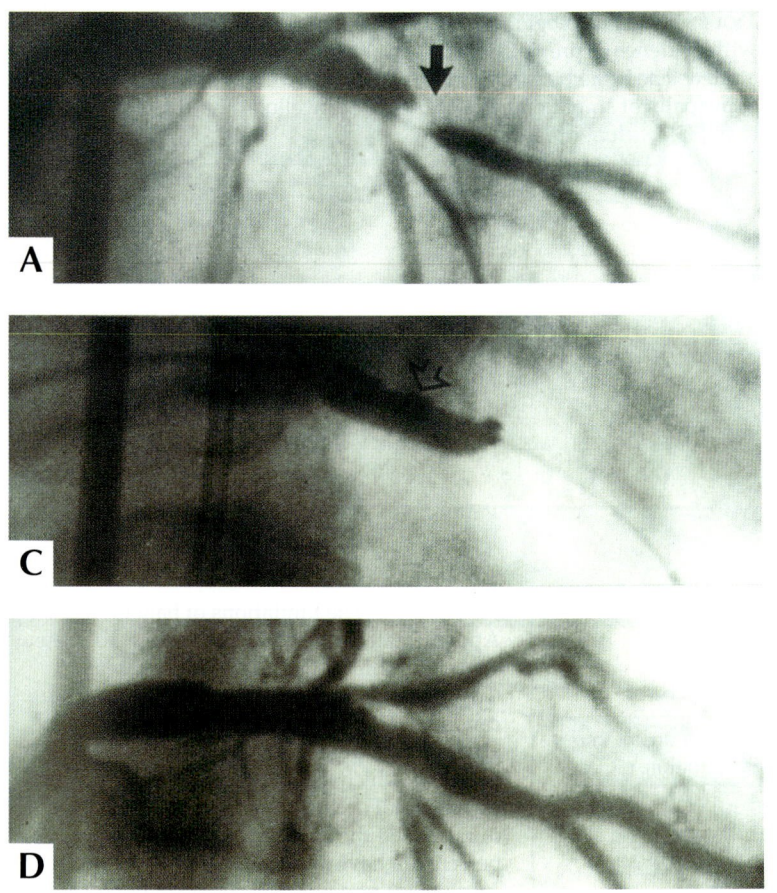

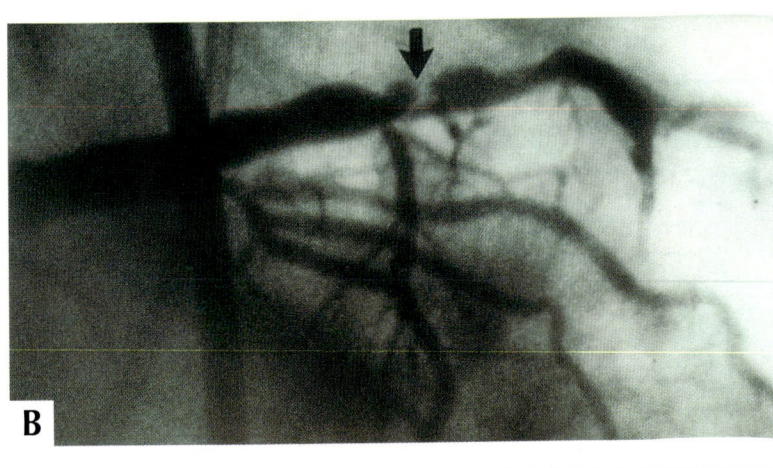

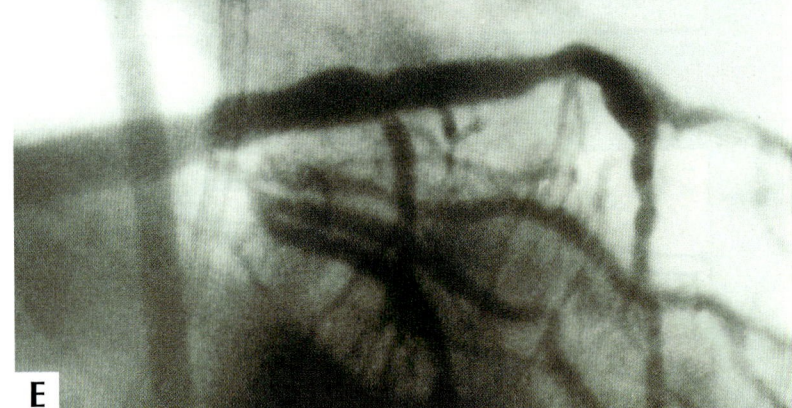

FIGURE 3-44. An example of directional atherectomy showing an extremely eccentric lesion in the middle left anterior descending artery. A and B, The lesion (*arrows*) can be seen. C, The atherectomy device is in place across the stenosis (*arrow*). D and E, The result demonstrates minimal residual stenosis. (*From* Fishman and Baim [37]; with permission.)

LASER ANGIOPLASTY

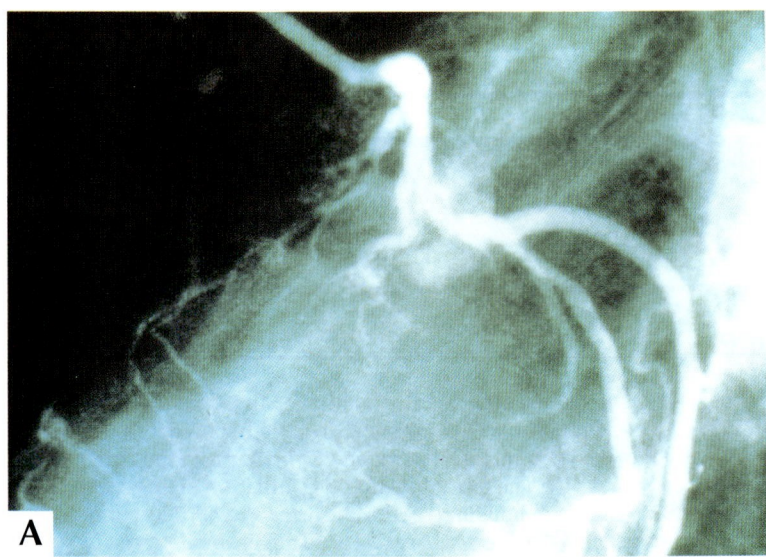

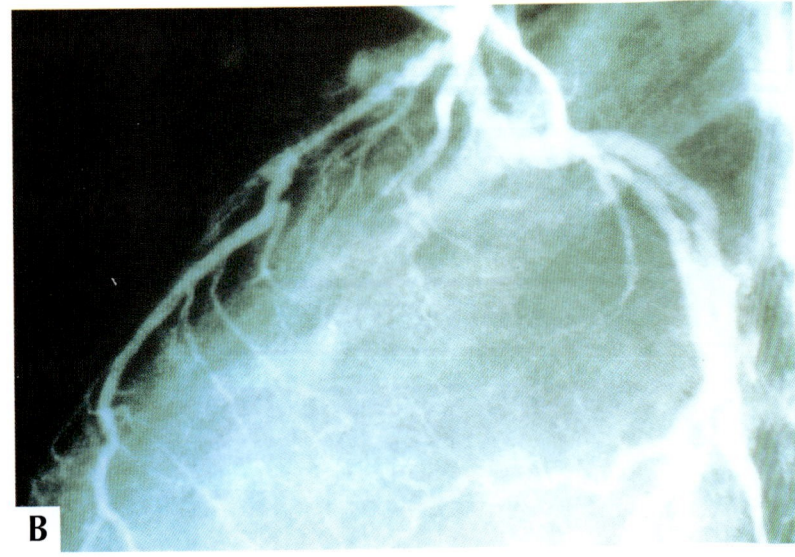

FIGURE 3-45. Laser PTCA. A, An occluded stenosis of the left anterior descending (LAD) artery is evident. B, A guidewire was passed through the stenosis and was followed by laser PTCA of the long proximal occlusion of the LAD artery. (*continued*)

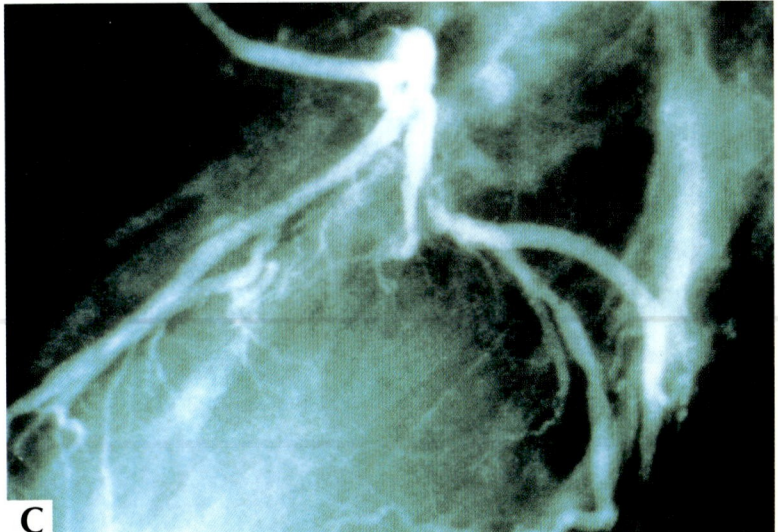

FIGURE 3-45 (*continued*) **C,** This procedure was followed by successful balloon PTCA with minimal residual stenosis [38]. (*Courtesy of* Advanced Interventional Systems, Inc., Irvine, CA.)

STENTS

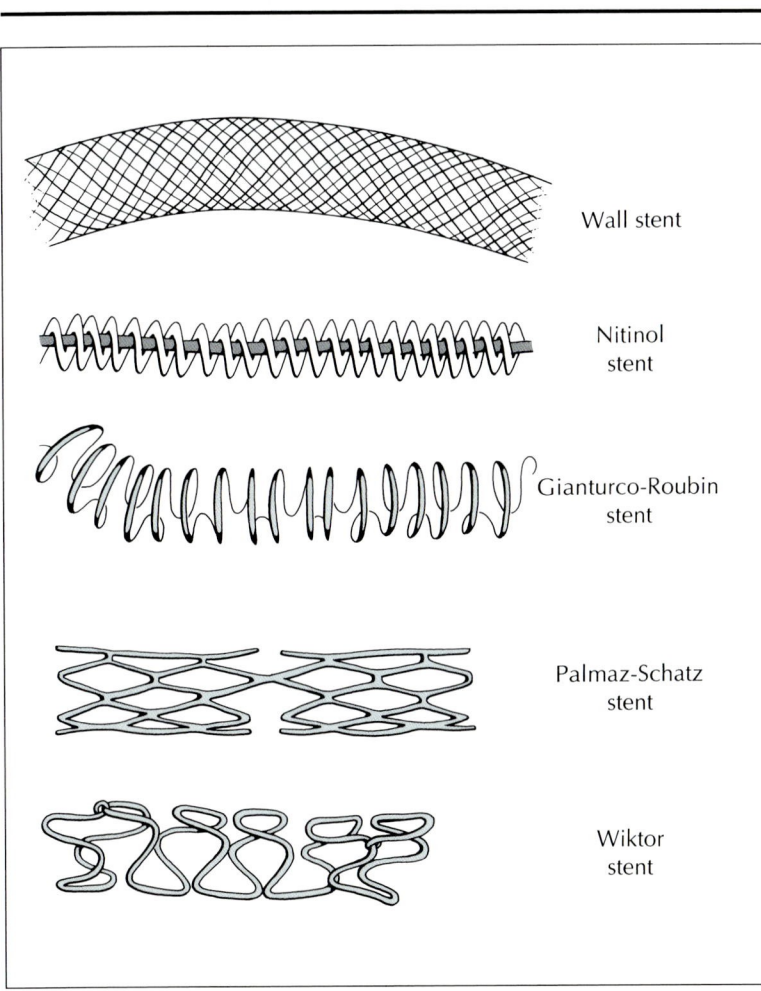

Wall stent

Nitinol stent

Gianturco-Roubin stent

Palmaz-Schatz stent

Wiktor stent

FIGURE 3-46. Various types of commonly used intracoronary stents. The wall stent was the first to be introduced. The most commonly used stents are balloon-expandable and include the Gianturco-Roubin stent, the Palmaz-Schatz stent, and the Wiktor stent. Others include Strecker, Cordis, and ACS stents (not shown). The configuration and amount of metal used in the design contribute to the physical properties and strength of a stent.

VENTRICULAR REMODELING

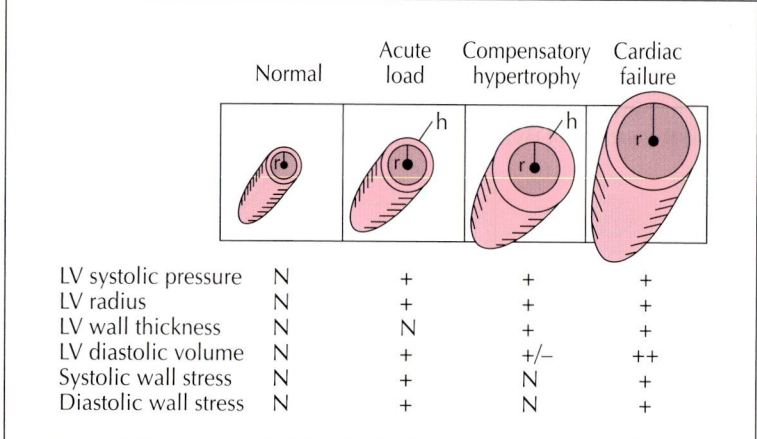

	Normal	Acute load	Compensatory hypertrophy	Cardiac failure
LV systolic pressure	N	+	+	+
LV radius	N	+	+	+
LV wall thickness	N	N	+	+
LV diastolic volume	N	+	+/–	++
Systolic wall stress	N	+	N	+
Diastolic wall stress	N	+	N	+

FIGURE 4-7. Hemodynamic overload is the most common stimulus for myocardial hypertrophy and remodeling. A frequent cause of hemodynamic overload is an increase (+) in left ventricular (LV) systolic pressure, as may occur in patients with hypertension or aortic stenosis. The normal (N) relationship between LV wall thickness (h) and chamber radius (r) is shown (*first panel*). An acute increase in systolic pressure causes an increase in systolic wall stress, which can be approximated by the equation $P \times r/h$, where P is LV systolic pressure. Diastolic wall stress is also increased when there is chamber dilatation or when diastolic pressure is elevated (*second panel*). If sufficient compensatory hypertrophy occurs, the increase in ventricular wall thickness may normalize the systolic and diastolic wall stresses (*third panel*). However, if additional chamber dilatation occurs or the increase in wall thickness is insufficient, systolic and diastolic wall stresses remain abnormally elevated. In this situation, further chamber dilatation may occur in association with hemodynamic failure (*fourth panel*). (*Adapted from* Swynghedauw *et al.* [6].)

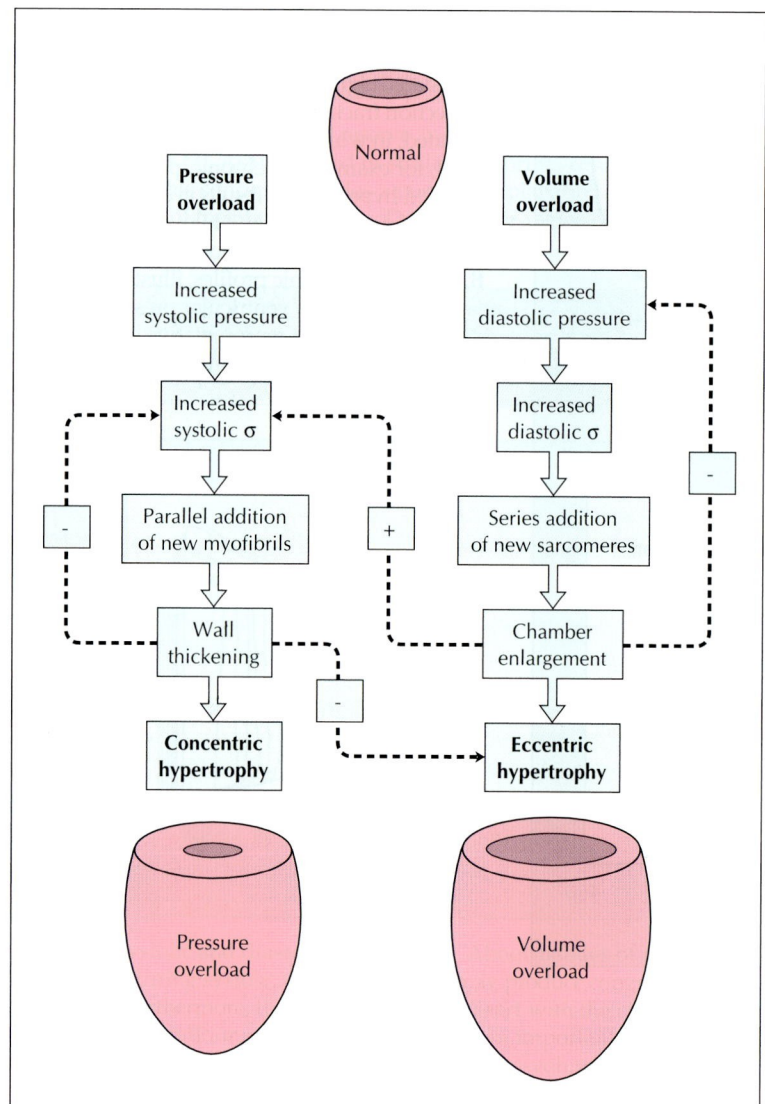

FIGURE 4-8. Patterns of ventricular hypertrophy. Specific patterns of ventricular remodeling occur in response to the imposed augmentation in workload. A pattern of hypertrophic growth characterized as concentric, in which increased mass is out of proportion to chamber volume, is particularly effective in reducing systolic wall stress (σ) under conditions of heightened pressure load. In contrast, in volume overload conditions, in which the major stimulus is diastolic loading, a predominant finding is an increase in the cavity size or volume. Although there can be extensive increases in mass, the relationship between mass and volume is either preserved or, in severe cases, reduced. The fundamental response is generated by cellular hypertrophy. However, the configuration of the new contractile tissue is specific and is related to the type of mechanical stimulus. (*Adapted from* Grossman *et al.* [7].)

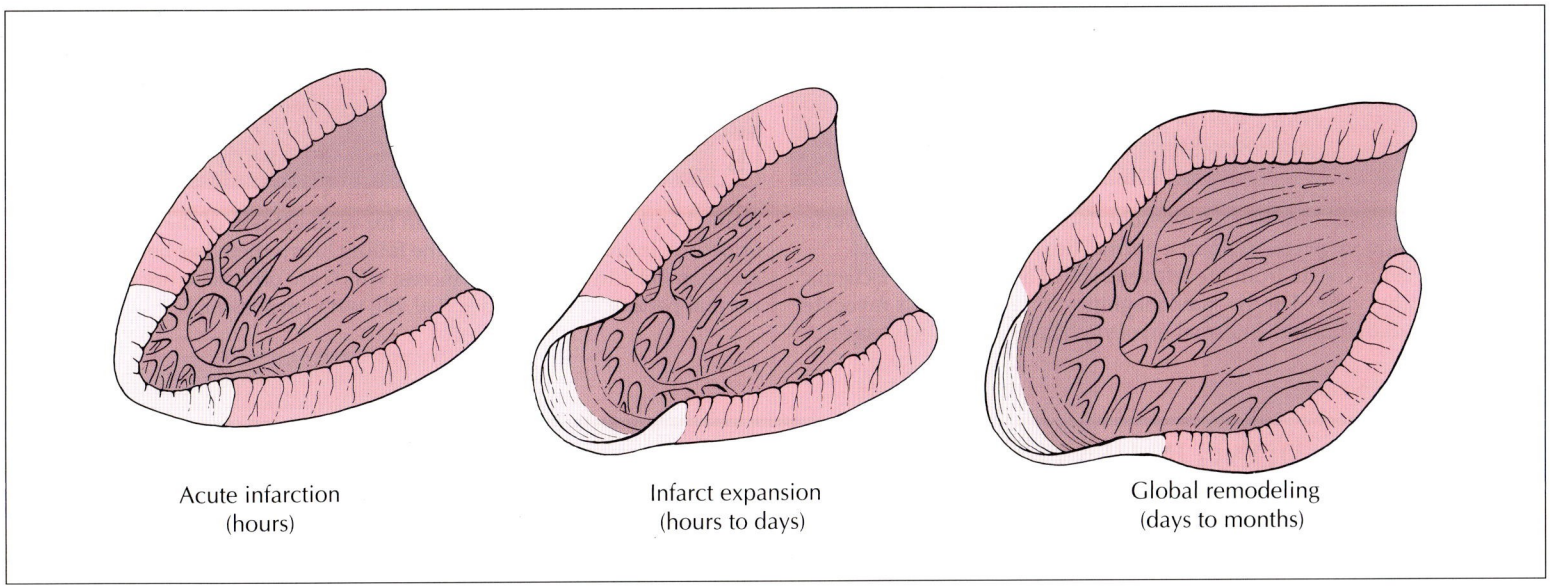

Acute infarction
(hours)

Infarct expansion
(hours to days)

Global remodeling
(days to months)

FIGURE 4-9. Left ventricular remodeling after myocardial infarction (MI). During the critical initial hours after MI when acute ischemia progresses to true necrosis, regional systolic dysfunction is already present. However, in this particularly crucial period measures to restore the balance between O_2 demand and delivery can lead to salvage of contractile tissue. Once cell death has occurred, and particularly if there is a transmural infarction involving the ventricular apex, there is a high likelihood that this will lead to infarct expansion. The distorted ventricle undergoes further remodeling as a consequence of heightened wall stress on the remaining viable myocardium, which leads to further cavity enlargement and shape distortion. The latter insidious process is associated with a greater likelihood of cardiovascular morbidity and mortality.

MOLECULAR AND CELLULAR MECHANISMS OF MYOCARDIAL REMODELING

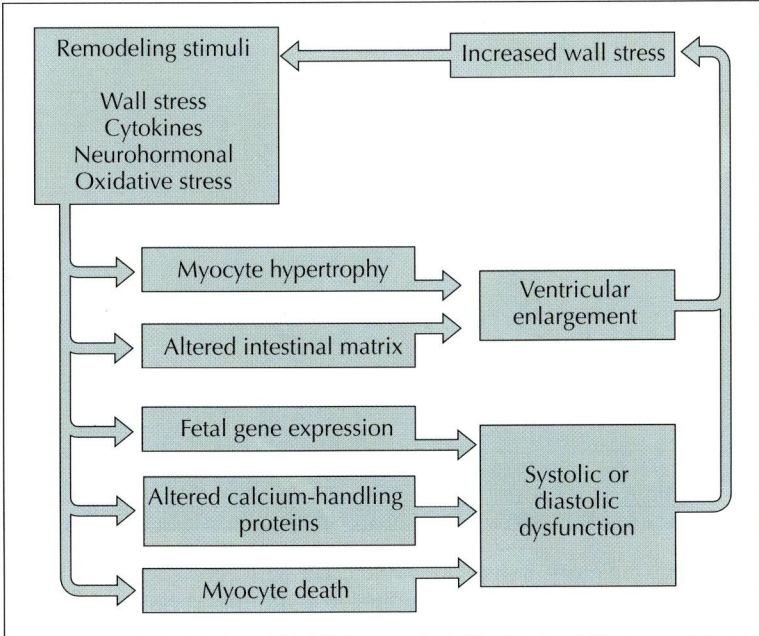

FIGURE 4-10. Remodeling stimuli. Chronic hemodynamic stimuli such as pressure and volume overload lead to ventricular remodeling through increases in myocardial wall stress, cytokines, signaling peptides, neuroendocrine signals, and perhaps, oxidative stress. The myocardium responds with adaptive as well as maladaptive changes. Re-expression of fetal contractile proteins and calcium handling proteins may contribute to impaired contraction and relaxation. Myocytes unable to adapt might be triggered to undergo programmed cell death (apoptosis). The net result of these changes is further impairment in pump function and increased wall stress, thus completing a vicious cycle that leads to further progression of the myocardial dysfunction.

THE RENIN-ANGIOTENSIN-ALDOSTERONE SYSTEM

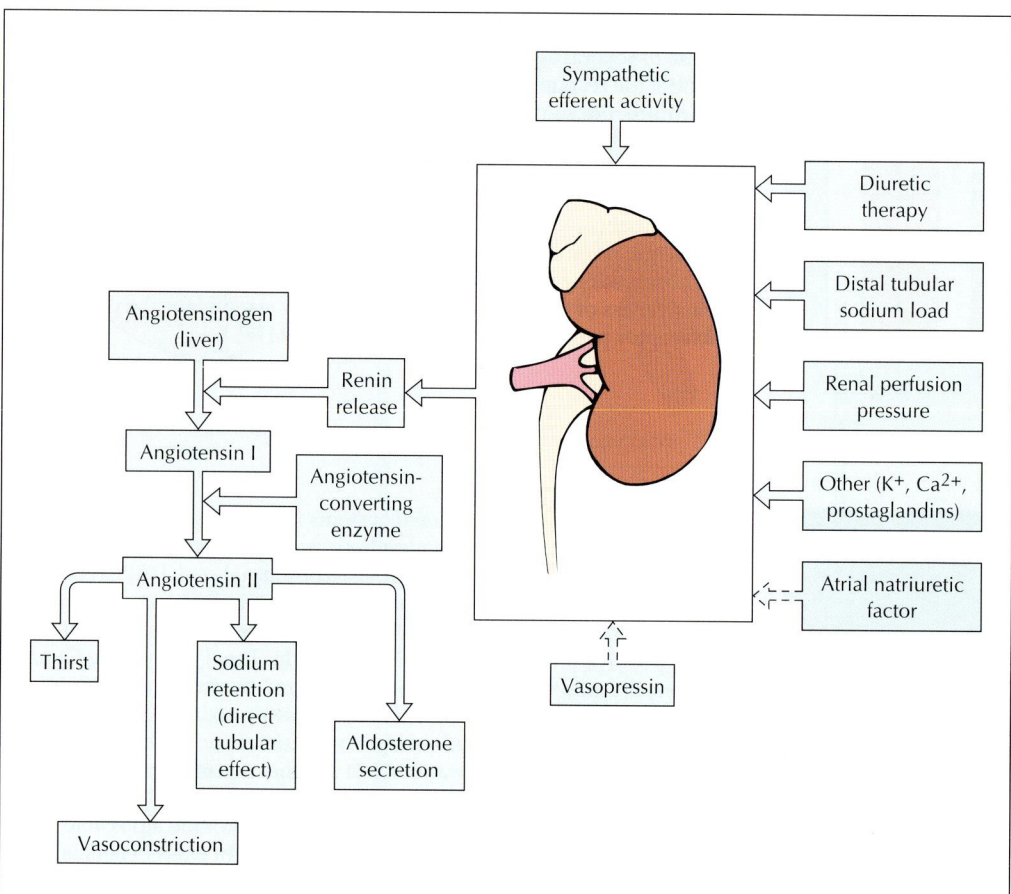

FIGURE 4-20. The renin-angiotensin system is activated in patients with congestive heart failure. The major site of release of circulating renin is the juxtaglomerular apparatus of the kidney, where multiple stimuli may contribute to renal release of renin into the systemic circulation, including increased renal sympathetic efferent activity, decreased distal tubular sodium delivery, reduced renal perfusion pressure, and diuretic therapy. Atrial natriuretic factor and vasopressin (*dashed arrows*) may inhibit the release of renin. Renin enzymatically cleaves angiotensinogen, a tetrapeptide produced in the liver, to form the inactive decapeptide angiotensin I. Angiotensin I is converted to the octapeptide angiotensin II by the angiotensin-converting enzyme. Angiotensin II is a potent vasoconstrictor; it promotes sodium reabsorption by increasing aldosterone secretion and by a direct effect on the tubules, and it stimulates water intake by acting on the thirst center. Angiotensin II causes vasoconstriction directly and may also facilitate the release of norepinephrine by acting on sympathetic nerve endings. (*Adapted from* Paganelli *et al.* [14].)

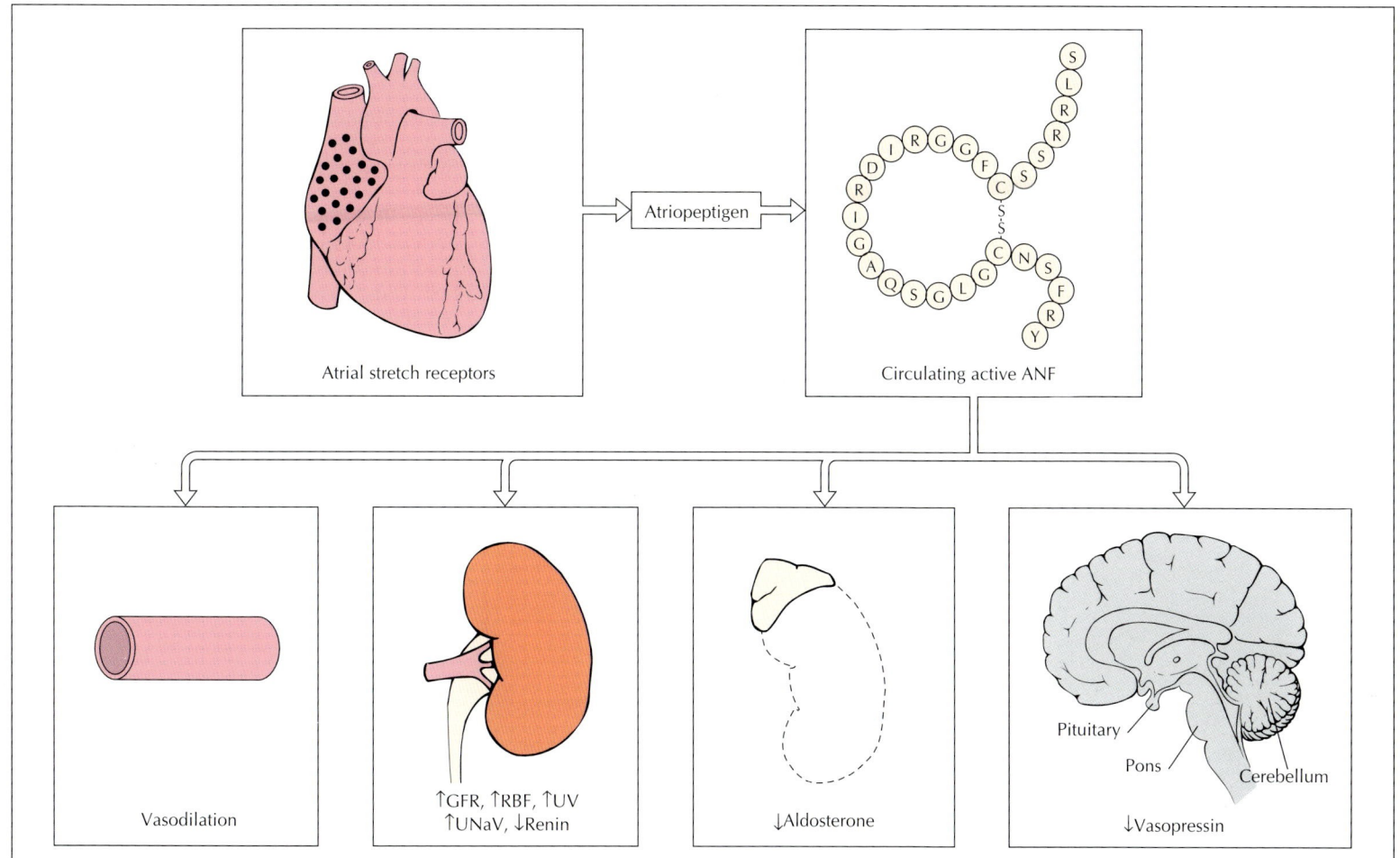

FIGURE 4-21. Regulation of the atrial natriuretic factor (ANF) hormonal system. ANF is a vasorelaxant peptide hormone that is secreted primarily from atrial myocytes in the circulation. The 126–amino acid prohormone atriopeptigen is stored in granules in perinuclear atrial cardiocytes. Increases in cardiac filling pressures are detected by right and left atrial stretch receptors, leading to its release. ANF binds to specific receptors and increases intracellular cGMP, producing a potent natriuretic and vasodilator action. Specific ANF receptors have been localized in vascular smooth muscle, endothelial cells, platelets, the adrenal glomerulosa, and the kidney. In the kidney, ANF increases glomerular filtration rate (GFR), renal blood flow (RBF), urine volume (UV), and sodium excretion (UNaV), and decreases the release of renin. Natriuresis and diuresis are due to suppression of the release of renin, aldosterone, and arginine vasopressin. Abnormalities in both the secretion of ANF and the response of target organs have been observed in congestive heart failure. In the failing heart, both ANF released from the distended atria and the synthesis of ANF by ventricular myocytes contribute to elevated circulating levels. (*Adapted from* Needleman and Greenwald [18].)

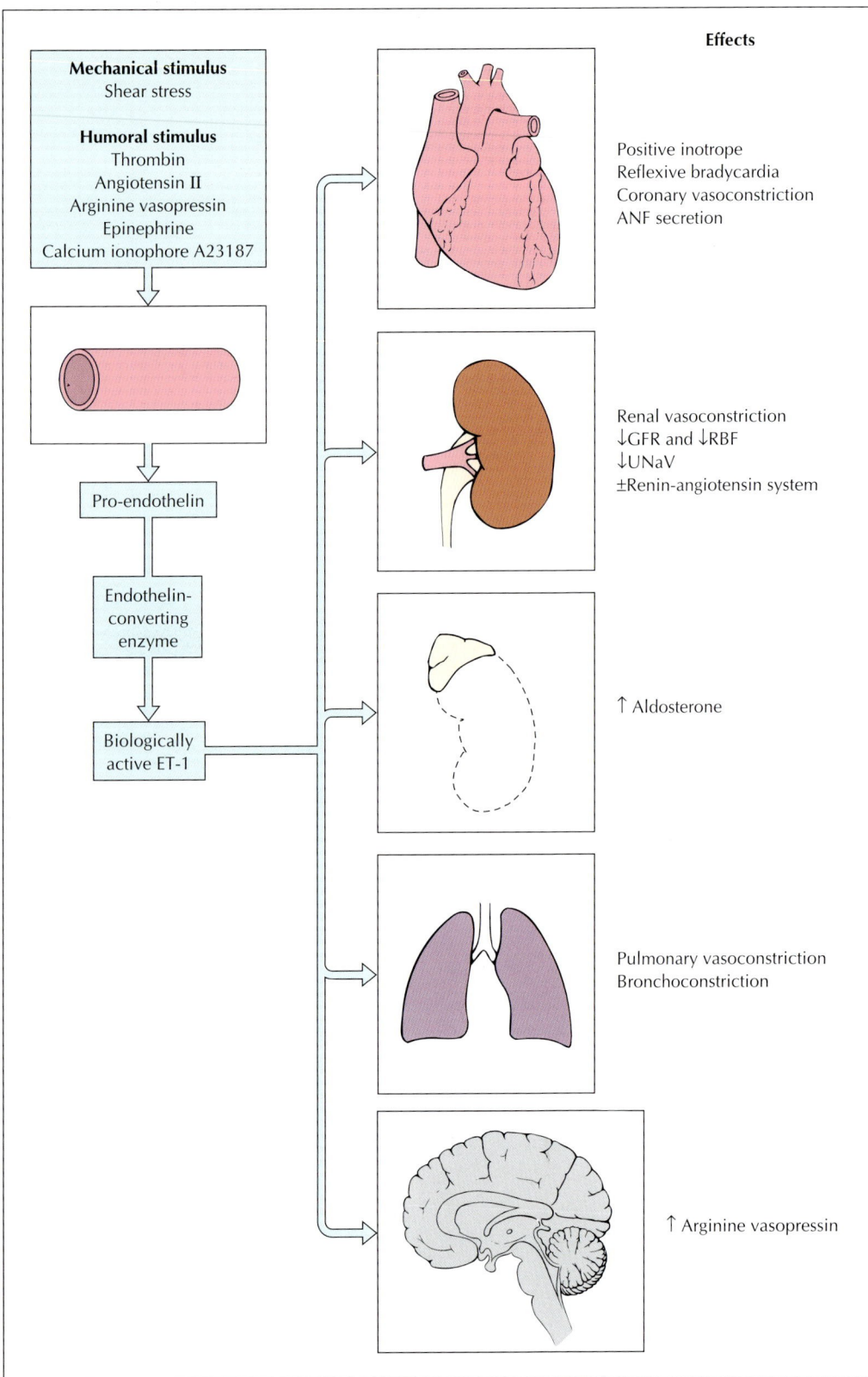

FIGURE 4-22. Summary of the stimuli for endothelin secretion and effects of endothelin in several organs. Mechanical (shear stress) and humoral (thrombin, angiotensin II, vasopressin, epinephrine, calcium ionophore A23187) stimuli may cause the release of endothelin-1 (ET-1). Endothelin increases circulating levels of atrial natriuretic factor (ANF), vasopressin, and aldosterone. It also modulates renin release. Endothelin has a positive inotropic effect and produces coronary and systemic vasoconstriction. These responses produce an increase in blood pressure that is associated with a reflex decrease in heart rate. ET-1 constricts human pulmonary resistance vessels and has a potent bronchoconstrictor effect. Furthermore, ET-1 causes renal vasoconstriction, leading to a reduction in renal blood flow (RBF) and glomerular filtration rate (GFR) and a decrease in urinary sodium excretion (UNaV). (*Adapted from* Underwood *et al.* [19].)

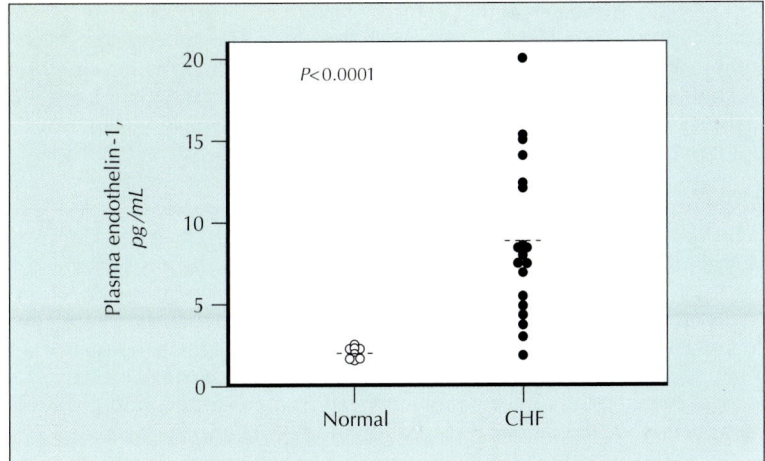

FIGURE 4-23. Cody *et al.* [20] measured immunoreactive circulating endothelin-1 in 12 normal control subjects and in 20 patients with congestive heart failure (CHF). Plasma endothelin-1 was 3.7±0.6 pg/mL in the control group and 9.1±4.1 pg/mL in the CHF group. Increased endothelin synthesis by angiotensin I and vasopressin stimulation and decreased endothelin clearance may contribute to the increased plasma endothelin levels in CHF. Of note, there was a strong positive correlation between endothelin levels and the severity of reactive pulmonary hypertension. (*Adapted from* Cody *et al.* [20].)

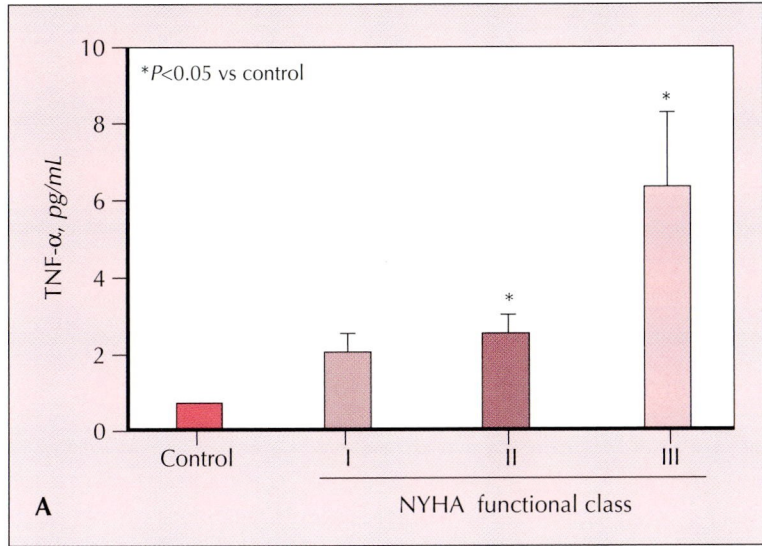

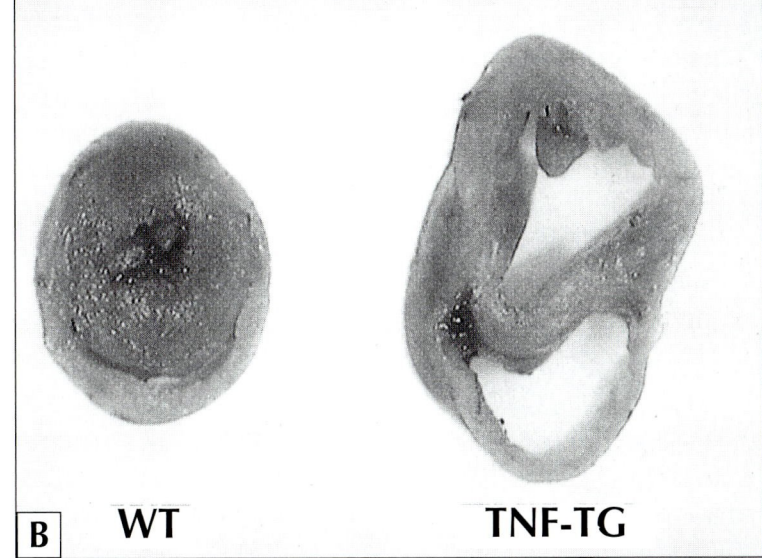

FIGURE 4-24. Proinflammatory cytokines such as tumor necrosis factor-α (TNF-α), interleukin-1β, (IL-1β), and interleukin-6 (IL-6) may play an important pathyphysiologic role in the progression of myocardial failure. The circulating levels of TNF-α and IL-6 were analyzed in randomly selected plasma samples from 63 patients in functional classes I to III enrolled in the neurohormonal substudies of the SOLVD trial. Compared with age-matched controls, patients with left ventricular dysfunction had elevated TNF-α levels (**A**) in direct proportion to functional class. Interestingly, this decrease in LV function was completely reversed 30 days after the infusion was stopped. When Bryant *et al.* [21] caused overexpression of TNF-α in transgenic mice, there was ventricular dilation and impaired survival of mice that was related to the intensity of TNF-α expression (**B**). TG—transgenic; WT—wild type. (Part A *adapted from* Torre-Amione *et al.* [22]; part B *from* Bryant *et al.* [21]; with permission.)

CLINICAL FEATURES

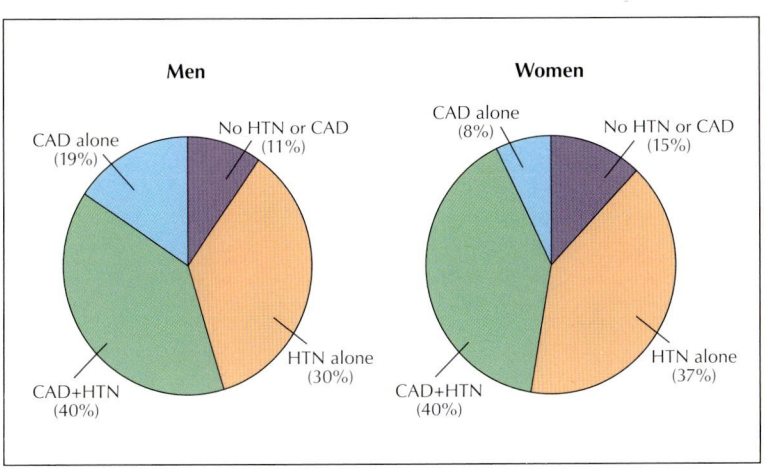

FIGURE 4-25. The epidemiology of congestive heart failure in the United States. The Framingham Heart Study, which followed a cohort of 9405 Americans over a 40-year period, has provided valuable information regarding the etiologic basis of congestive heart failure in the United States [23]. Of 331 men and 321 women who developed heart failure, the majority had coronary artery disease (CAD) with or without hypertension (HTN), and approximately one third had HTN alone. At present, idiopathic dilated cardiomyopathy has replaced HTN as the second most important etiologic factor in the development of heart failure. CAD continues to be the most common risk factor for the development of heart failure in the United States. (*Adapted from* Ho *et al.* [23].)

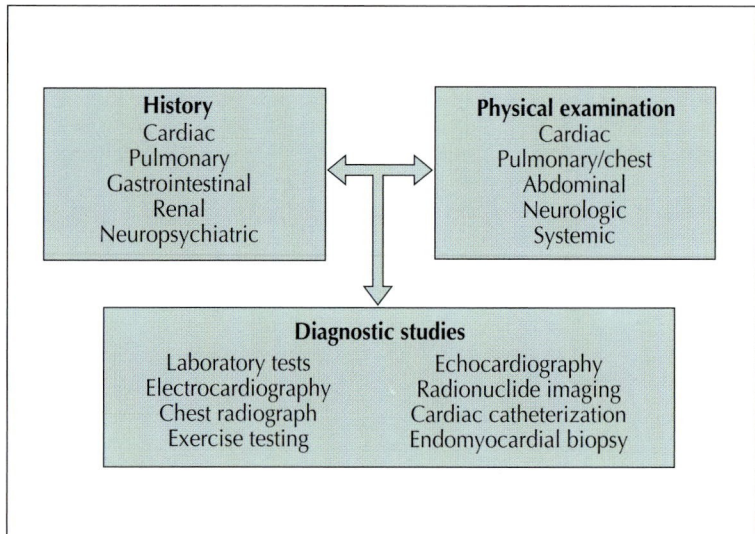

History
Cardiac
Pulmonary
Gastrointestinal
Renal
Neuropsychiatric

Physical examination
Cardiac
Pulmonary/chest
Abdominal
Neurologic
Systemic

Diagnostic studies

Laboratory tests
Electrocardiography
Chest radiograph
Exercise testing

Echocardiography
Radionuclide imaging
Cardiac catheterization
Endomyocardial biopsy

Figure 4-26. Approach to the problem of assessing heart failure. To adequately assess patients with heart failure, historical information, data from the physical examination, and diagnostic study information should be obtained and integrated. It should be emphasized that although information from all three categories may be used in the evaluation, not every test needs to be, or should be, performed. In most patients, an electrocardiogram, a chest radiograph, and an echocardiogram are performed. Additional diagnostic studies should be tailored to the patient. Echocardiography could include M-mode, two-dimensional, and Doppler studies. Radionuclide examination might consist of perfusion, performance, or positron-emission tomographic studies. Cardiac catheterization could include angiography, hemodynamics, or endomyocardial biopsy in certain circumstances. Computed tomography and magnetic resonance imaging are sometimes useful, as is determination of maximal exercise oxygen consumption. Information obtained from the history and physical examination should dictate the need for and type of ancillary testing.

FRAMINGHAM CRITERIA FOR DIAGNOSIS OF CONGESTIVE HEART FAILURE

MAJOR CRITERIA

Paroxysmal nocturnal dyspnea

Neck vein distention

Rales

Cardiomegaly

Acute pulmonary edema

S_3 gallop

Increased venous pressure (>16 cm H_2O)

Positive hepatojugular reflux

MINOR CRITERIA

Extremity edema

Night cough

Dyspnea on exertion

Hepatomegaly

Pleural effusion

Vital capacity reduced by one third from normal

Tachycardia (≥120 bpm)

MAJOR OR MINOR

Weight loss ≥4.5 kg over 5 days' treatment

Figure 4-27. A constellation of symptoms and abnormal physical findings should be used in making the diagnosis of congestive heart failure. The Framingham Study, for example, suggested that several specific clinical criteria be combined and weighted. To establish a clinical diagnosis of congestive heart failure by this method, at least one major and two minor criteria are required [24–26].

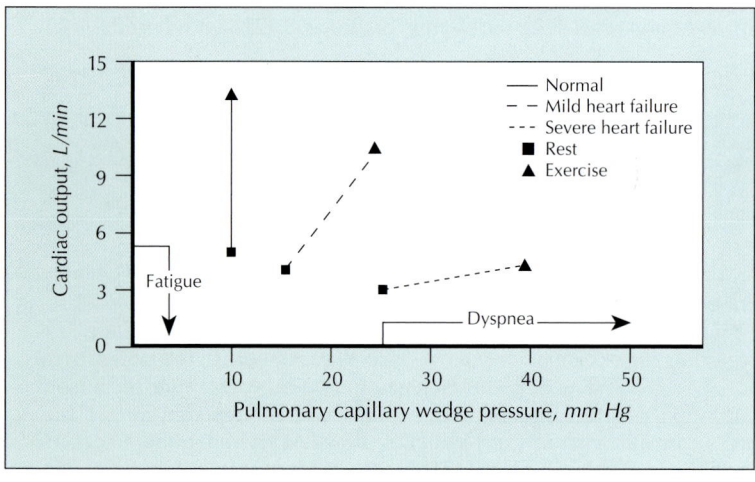

Figure 4-28. Symptoms of heart failure are related to pathophysiology. Exercise testing is important in patients with heart failure because it may unmask significant symptomatology. In patients with significant systolic ventricular dysfunction, the cardiac output fails to increase normally under the physiologic stress of exertion, and the pulmonary pressures become disproportionately elevated.

A

PARAMETERS	SYSTOLIC	DIASTOLIC
History		
Coronary heart disease	++++	+
Hypertension	++	++++
Diabetes	+++	+
Valvular heart disease	++++	-
Paroxysmal dyspnea	++	+++
Physical examination		
Cardiomegaly	+++	+
Soft heart sounds	++++	+
S_3 gallop	+++	+
S_4 gallop	+	+++
Hypertension	++	++++
Mitral regurgitation	+++	+
Rales	++	++
Edema	+++	+
Jugular venous distention	+++	+

B

PARAMETERS	SYSTOLIC	DIASTOLIC
Chest roentgenogram		
Cardiomegaly	+++	+
Pulmonary congestion	+++	+++
Electrocardiograms		
Low voltage	+++	-
Left ventricular hypertrophy	++	++++
Q waves	+++	+
Echocardiograms		
Low ejection fraction	++++	-
Left ventricular dilation	+++	-
Left ventricular hypertrophy	++	++++

FIGURE 4-29. **A** and **B**, Although it is common, congestive heart failure in which diastolic dysfunction is preponderant (vs systolic dysfunction) may be difficult to diagnose [27]. It is important to remember that the clinical features of heart failure may be similar whether left ventricular systolic function is normal or is substantively depressed [28]. The pathophysiology of heart failure with normal systolic ventricular function is different, however, from that noted in patients with depressed left ventricular ejection fraction [29,30]. Furthermore, certain aspects of the history and physical examination (*panel A*), along with clinical measurements (*panel B*), help to distinguish diastolic problems from those more often associated with systolic failure. Patients with hypertensive heart disease, for example, particularly severe left ventricular hypertrophy, often experience heart failure because of diastolic dysfunction. *Plus signs* indicate "suggestive" (the number reflects relative weight). *Minus signs* indicate "not very suggestive."

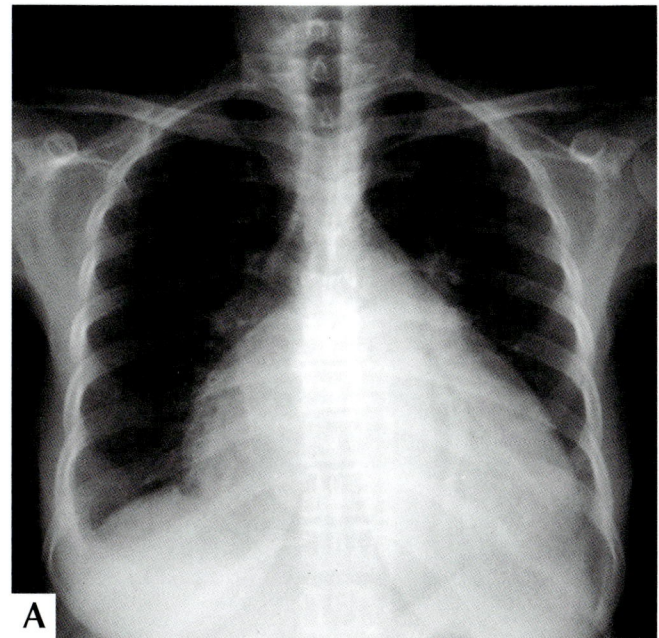

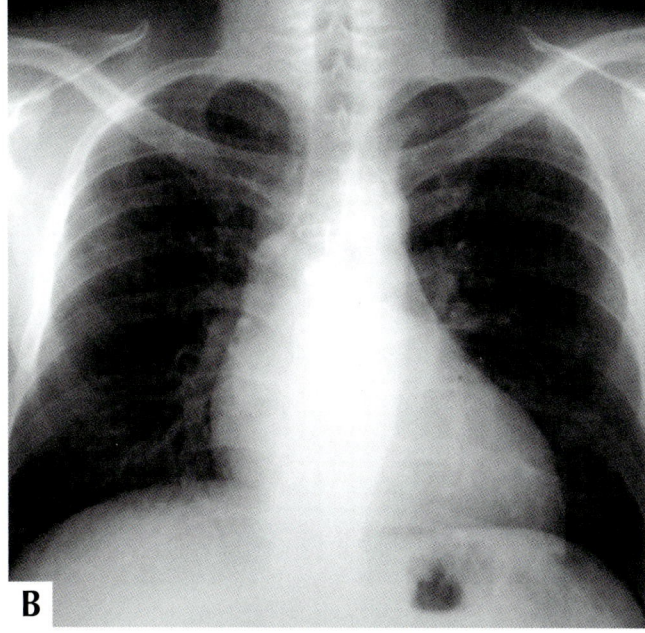

FIGURE 4-30. Chest roentgenograms of patients with heart failure. **A,** Congestive heart failure with cardiomegaly. This roentgenogram demonstrates cardiomegaly (cardiothoracic ratio 0.77), pulmonary congestion, and bilateral pleural effusions (note blunted costophrenic angles). The cardiac silhouette may indicate the existence of a pericardial effusion. Also note the thin chest wall and osteopenia suggesting cachexia.

B, Congestive heart failure with left ventricular hypertrophy. This roentgenogram demonstrates mild pulmonary congestion with a high-normal cardiothoracic ratio of 0.53. These roentgenographic findings are typical of patients with hypertensive heart disease or hypertrophic cardiomyopathy resulting in diastolic dysfunction in the presence of a normal ejection fraction.

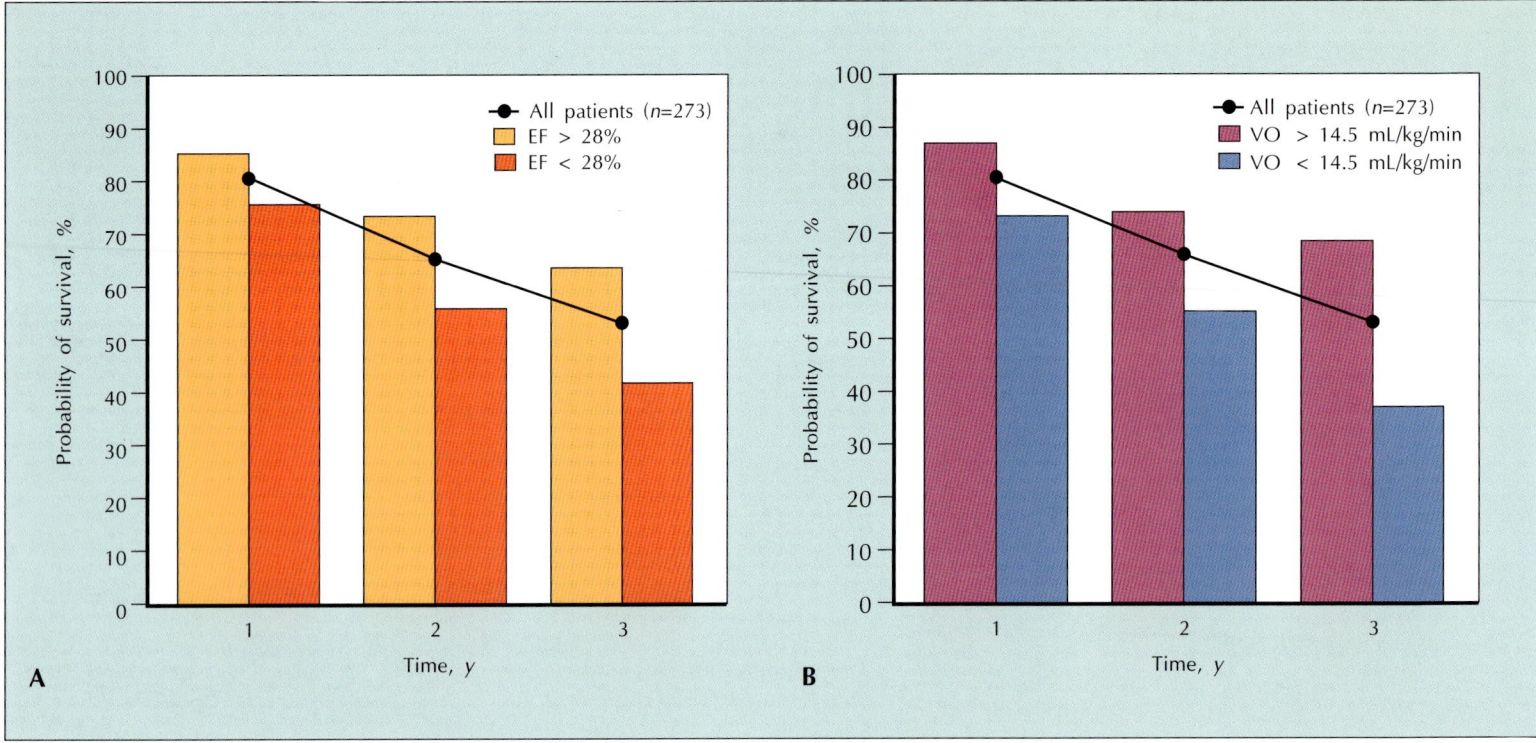

FIGURE 4-31. Examples of the prognostic information available from measurement of the left ventricular ejection fraction (EF; **A**) and peak oxygen consumption (VO₂; **B**) in the Vasodilator Heart Failure Trial (V-HeFT I). These data from the placebo group (patients treated with digoxin and diuretic) [31] indicate that the probability of survival over 3 years in different risk strata can differ by 20% to 30%. Strata were defined arbitrarily by the median values in this sample and may not represent the most discriminating cutpoints for these prognostic variables.

MANAGEMENT OF HEART FAILURE

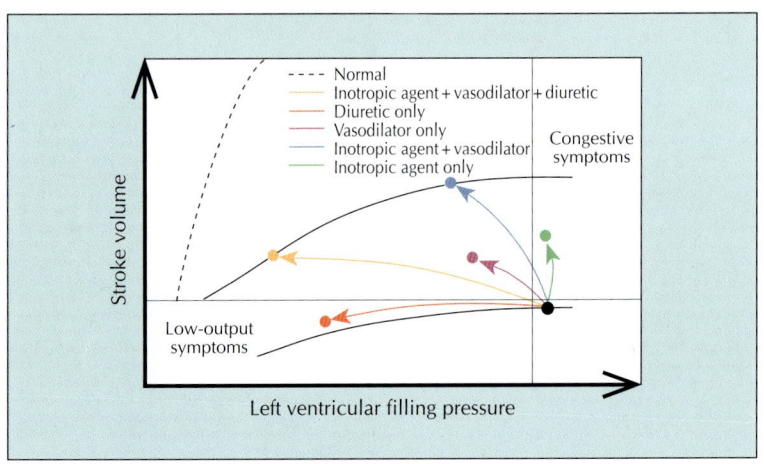

FIGURE 4-32. Physiologic response to pharmacologic intervention in heart failure. These curves represent the Frank-Starling relationship between left ventricular end-diastolic filling pressure and stroke volume for a normal heart and for the patient with heart failure symptoms resulting from predominant systolic dysfunction before and after treatment with digoxin or diuretics, alone or in combination with a vasodilator. Note that only positive inotropic agents, such as digoxin, and vasodilators shift the patient's hemodynamic profile upward and leftward to a more favorable ventricular function curve, resulting in an improvement in cardiac output despite a reduction in ventricular filling pressure. Diuretics reduce heart failure symptoms by lowering ventricular filling pressures, but they may cause a reduction in cardiac output in patients who have decompensated heart failure and marginal systolic reserve.

DIURETICS

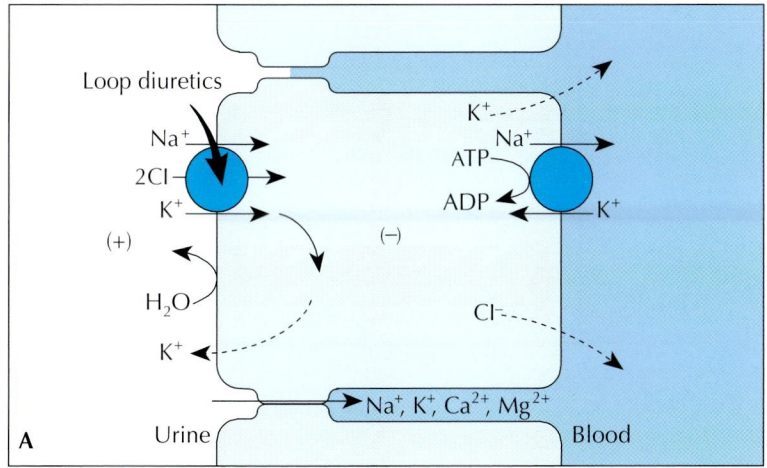

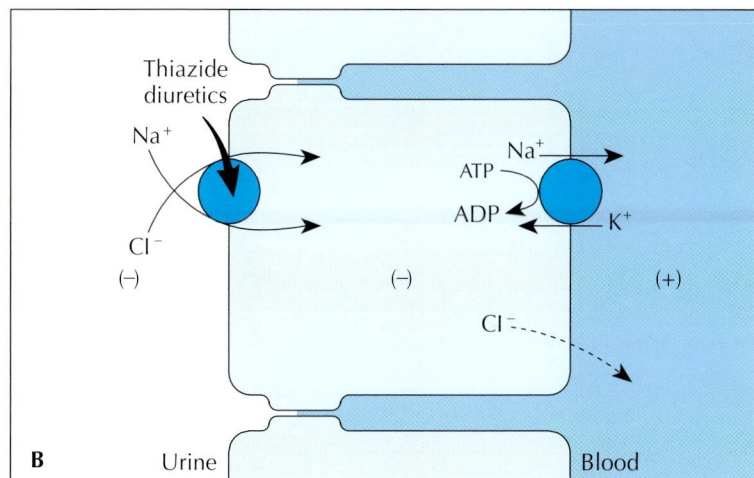

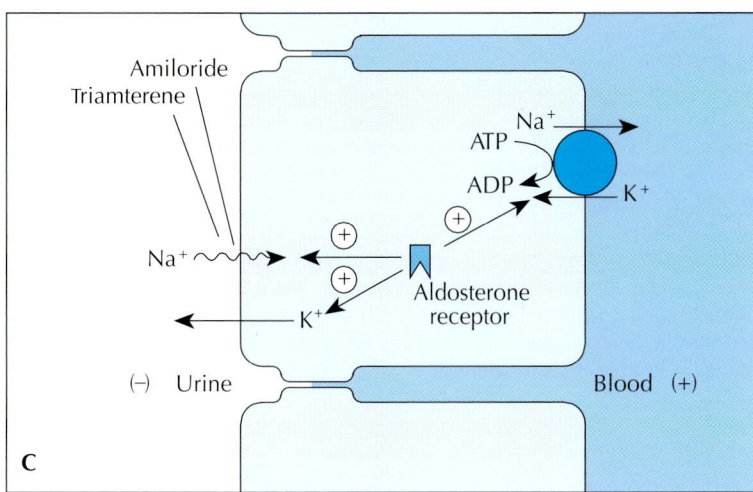

Figure 4-33. Loop diuretics in heart failure. **A,** The introduction in the 1960s of diuretics that act within the loop of Henle, so-called "high-ceiling" or "loop" diuretics, dramatically affected the ability of clinicians to improve symptoms of congestive heart failure with minimum toxicity and predictable efficacy compared with other drugs available at that time. These diuretics act on a specific transport protein, the $Na^+K^+/2Cl^-$ cotransporter, located on the apical membrane of renal epithelial cells in the ascending limb of Henle's loop. Ions transported into the cell are then transferred out of the cell by Na^+K^+-ATPase (the "sodium pump") on the basolateral membranes of these cells. Loop diuretics also decrease the absorption of Ca^{2+} and Mg^{2+} in this portion of the nephron, cations whose absorption is indirectly linked to NaCl uptake. Thus, hypocalcemia and hypomagnesia, as well as hypokalemia and volume depletion, may result from prolonged use of these drugs.

Loop diuretics also reduce the tonicity of the medullary interstitium by preventing the normal uptake of solute in the absence of water in the thick ascending limb of Henle's loop. This limits the kidney's ability to concentrate the urine and may contribute to the development of hyponatremia. The loop diuretics are clearly the most useful diuretics as single agents for patients with decompensated congestive failure, in large part because of the magnitude of the natriuresis that can be achieved over a short period, which can reach as high as 20% of the filtered load of sodium. Typically, the fraction of NaCl filtered at the glomerulus and reabsorbed in the ascending limb of the loop of Henle declines from about 20% to 13% with a loop diuretic, resulting in a 1% to 2% increase in the fractional excretion of sodium over 24 hours [32].

B, Thiazide diuretics. In general, the thiazide diuretics are not useful as single drugs for the therapy of volume retention in heart failure patients, largely because their site of action in the distal convoluted tubule permits rapid adjustment of water and solute absorption in other more proximal nephron segments. Interestingly, the target renal tubular protein of the thiazide class of diuretics, the electroneutral Na^+Cl^- cotransporter, has recently been cloned and sequenced. This is the last of the known diuretic-responsive renal epithelial cell transport proteins to be identified. Many other tissues also express this transport protein, which may have important implications for understanding the effectiveness of these drugs in the treatment of hypertension as well as their less desirable metabolic effects on lipid and glucose metabolism. Unlike loop diuretics, thiazides enhance calcium reabsorption but not that of magnesim, although magnesium wasting is much more pronounced with loop diuretics [32].

C, Potassium-sparing diuretics. The potassium-sparing diuretics fall into two categories: agents such as amiloride and triamterene, which reduce Na^+ conductance through an apical membrane sodium channel; and aldosterone antagonists, which, by inhibiting the actions of aldosterone at its intracellular receptor in renal epithelial cells of the distal collecting duct, reduce Na^+ uptake from the tubular lumen and decrease K^+ secretion by several mechanisms. Aldosterone antagonists also limit the kidney's ability to acidify the urine by inhibiting the action of aldosterone on a renal tubular proton pump. Although none of these diuretics is effective as a single agent in the treatment of heart failure, they play a useful role in diminishing renal K^+ wasting. When combined with loop or thiazide diuretics, the aldosterone antagonists also prevent Mg^{2+} depletion. Because ACE inhibitors increase the serum K^+ concentration, an effect that may be magnified by β-blockers and NSAIDs, potassium-sparing diuretics should be prescribed cautiously for patients who are already receiving vasodilators of this class [32].

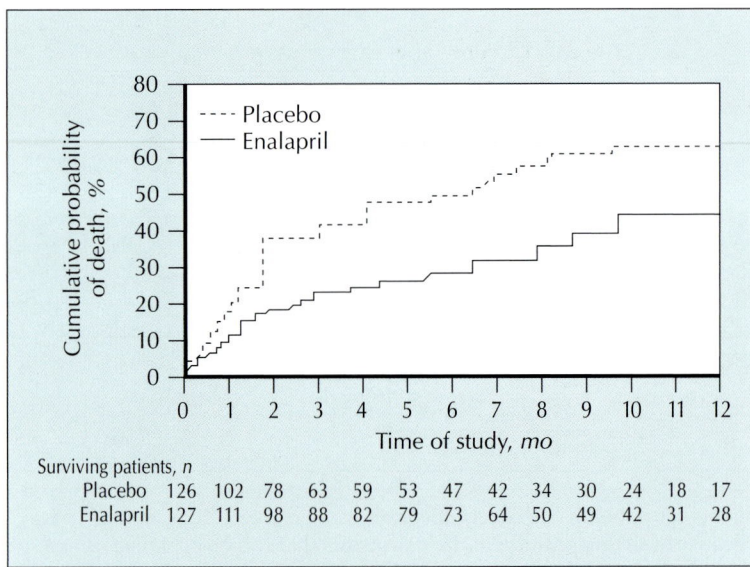

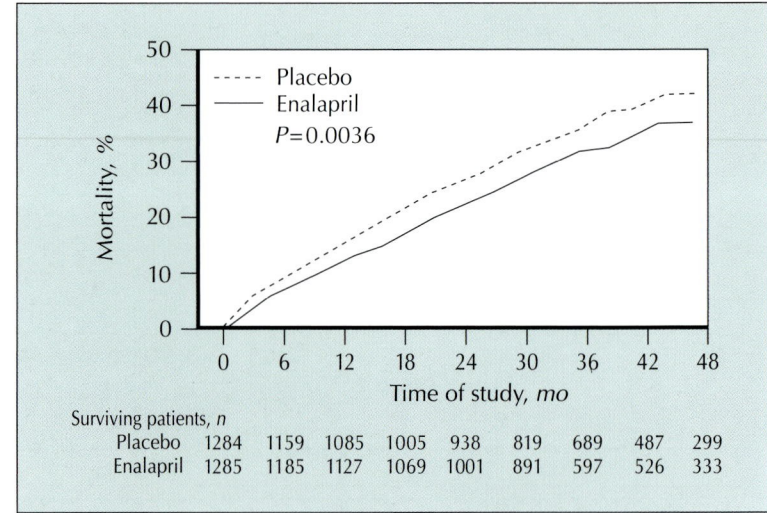

FIGURE 4-34. The CONSENSUS (Cooperative North Scandinavian Enalapril Survival Study) trial, the first mortality study of an angiotensin-converting enzyme (ACE) inhibitor in patients with congestive heart failure, demonstrated that an ACE inhibitor improved mortality compared with placebo. A lesser-known aspect of the study was that the mean age of the patients at randomization was 70 years. In addition, the majority of patients were elderly and belonged to New York Heart Association functional class IV despite digoxin and diuretic therapy. Approximately 25% of the patients in this trial were also receiving other vasodilators, such as nitrates, before randomization. Early diagnosis of the placebo and enalapril treatment groups prompted early termination of the study. The mean dose of enalapril was just under 20 mg/d. Careful dose titration obviated the excess hypotension observed in early stages of the study. (*Adapted from* CONSENSUS Trial Study Group [33].)

FIGURE 4-35. The SOLVD (Studies of Left Ventricular Dysfunction) treatment subgroup demonstrated mortality benefit in moderate heart failure. The treatment subgroup included patients who already had symptomatic congestive heart failure and were randomized to either placebo or enalapril therapy. Criteria for randomization were a baseline ejection fraction of 35% or less and symptomatic heart failure. The majority of patients in this study had functional class II congestive heart failure. Enalapril was associated with a significant reduction in mortality compared with placebo in these patients. This mortality benefit was primarily the result of reducing mortality due to congestive heart failure. Mortality due to presumed arrhythmic death was not significantly different from placebo. (*Adapted from* the SOLVD Investigators [34].)

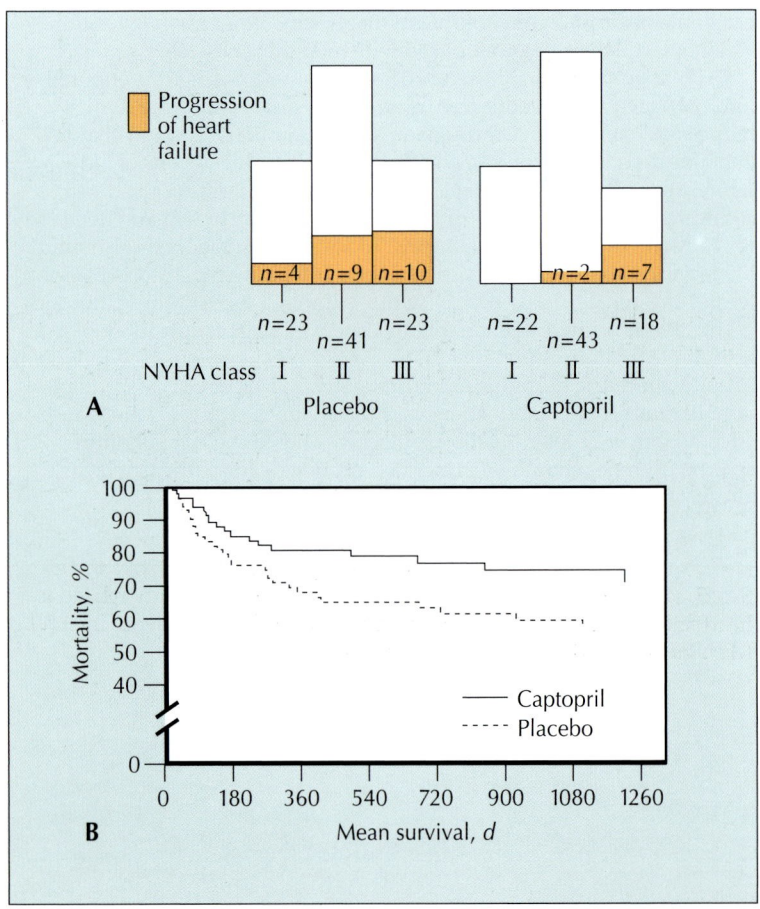

FIGURE 4-36. The Munich Mild Heart Failure Study prospectively determined whether an ACE inhibitor would alter the natural outcome in heart failure by reducing the progression to severe heart failure from milder heart failure. **A,** Patients were randomized to placebo or captopril, and subclassified according to New York Heart Association (NYHA) functional class I, II, or III. The majority of patients in this study were either asymptomatic (NYHA functional class I) or mildly symptomatic (NYHA functional class II), although patients with more severe heart failure (NYHA functional class III) contributed to both treatment groups. In the placebo group, 23 of 87 patients demonstrated progression of heart failure. In the captopril group, only nine of 83 patients demonstrated progression of heart failure. **B,** The mean survival time until the development of progressive heart failure was 223 days longer in the captopril group compared with placebo. Patients treated with the ACE inhibitor could anticipate a greater interval without progression of their heart failure symptoms once the ACE inhibitor had been initiated, compared with the placebo. However, total mortality in the study for the two treatment groups was virtually identical. Twenty-two of the 83 patients receiving captopril died, compared with 22 of the 87 patients receiving placebo. (*Adapted from* Kleber *et al.* [35].)

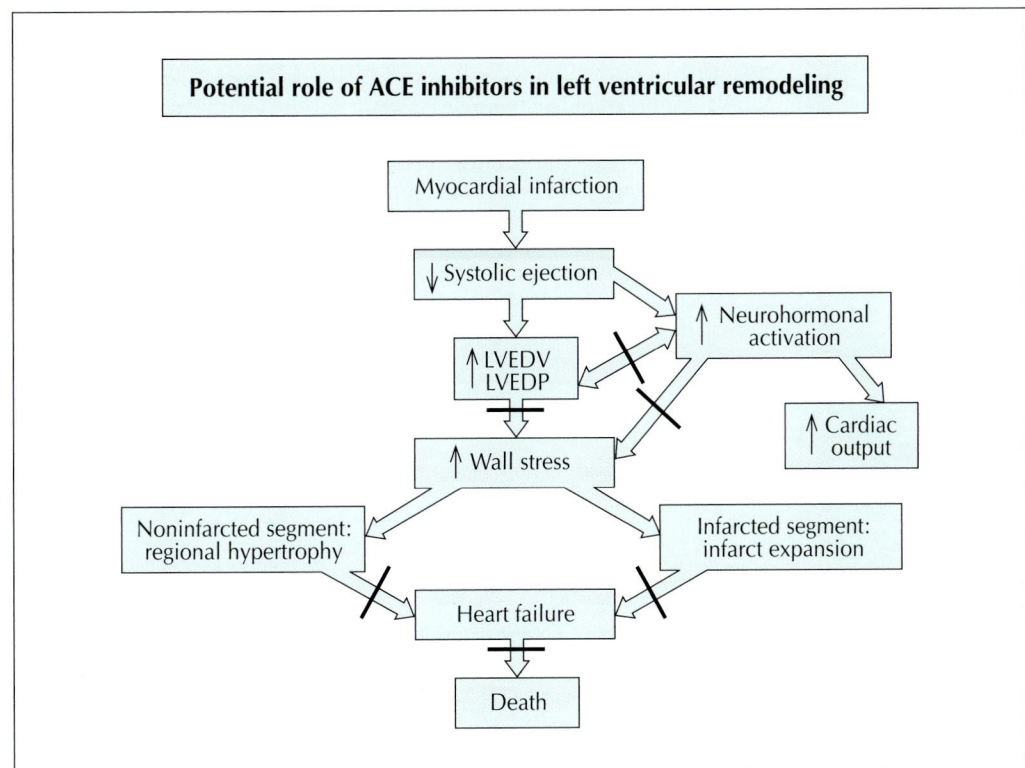

Potential role of ACE inhibitors in left ventricular remodeling

FIGURE 4-37. Although the pathophysiology of infarct healing is complex, there are several potential mechanisms by which an angiotensin-converting enzyme (ACE) inhibitor may favorably improve left ventricular remodeling. Shown with *intersecting bars* are sites at which an ACE inhibitor may interrupt an adverse consequence of myocardial infarction that would contribute to heart failure or death. LVEDP—left ventricular end-diastolic pressure; LVEDV—left ventricular end-diastolic volume. (*Adapted from* McKay *et al.* [36].)

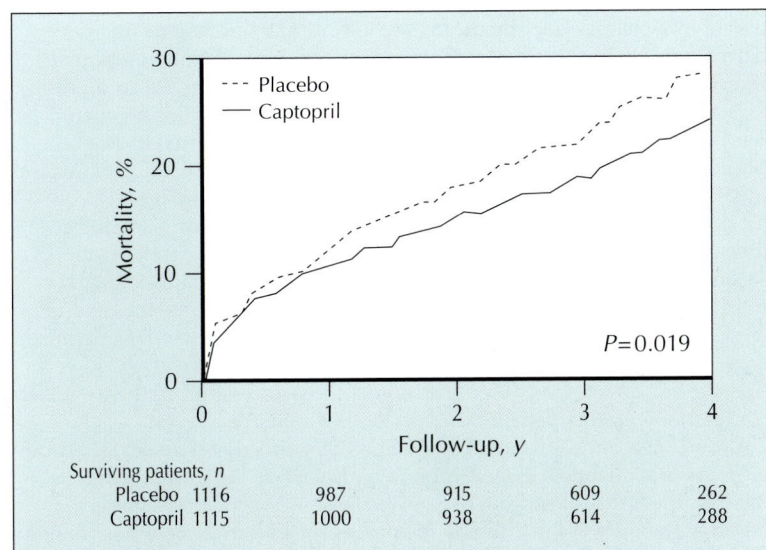

Surviving patients, *n*				
Placebo 1116	987	915	609	262
Captopril 1115	1000	938	614	288

FIGURE 4-38. The results of the SAVE (Survival and Ventricular Enlargement) study demonstrated that an angiotensin-converting enzyme (ACE) inhibitor given to the high-risk anterior myocardial infarction subgroup was associated with a 19% reduction in all-cause mortality. There was no effect of captopril compared with placebo on short-term mortality during the first year of follow-up. After 1 year of follow-up, mortality reduction was evident in the captopril group. This suggested that the reduction may be due to a decrease in deaths related to the development of heart failure. (*Adapted from* Pfeffer *et al.* [37].)

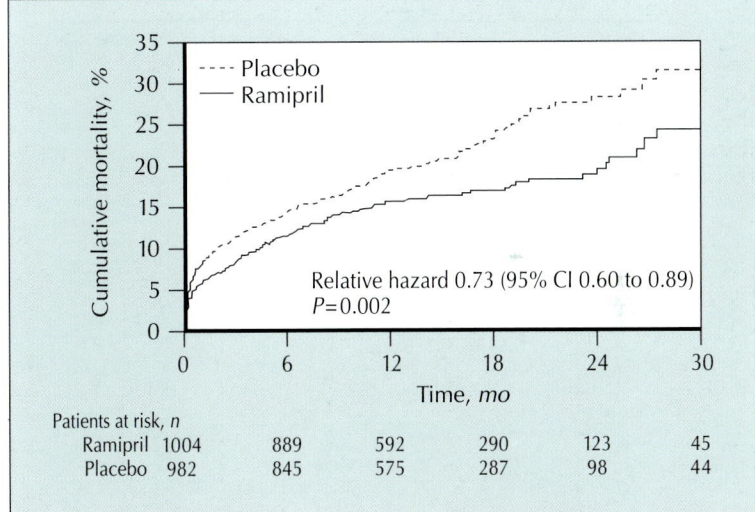

Patients at risk, *n*					
Ramipril 1004	889	592	290	123	45
Placebo 982	845	575	287	98	44

FIGURE 4-39. The outcome of the all-cause mortality primary endpoint in the AIRE (Acute Infarction Ramipril Evaluation) trial, based on intention to treat. It is instructive to compare this figure with the results of the SAVE (Survival and Ventricular Enlargement) trial in Figure 4-38. In AIRE there is an early divergence of survival benefit for ramipril, which is not apparent in SAVE. Many believe that this reflects the greater clinical severity of heart failure in AIRE, whereas patients in SAVE had asymptomatic left ventricular dysfunction. In fact, clinical evidence of heart failure excluded patients from SAVE. In AIRE, this early survival benefit persisted throughout follow-up, as the survival curves continue to diverge. This suggests that, in contrast to SAVE, early survival benefit results from reduction of mortality related to heart failure, which continues through follow-up. CI—confidence interval. (*Adapted from* AIRE Study Investigators [38].)

VASODILATORS

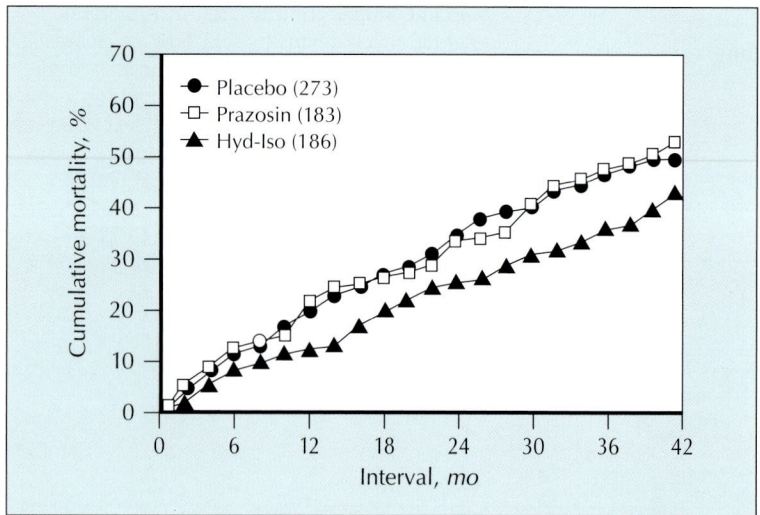

FIGURE 4-40. In addition to short-term hemodynamic improvement, the VHeFT (Veterans Administration Vasodilator in Heart Failure Trial) I study demonstrated a favorable effect on survival with the combination of hydralazine and isosorbide dinitrate (Hyd-Iso). As shown here, the α-adrenergic blocking agent prazosin did not significantly reduce mortality. In fact, the VHeFT I study provided the final data that led to the discontinuation of α-adrenergic blocking agents for treatment of heart failure. In contrast, the combination of hydralazine and isosorbide dinitrate significantly reduced mortality. This was the first published, prospective, placebo-controlled, randomized survival study in heart failure to demonstrate an improved survival outcome for the pharmacologic treatment of congestive heart failure. (*Adapted from* Cohn *et al.* [39].)

POSITIVE INOTROPIC AGENTS

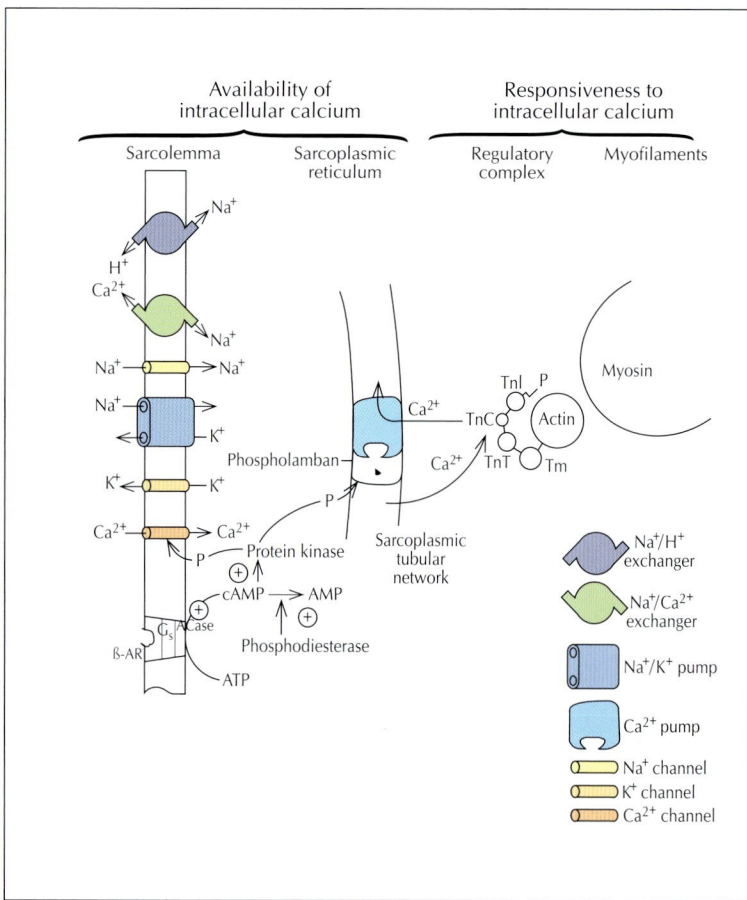

FIGURE 4-41. The contractile state of the myocardium is determined by the interaction of calcium with the contractile apparatus. Essentially all positive inotropic drugs act by increasing the amount of calcium available to the contractile apparatus, by increasing the sensitivity of the contractile

apparatus to calcium, or by a combination of these mechanisms. Shown here are the major biochemical pathways involved in the action of positive inotropic drugs. Digitalis inhibits the Na^+/K^+ pump, thereby favoring the accumulation of intracellular Na^+ and secondarily leading to the accumulation of intracellular Ca^{2+} by means of the Na^+/Ca^{2+} exchanger. β-Adrenergic agonists such as dobutamine, isoproterenol, and norepinephrine, the natural sympathetic neurotransmitter in the heart, act by binding to β-adrenergic receptors (β-AR) on the surface of the cardiac myocyte. The β-adrenergic receptor is coupled to a second protein, referred to as a G-protein (G_s), which activates the enzyme adenylate cyclase (ACase). ACase mediates the synthesis of cAMP, an important intracellular second messenger that acts on the voltage-dependent calcium channel to increase the amount of calcium that enters the myocyte with each depolarization. A second class of positive inotropic agents, which includes amrinone and milrinone, acts by preventing degradation of cAMP and, like the β-adrenergic agonists, increases the intracellular level of cAMP. However, because these phosphodiesterase inhibitors act distally to the β-adrenergic receptor, they are less affected by desensitization of the β-adrenergic pathway, which commonly occurs in patients with severe heart failure.

A third class of positive inotropic agents acts directly on myocyte sodium or potassium channels. For example, agents such as vesnarinone may increase the influx of sodium by so-called *fast sodium channels*, thereby favoring the influx of calcium by the process of sodium/calcium exchange (Na^+/Ca^{2+} exchanger). Vesnarinone may also block the efflux of potassium via outward-rectifying potassium channels, thereby lengthening the period of cellular depolarization and enabling more calcium to enter the cell by way of voltage-dependent calcium channels. A fourth and particularly interesting positive inotropic mechanism is an increase of the *sensitivity* of the contractile apparatus to calcium. An increasing number of agents, including pimobendan and levosimendan, act directly on the contractile apparatus to increase the contractile response without altering the intracellular concentration of calcium. In theory, these agents are attractive because they might allow dissociation of the drug's positive inotropic effect from increases in cAMP and calcium, which can cause tachycardia and arrhythmias. Tm—tropomyosin; TnC—troponin C; TnI—troponin I; TnT—troponin T. (*Adapted from* Morgan [40].)

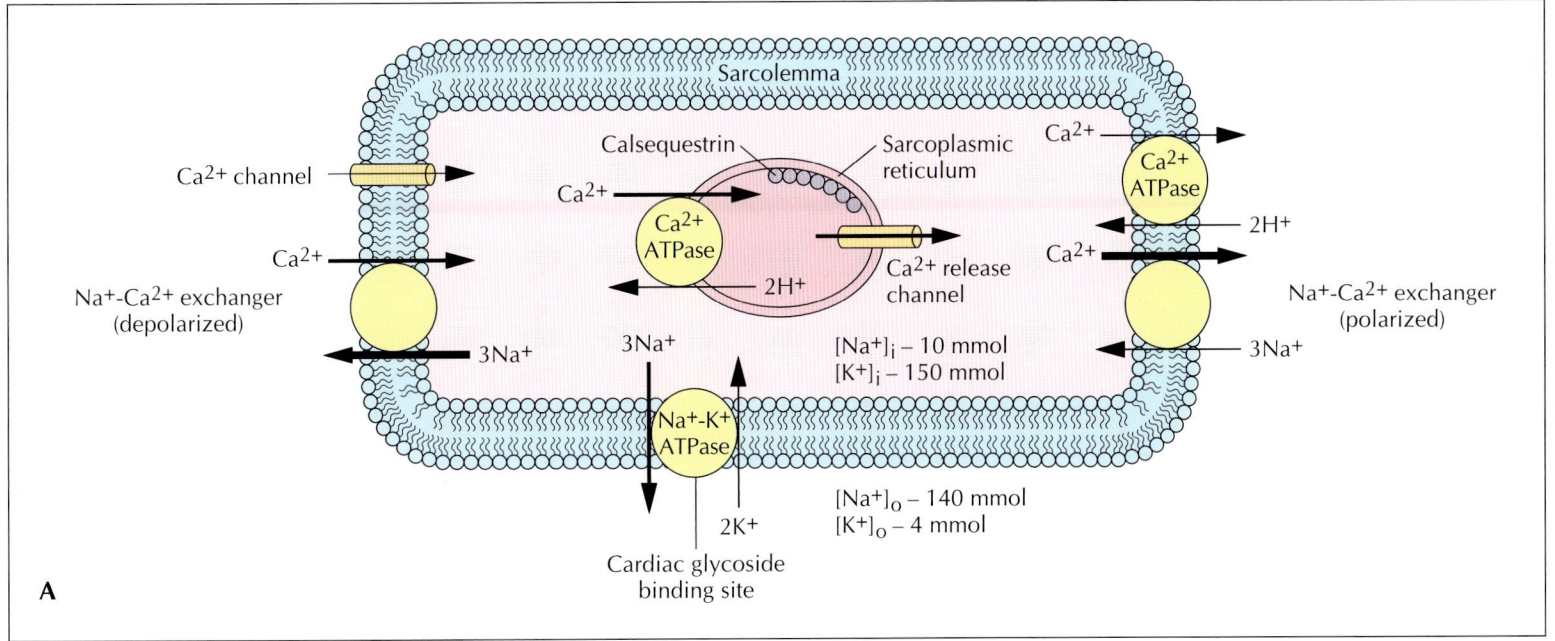

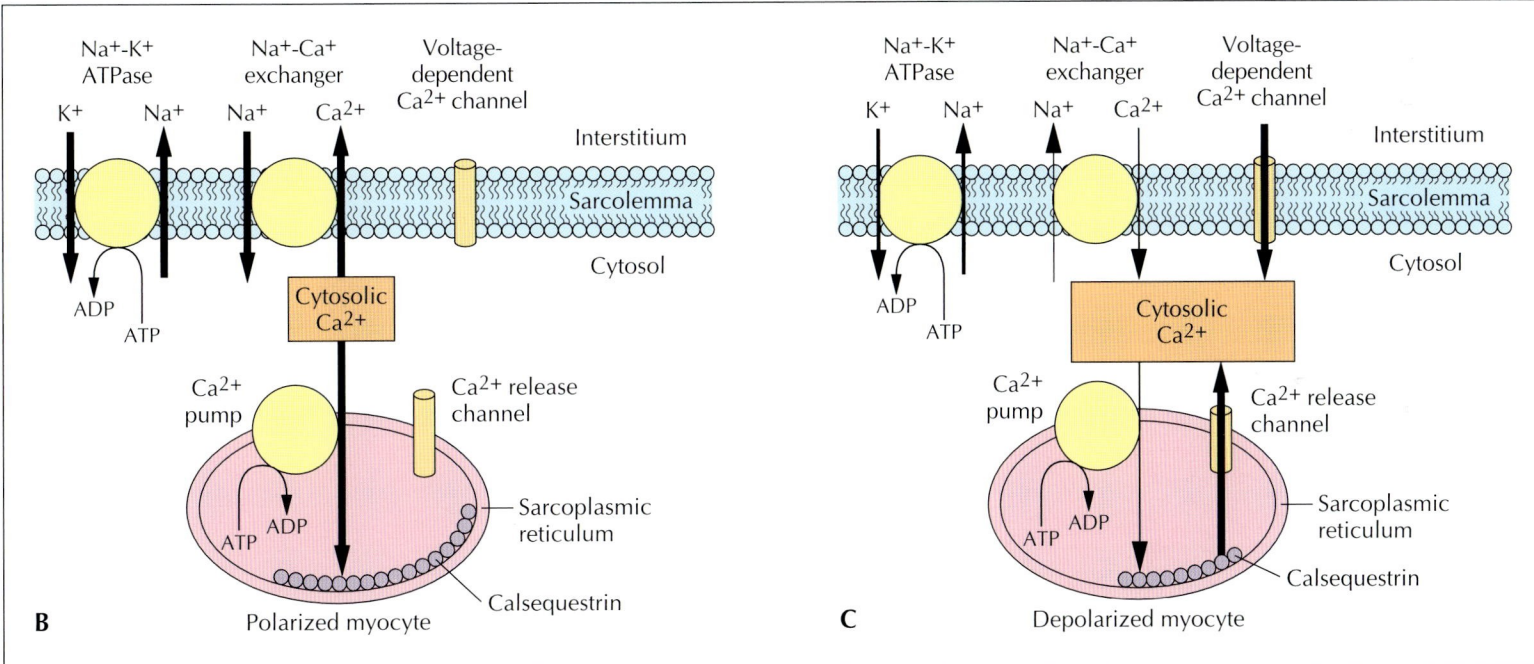

FIGURE 4-42. Sodium pump inhibition by cardiac glycosides. The present understanding of the mechanism by which the cardiac glycosides induce a positive inotropic effect in cardiac muscle is based on the specificity of these drugs for Na^+K^+-ATPase (or the "sodium pump"), a cell membrane protein responsible for the active (ie, ATP-consuming) transport of the monovalent cations Na^+ and K^+.

A, Both Na^+ and Ca^{2+} ions enter cardiac muscle cells during each cycle of depolarization, contraction, and repolarization. Ca^{2+} is also released from internal stores in an intracellular compartment called the sarcoplasmic reticulum (SR), where it is bound to the protein calsequestrin. During cellular repolarization, Na^+ is actively extruded by Na^+K^+-ATPase, while Ca^{2+} is

either pumped back into the SR by a Ca^{2+}-ATPase or is removed from the cell by a cell membrane transport protein that exchanges Na^+ for Ca^{2+}. This Na^+ for Ca^{2+} exchanger transports three Na^+ ions in for every Ca^{2+} ion out when the cell is polarized, using the favorable chemical and electrical potential of Na^+ to drive the exchange reaction. **B,** The direction and magnitude of Na^+ and Ca^{2+} transport during diastole (polarized myocyte).

C, The direction and magnitude of Na^+ and Ca^{2+} transport during systole (depolarized myocyte). Note that the exchanger may briefly run in reverse during cell depolarization when the electrical gradient across the plasma membrane is transiently reversed. The capacity of the exchanger to extrude Ca^{2+} from the cell depends critically on the intracellular Na^+ concentrations.

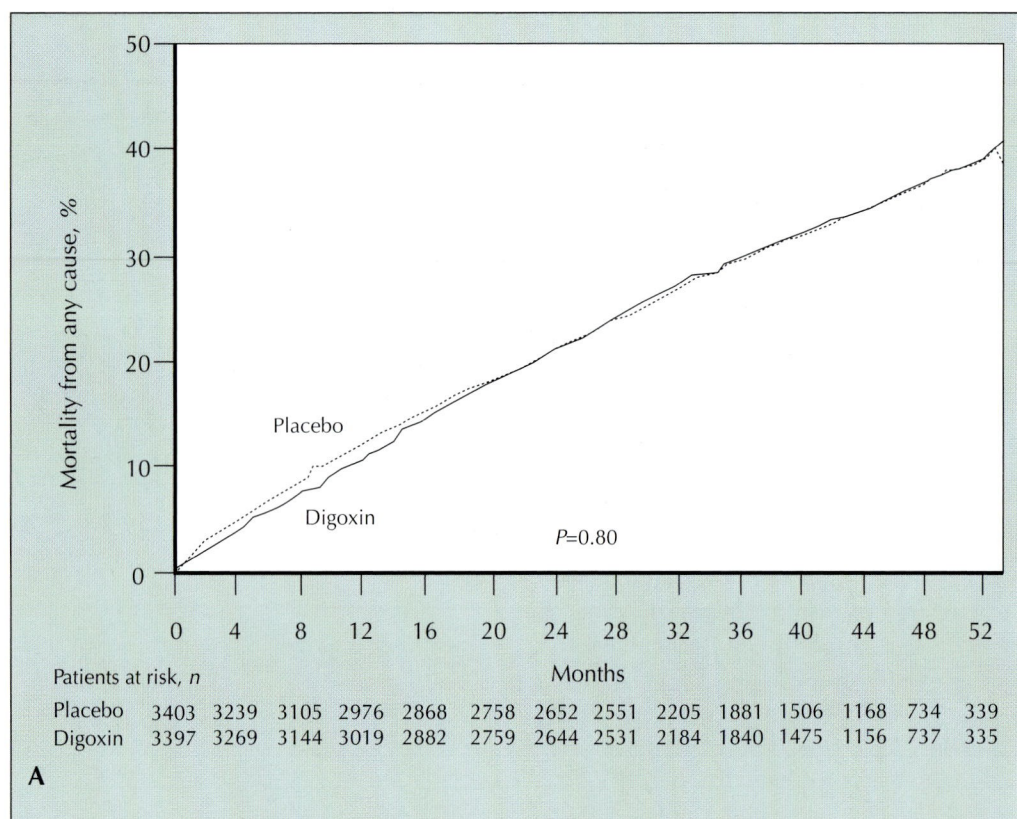

FIGURE 4-43. The Digitalis Investigation Group (DIG) trial evaluated the effects of digoxin on survivial in 6800 patients. The average follow-up was 37 months. Digoxin did not increase or decrease overall mortality (**A**). However, digoxin-treated patients had a reduction in the overall rate of hospitalization and also the rate of hospitalization for worsening heart failure (**B**). There was no increased risk of ventricular arrhythmias in the digoxin-treated group. (*Adapted from* Digitalis Investigation Report [41].)

Patients at risk, n

	0	4	8	12	16	20	24	28	32	36	40	44	48	52
Placebo	3403	3239	3105	2976	2868	2758	2652	2551	2205	1881	1506	1168	734	339
Digoxin	3397	3269	3144	3019	2882	2759	2644	2531	2184	1840	1475	1156	737	335

A

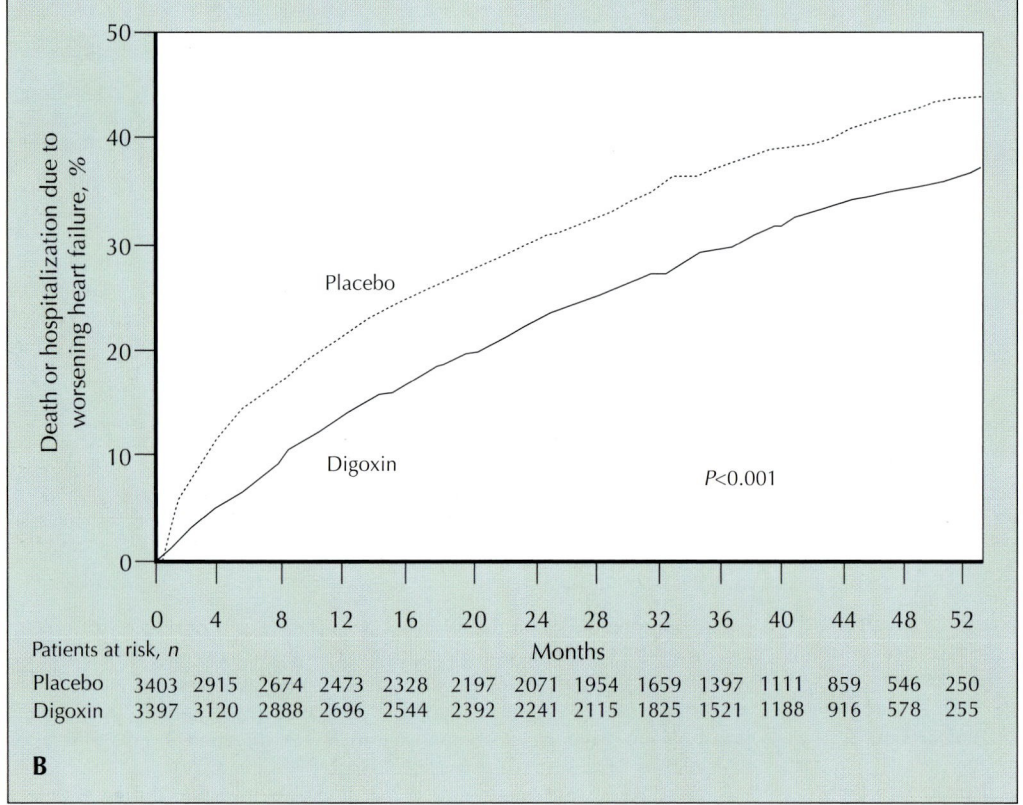

Patients at risk, n

	0	4	8	12	16	20	24	28	32	36	40	44	48	52
Placebo	3403	2915	2674	2473	2328	2197	2071	1954	1659	1397	1111	859	546	250
Digoxin	3397	3120	2888	2696	2544	2392	2241	2115	1825	1521	1188	916	578	255

B

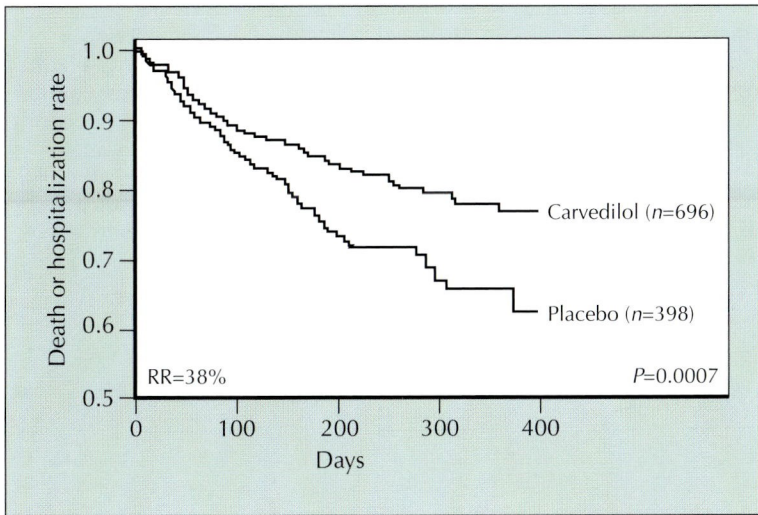

FIGURE 4-44. United States Carvedilol Heart Failure Trials Program: effect on major clinical events. In 1997, the US Food and Drug Administration approved carvedilol, a nonselective β-adrenergic antagonist with α_1-adrenergic receptor blocking and antioxidant properties, as adjunctive therapy for patients with mild to moderate heart failure. This decision was based in large part on the results of the US Carvedilol Heart Failure Trials Program, which randomized 1094 patients with chronic heart failure and a left ventricular ejection fraction of 35% or less to placebo or carvedilol in addition to conventional therapy with digoxin, diuretics, and an agiotensin-converting enzyme inhibitor. Patients were assigned to one of four treatment protocols based on exercise capacity as assessed by a 6-minute walk test. After a mean follow-up of 7 months, carvedilol resulted in a 27% reduction in the risk of cardiovascular hospitalization ($P=0.036$) and a 38% reduction in the combined endpoint of death or cardiovascular hospitalization. (*Adapted from* Packer *et al.* [42].)

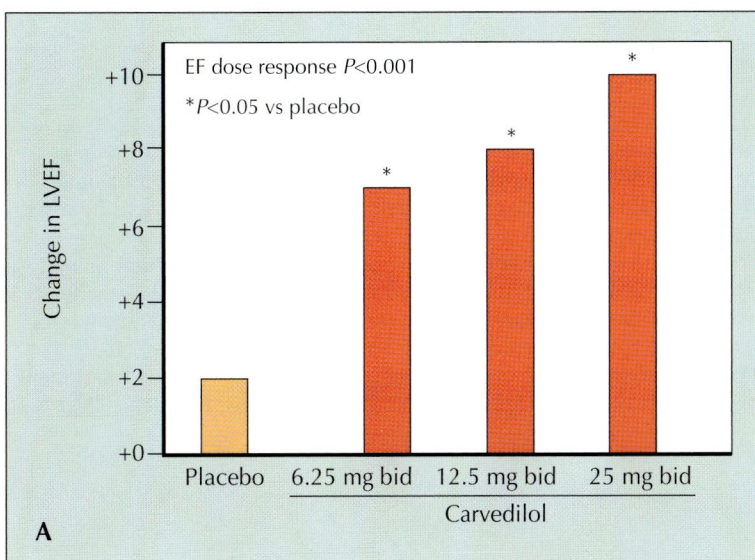

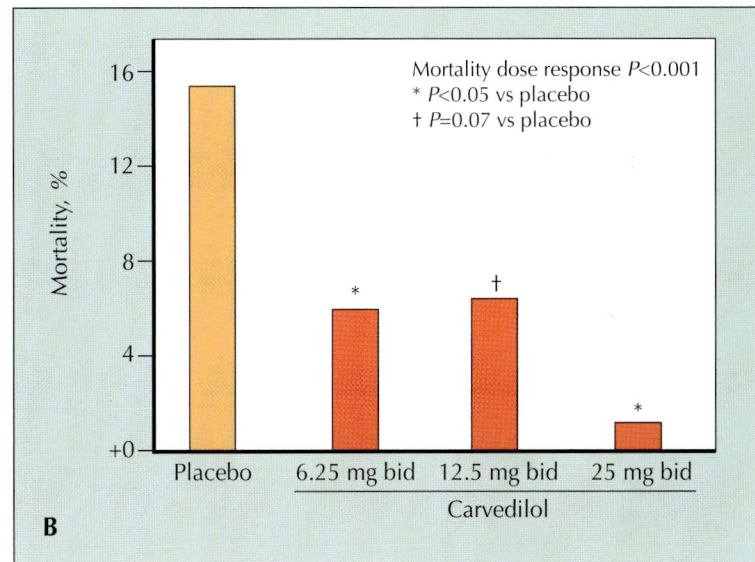

FIGURE 4-45. Effect of carvedilol on ejection fraction and mortality in the Multicenter Oral Carvedilol Heart Failure Assessment (MOCHA) trial. The MOCHA trial, a component of the US Carvedilol Heart Failure Trials Program, tested whether the effects of carvedilol were dose-related. Patients (n=345) with mild to moderate heart failure were randomly assigned to treatment with placebo or carvedilol in one of three target doses: 6.25 mg twice a day (low-dose group), 12.5 mg twice a day (medium-dose group), or 25 mg twice a day (high-dose group). Although carvedilol had no effect on the primary endpoint of submaximal exercise, there were significant dose-related improvements in left ventricular function (**A**) and all-cause mortality (**B**). In this study, carvedilol also lowered the hospitalization rate by approximately 60%. bid—twice a day. (*Adapted from* Bristow *et al.* [43].)

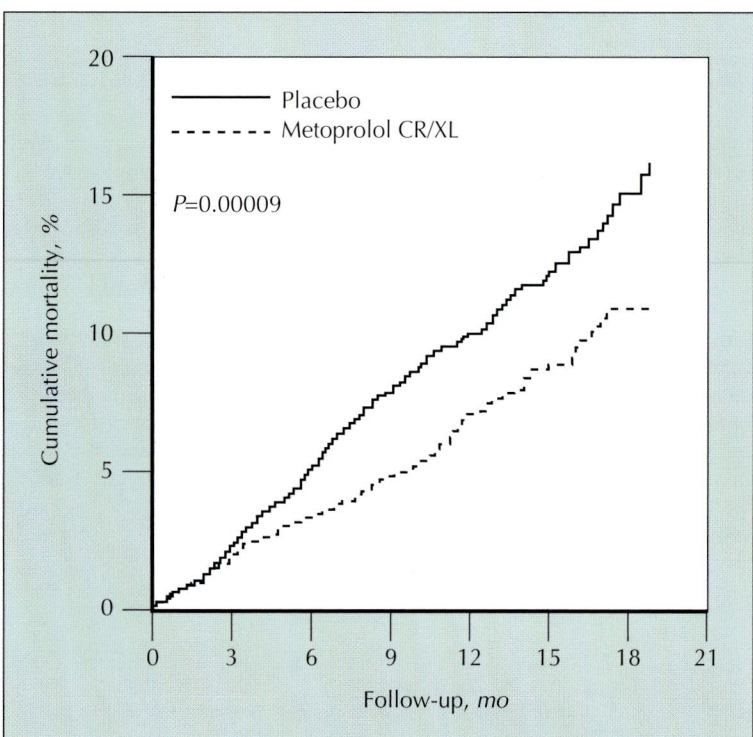

FIGURE 4-46. Effect of metoprolol on all-cause mortality, sudden death, and death due to worsening heart failure in the Metoprolol CR/XL Randomized Intervention Trial in Congestive Heart Failure (MERIT-HF) Trial. In this trial 3991 patients with New York Heart Association (NYHA) functional class II, III, or IV heart failure and a left ventricular ejection fraction below 40% were randomized to treatment with metoprolol controlled release/extended release (CR/XL) or placebo, in addition to optimal standard therapy. Metoprolol CR/XL was begun in a dose of 12.5 mg per day (NYHA III and IV patients) or 25 mg per day (NYHA class II patients), and titrated to a target dose of 200 mg per day over 8 weeks. After a mean follow-up of 1 year, metoprolol CR/XL decreased all-cause mortality by 34% ($P=0.00009$). The risk of sudden death was decreased by 41% and the risk of death due to worsening heart failure was reduced by 49%. (*Adapted from* MERIT-HF Study Group [44].)

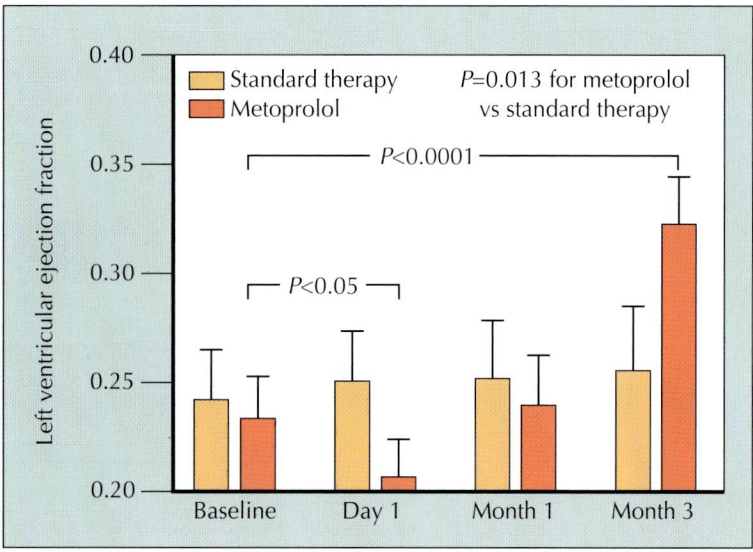

FIGURE 4-47. Time course of the effect of beta-adrenergic blockade on left ventricular ejection fraction in patients with heart failure. Twenty-six patients with dilated cardiomyopathy and a reduced ejection fraction were treated with standard therapy or metoprolol and followed by serial echocardiograms for 18 months. In standard therapy patients there was no change in ejection fraction over time. In patients treated with metoprolol, ejection fraction initially declined at 1 day, returned to baseline at 1 month, and increased markedly above baseline at 3 months. At 18 months, there were decreases in left ventricular mass and sphericity. These observations demonstrate that beta-blockade causes a time-dependent reversal of pathologic remodeling. (*Adapted from* Hall *et al.* [45].)

STEPS IN CLINICAL AND HEMODYNAMIC STABILIZATION OF ACUTE HEART FAILURE

1. Administer oxygen ($\uparrow$ F_iO_2)

2. When accompanied by fluid volume overload or a "congestive" component

    Sublingual nitroglycerin

    Intravenous furosemide

    Consider morphine sulfate

    Consider additional preload-afterload reduction

3. Evaluate early for

    Readily reversible causes of acute heart failure (*eg*, cardiac dysrhythmias, pericardial tamponade). If present initiate appropriate intervention

    Myocardial ischemia-infarction. If present, promptly initiate appropriate interventions (*eg*, thrombolytic therapy)

4. If patient is refractory to above therapies, hypotensive, or in cardiogenic shock

    Consider fluid or intravenous inotropic and/or vasopressor agents

    Consider catheterization (pulmonary and systemic arterial)

    Obtain echocardiogram to assist in diagnosis, evaluation, and reparability of the culprit lesion or condition

    Consider need for mechanical circulatory assistance (intra-aortic balloon counterpulsation)

5. Proceed to definitive diagnostic and interventional procedures

FIGURE 4-48. The major steps in the initial management of acute heart failure are presented [46–65]. The interventions are arranged in the general order of application and according to the general types of acute heart failure encountered.

1) When possible, it is informative to obtain arterial blood for gas analysis before oxygen administration.

2) Sublingual nitroglycerin can be administered at a dose of 1 tablet (1 or 2 sprays) every 5 minutes three or four times until intravenous nitroglycerin or nitroprusside can take effect. Furosemide is usually administered in a dose range of 20 to 80 mg intravenously. Preload-afterload reduction beyond sublingual nitroglycerin is best achieved by intravenous administration of nitroglycerin or nitroprusside.

3) The medical history and electrocardiogram are obtained early in the evaluation of the patient with acute heart failure to determine whether myocardial ischemia-infarction is the underlying cause for the acute event and whether the patient is a candidate for acute intervention (*eg*, thrombolytic therapy, coronary angioplasty).

4) Dobutamine, dopamine, and norepinephrine represent the principal inotropic and/or vasopressor agents used in this clinical setting.

5) Once the patient's condition is stabilized, diagnostic and interventional procedures can be performed.

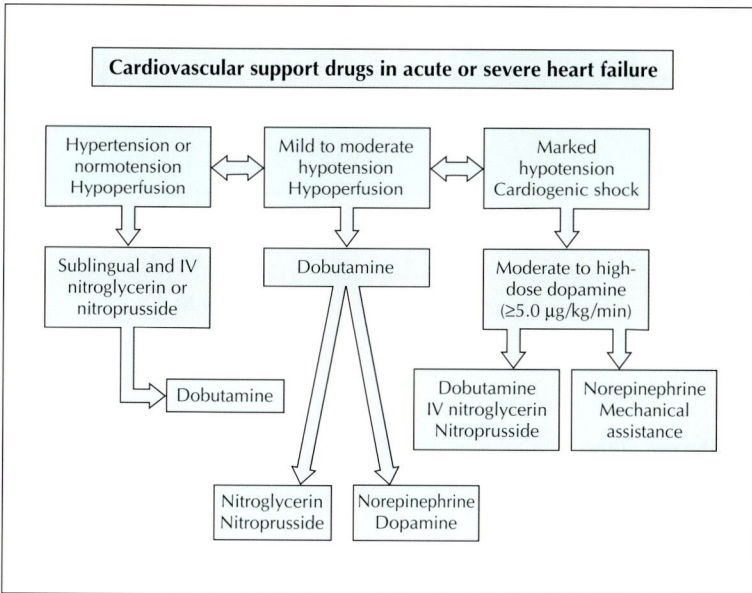

FIGURE 4-49. A practical working diagram of the cardiovascular support drugs commonly employed in the initial short-term management of acute or severe heart failure. It is assumed that patients who require these support drugs have adequate to high left ventricular diastolic filling pressures ($\geq$ 18 mm Hg) or clinical evidence of fluid volume overload. Systemic hypoperfusion and hypotension in a patient without evidence of volume overload or with filling pressures of less than 18 mm Hg should be approached with a fluid volume challenge as the first step. On the basis of the clinical presentation and the state of systemic perfusion and blood pressure, the initial drug of choice is selected and its dosage is increased until clinical or hemodynamic endpoints are achieved or adverse effects appear. At this point, inadequate improvement of clinical status usually requires either the addition of a second agent as combination therapy or mechanical assistance. IV—intravenous.

ASSESSMENT OF DONOR FOR HEART TRANSPLANTATION

Brain death

Age
  Up to 60 y
  Angiography performed
    after age 40–50 y

Cardiac function
  History of risk factors
  Recent insult
    Cause of death
    Anoxia
    Prolonged CPR
  Echocardiographic function
  Need for pressor support

Potential infection
  Acute infection
  Risk factors for AIDS
  Hepatitis
  CMV status

Compatibility with recipient
  Blood type
  Circulating antibodies
  Size

FIGURE 4-57. Considerations in the evaluation of a donor for heart transplantation [72]. Definitions of brain death vary among states. Age restrictions are being liberalized to expand the pool of donor hearts. A history of hypertension or smoking is a greater cause for concern in the older heart,

particularly in male donors. Angiography is frequently performed in the older hearts to determine the presence of coronary artery disease, for which hearts may be rejected; or, in cases of urgent candidate need, bypasses can sometimes be performed at the time of implantation. In the setting of brain injury and death, left ventricular function may be abnormal either globally or regionally, attributable to catecholamine surges and other endocrine derangement, and does not always recover. Cardiac abnormalities may be more often reversible in younger patients and in those with intracranial hemorrhage as opposed to head trauma.

Many potential donors require moderate support with dopamine or dobutamine, usually not exceeding 5 to 10 µg/kg/min, but the need for higher doses may indicate more severe cardiac injury, assuming that fluid replacement has been monitored adequately in the setting of the central diabetes insipidus that often occurs. Hearts from donors with active infection, such as bacteremia or pneumonia, may occasionally be accepted for a critically ill recipient. Risk factors for acquired immunodeficiency syndrome (AIDS) are usually contraindications. Hepatitis B infection is also a contraindication, but decisions regarding hepatitis C infection are still controversial. Evidence of previous cytomegalovirus (CMV) infection is common in both donors and recipients, who may be matched in the future for CMV status. Blood types between donor and recipient are matched as for transfusions. Except in rare cases of multiple sensitization, a donor heart is not given to a recipient with specific preformed antibodies against lymphocytes from that donor. Size matching remains controversial, usually within 20% body weight, depending on the urgency, relative heights of donor and recipient, and recipient cardiomegaly. CPR—cardiopulmonary resuscitation.

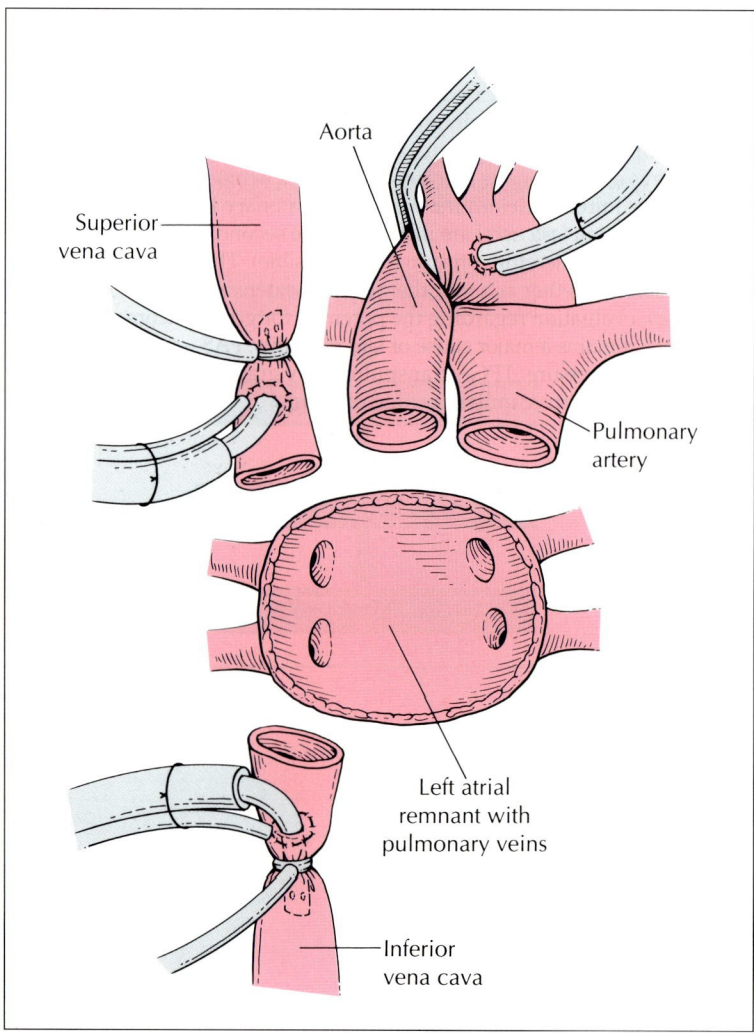

FIGURE 4-58. Recipient heart explantation in preparation for bicaval anastomoses rather than biatrial anastomoses, which have frequently been employed. The atrial septum and right atrium are resected with the ventricles of the diseased heart, leaving only a small cuff at the origin of the venae cavae. The left atrium is further resected, leaving a cuff of tissue around the ostia of the pulmonary veins. (*Adapted from* Kapoor and Laks [73].)

Aorta

Superior vena cava

Pulmonary artery

Left atrial remnant with pulmonary veins

Inferior vena cava

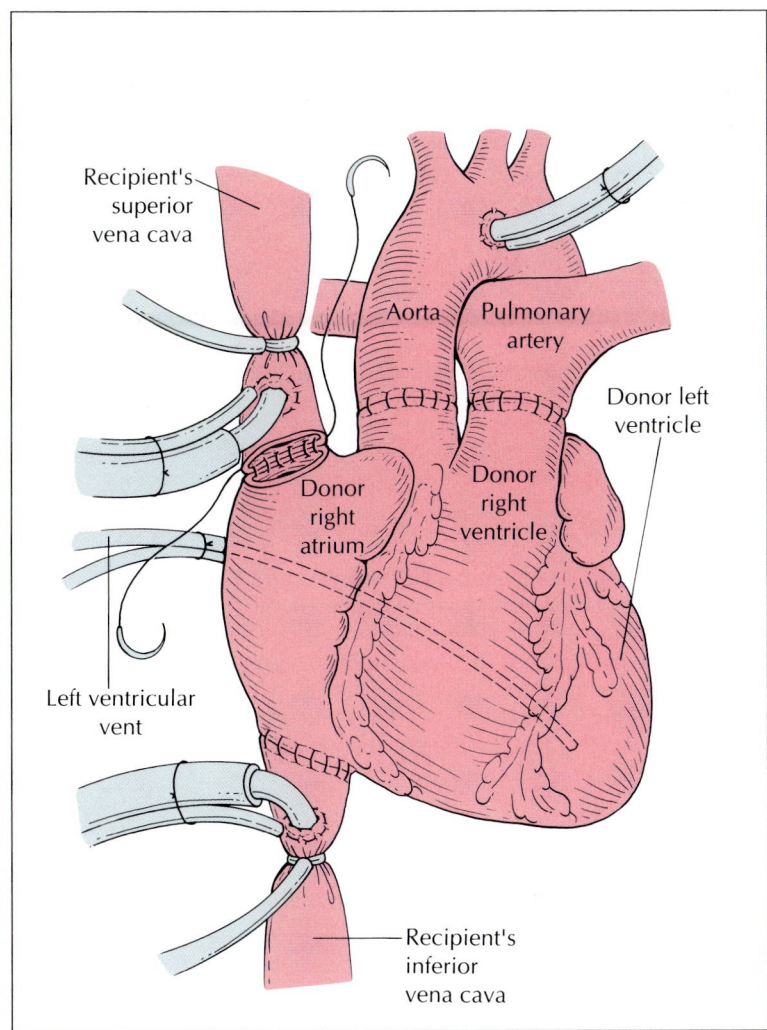

FIGURE 4-59. The left atrial anastomosis is completed and a left ventricular vent is inserted through the suture line. After the recipient and donor pulmonary artery anastomosis is completed except for the anterior part, the aortic anastomosis is completed. The heart is de-aired and modified reperfusion is instituted. During reperfusion the inferior vena caval anastomosis is performed. The heart is then de-aired and the cross-clamp is released. The superior vena caval anastomosis is then completed while the heart is beating. (*Adapted from* Kapoor and Laks [73].)

MANAGEMENT OF THE TRANSPLANT PATIENT

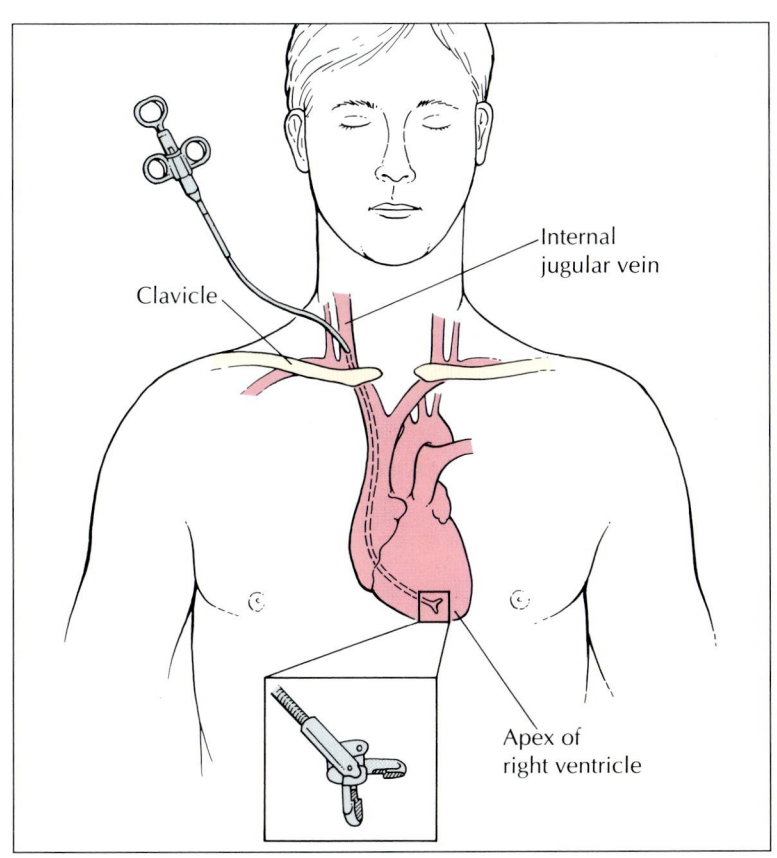

FIGURE 4-60. Bioptome and access route for right ventricular endomyocardial biopsies from the superior vena cava. Improvements in disposable bioptomes, the instruments used to obtain biopsy specimens, now yield sample quality comparable to that of other bioptomes that require sterilization and sharpening. The majority of biopsies are performed through the right internal jugular approach, but scarring, thrombosis, and other technical problems sometimes necessitate the use of the left internal jugular, subclavian, or femoral veins. With repeated biopsies, some tissue specimens reveal only fibrosis from old biopsy sites. Three to four pieces containing at least 50% myocytes are required for 90% to 95% confidence in the interpretation [74].

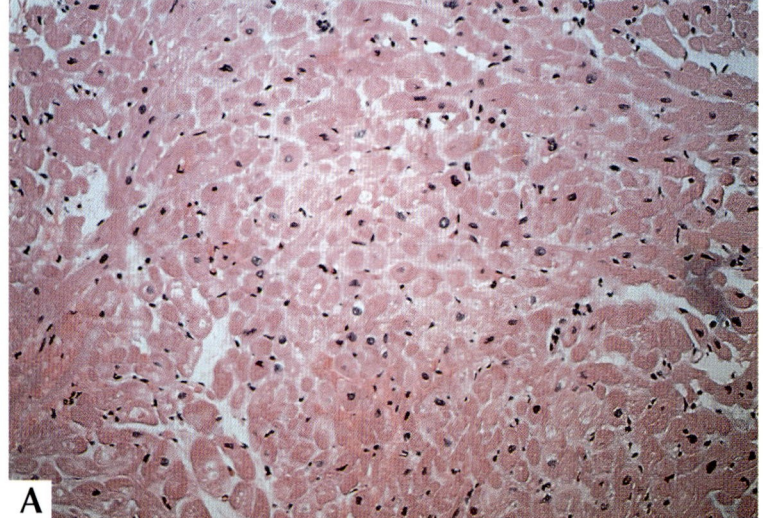

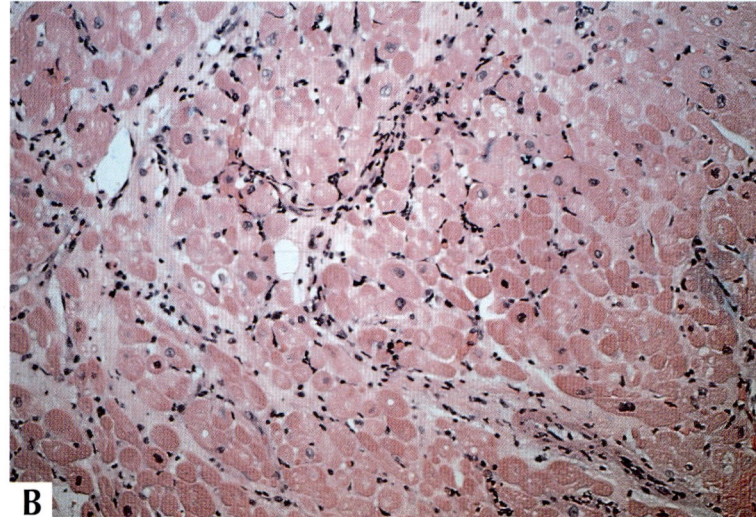

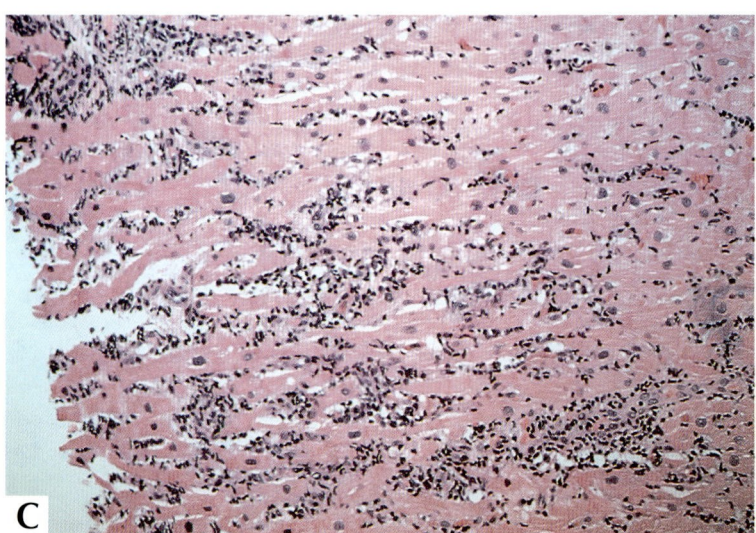

FIGURE 4-61. A–C, Right ventricular endomyocardial biopsy specimens stained with hematoxylin and eosin, demonstrating normal myocardium (**A**), mild rejection with focal lymphocyte infiltrate without evidence of myocyte necrosis (grade 1) (**B**), and moderate rejection demonstrating more intensive lymphocytic infiltration with evidence of myocyte vacuolization and loss (grade 3) (**C**). The refinements of grading relate to the extent of involvement in different areas and samples. (*Courtesy of* Jon A. Kobashigawa, Los Angeles, CA.)

SAMPLE REGIMEN OF MEDICATIONS AFTER TRANSPLANTATION

Cyclosporine	Clotrimazole troches
Azathioprine	Trimethoprim-sulfamethoxazole
Prednisone	HMG-CoA reductase inhibitor
Diltiazem or ACE inhibitor	Aspirin
Furosemide	Calcium carbonate
H$_2$-receptor blocker	Vitamin D

FIGURE 4-62. Typical regimen of medications for 4 months after cardiac transplantation. In addition to immunosuppressive medications, approximately 75% of patients require drug therapy for hypertension, often with diltiazem, which decreases the metabolism and cost of cyclosporine and may decrease coronary artery disease, and/or an angiotensin-converting enzyme (ACE) inhibitor. A loop diuretic is required to control fluid retention in most patients during the first 6 months and is less commonly required thereafter. Ranitidine or cimetidine is commonly given to decrease gastrointestinal side effects of prednisone. Clotrimazole troches are used to decrease mucosal candidiasis during the first 3 months. Trimethoprim-sulfamethoxazole may be given twice weekly to decrease the incidence of *Pneumocystis carinii* pneumonia during the first 6 months. Both prophylactic antibiotics may be resumed briefly after subsequent therapy for rejection. There is increasing interest in lowering cholesterol in transplant recipients, who respond well to HMG-CoA reductase inhibitors but require lower doses and careful monitoring to avoid rhabdomyolysis [75]. Aspirin is often used to decrease platelet aggregation as a potential factor in the vasculopathy. Calcium and vitamin D are recommended in postmenopausal women and other patients with decreased bone density, which can result from cyclosporine and corticosteroid use. HMG-CoA—hepatic hydromethylglutaryl coenzyme A; H$_2$—histamine$_2$.

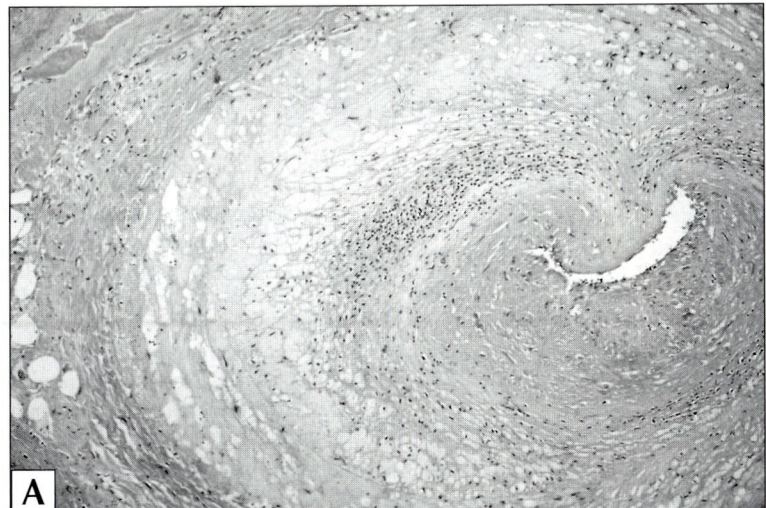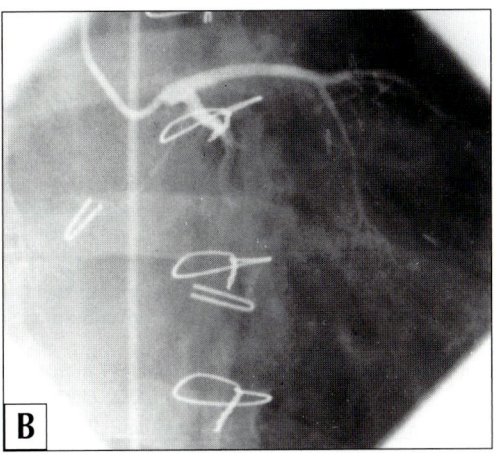

FIGURE 4-63. Transplantation coronary allograft disease (TCAD). The major cause of late death after cardiac transplantation is the development of TCAD, a unique, accelerated form of coronary artery disease. By 1 year posttransplant, about 30% of patients demonstrate some TCAD, and the incidence and severity continue to increase with time [76]. The pathogenesis of TCAD is thought to begin with immunologic and nonimmunologic injury to the arterial endothelium, with resultant loss of endothelial integrity [77]. Microthrombi, cellular proliferation, and plasma lipids accumulate at the site of the injured intima. **A,** This leads to further cellular proliferation and finally profound myointimal hyperplasia leding to diffuse coronary artery lumen narrowing. **B,** Selective left coronary angiography from a patient with severe TCAD, which shows diffuse tapering of the left anterior descending and circumflex arteries as well as pruning of all the secondary vessels. Immunologic mechanisms resulting in endothelial injury include both cellular and humoral factors [78]. Nonimmunologic risk factors also contribute to the development of cardiac allograft vasculopathy. Recipient age and gender, donor age and gender, obesity, hyperlipidemia, and donor ischemic time may impact on the development of vasculopathy [79]. An association has also been found between the presence of active cytomegalovirus infection and the development of vasculopathy [80]. Given the diffuse, concentric nature of this disease, percutaneous transluminal coronary angioplasty and coronary artery bypass grafting are not useful strategies for management. Unfortunately, patients with TCAD have a fivefold greater risk of cardiac events such as myocardial infarction, severe refractory heart failure, and sudden death. Presently retransplantation is the only treatment for severe TCAD; however survival after repeat transplantation is significantly reduced. Consequently, preventative strategies have assumed clinical importance. Hyperlipidemia management with HMG Co-A (3-hydroxy-3-methylglutaryl-coenzyme A) reductase inhibitors and routine aspirin use are two such approaches.

SURVIVAL

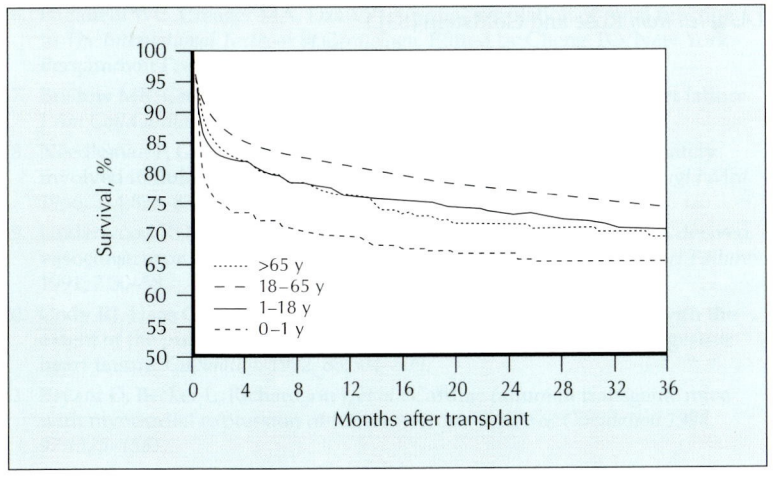

FIGURE 4-64. Actuarial survival according to recipient age, calculated from 15,000 heart transplant recipients in the Registry from the International Society of Heart and Lung Transplantation [67]. Neonatal transplants are associated with a poorer survival, as are those performed in recipients over 65 years of age. Five-year survival for adults is now 68%. The first-year survival in the Registry may continue to improve as a greater proportion of patients followed have received cyclosporine from the time of transplantation. There will be less improvement in later survival, largely limited by transplant vasculopathy, which has *not* been noticeably decreased in the cyclosporine era [70]. (*Adapted from* Kaye [67].)

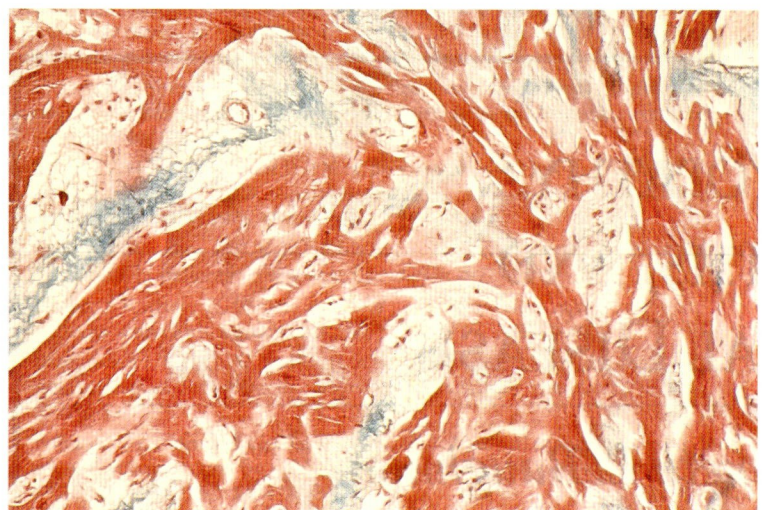

FIGURE 5-2. Myocardial fiber disarray. Microscopic section of the ventricular septum of a 28-year-old patient with HCM who died while jogging. This section shows a typical area of myocardial fiber disarray. The muscle cells are short and plump, and the nuclei are large and hyperchromatic. Note the extensive amount of loose intercellular connective tissue that may become transformed into diffuse myocardial fibrosis late in the disease (magnification, × 100). (*From* Wigle *et al.* [1]; with permission.)

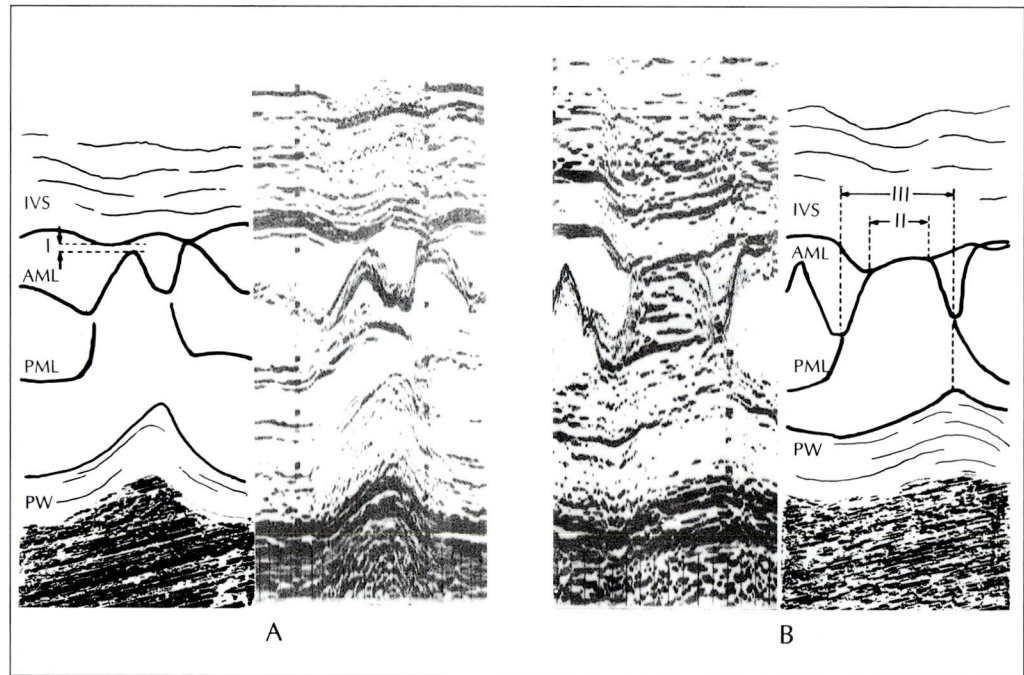

FIGURE 5-3. Determination of the degree of systolic anterior motion (SAM) of the anterior mitral leaflet (AML) in subaortic obstructive HCM. When there is no mitral leaflet–septal contact, the minimal distance between the left side of the interventricular septum (IVS) and the AML is measured (I in **A**). If that distance is 10 mm or more, the degree of mitral leaflet SAM is classified as mild. If that distance is less than 10 mm or there is brief mitral leaflet–septal contact, the degree of SAM is classified as moderate (**A**). If there is mitral leaflet–septal contact, the ratio of the duration of that contact (II in **B**) to total echocardiographic systole (III in **B**) is determined and expressed as a percentage. When the duration of mitral leaflet–septal contact is greater than 30% of echocardiographic systole, severe SAM is said to be present (**B**). The hemodynamic state of the patient is determined by the degree of mitral leaflet SAM. Thus patients with nonobstructive HCM have no or, at most, very mild SAM. Patients with subaortic obstructive HCM have severe SAM, and patients with latent subaortic obstruction will have mild or moderate SAM, which becomes severe on provocation. PML—posterior mitral leaflet; PW—posterior wall. (*From* Gilbert *et al.* [2]; with permission.)

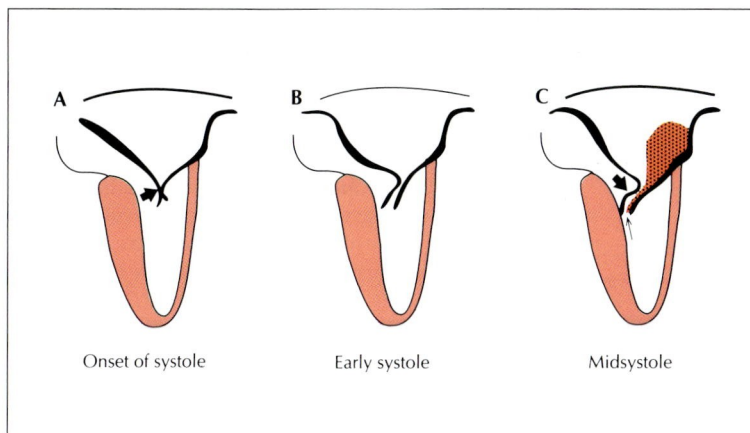

A B C

Onset of systole   Early systole   Midsystole

FIGURE 5-4. Functional anatomy of mitral leaflet systolic anterior motion and mitral regurgitation in subaortic obstructive HCM. Drawing of a transesophageal echocardiogram (frontal long-axis plane) demonstrating the anterior and superior motion of the anterior mitral leaflet to produce mitral leaflet–septal contact and failure of leaflet coaptation in midsystole. **A,** At the onset of systole, the coaptation point (*arrow*) is in the body of the anterior and posterior leaflets rather than at the tip of the leaflets, as in normal subjects [3,4]. The portion of the leaflets beyond the coaptation point is referred to as the residual length of the leaflet [3,4]. During early systole (**B**) and midsystole (**C**) there is anterior and superior movement of the residual length of the anterior mitral leaflet (*thick arrow* in *C*), with septal contact and failure of leaflet coaptation (*thin arrow* in *C*) with consequent mitral regurgitation directed posteriorly into the left atrium (*dotted area*). (*Adapted from* Grigg *et al.* [4].)

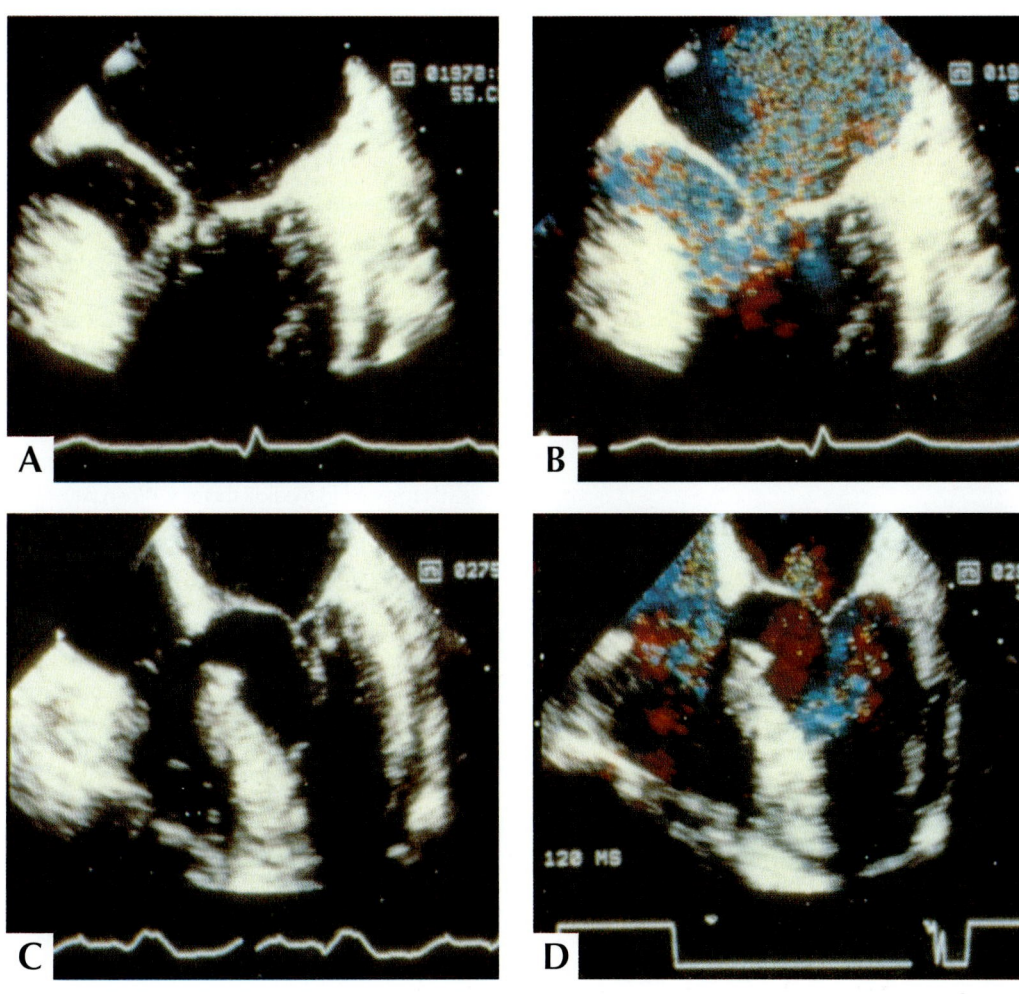

A   B   C   D

FIGURE 5-5. Obstruction and mitral regurgitation in subaortic obstructive HCM before and after myectomy. Intraoperative transesophageal echocardiographic and Doppler study (frontal long-axis plane) before (**A** and **B**) and after (**C** and **D**) myectomy. *Panel A* shows a two-dimensional systolic frame demonstrating systolic anterior motion of the residual length of the anterior mitral leaflet, with mitral leaflet–septal contact and failure of coaptation between the mitral leaflets. *Panel B* shows the same frame with Doppler color-flow imaging demonstrating turbulent left ventricular outflow as a result of the subaortic obstruction and a large jet of posteriorly directed mitral regurgitation arising from the funnel-shaped gap between the two mitral leaflets due to their failure to coapt. Note there is no evidence of left ventricular cavity obliteration at the time of subaortic obstruction and concomitant mitral regurgitation. *Panel C* is a two-dimensional systolic frame following myectomy demonstrating a widened left ventricular outflow tract and abolition of systolic anterior motion. *Panel D* is the same frame with Doppler color-flow imaging demonstrating nonturbulent left ventricular outflow with a marked reduction in the severity of the mitral regurgitation (which is now reflected only by a small residual central jet) [4].

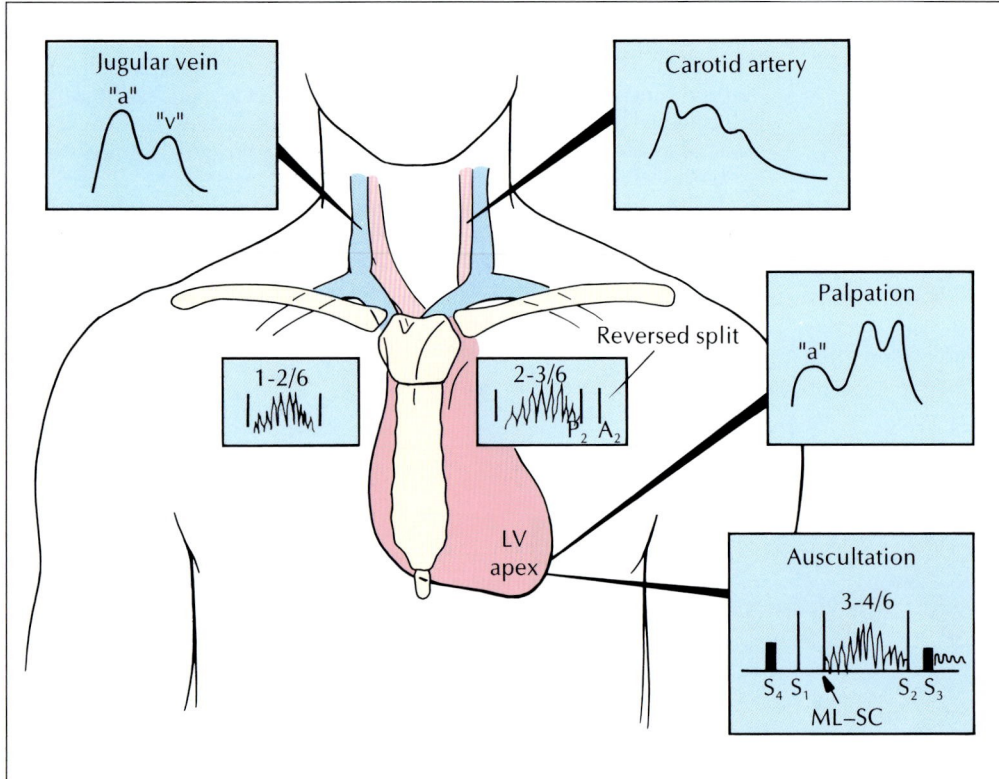

FIGURE 5-6. Physical examination in subaortic obstructive HCM. There are seven physical signs in subaortic obstructive HCM that are not found in nonobstructive HCM. On palpation, a spike-and-dome arterial pulse can often be felt in the carotid artery or in a peripheral pulse. On palpation of the left ventricular (LV) apex, there may be a triple apex beat caused by a palpable left atrial gallop and a double systolic

impulse—one impulse comes before the onset of obstruction and the other after. On auscultation, at or just medial to the LV apex, there is a late onset, diamond-shaped systolic murmur of grade 3 to 4/6 in intensity. This murmur is caused by both the subaortic obstruction and the concomitant mitral regurgitation, causing the murmur to radiate to both the left sternal border and to the axilla. Because of the mitral regurgitation, there is often a short diastolic inflow murmur after the third heart sound. Rarely, a mitral leaflet– septal contact (ML–SC) sound may be heard preceding the systolic murmur at the apex. Finally, if there is severe subaortic obstruction, reversed splitting of the second heart sound may occur. In nonobstructive HCM, there is often a third or fourth heart sound at the apex, depending on the type of diastolic dysfunction. If the fourth heart sound is palpable, there will be a double apex beat, which is quite different in timing and significance from the double *systolic* apex beat that occurs in subaortic obstructive HCM. In nonobstructive HCM, there is either no apical systolic murmur or at most a grade 1 to 2/6 murmur of mitral regurgitation. In any type of HCM, a grade 1 to 3/6 systolic ejection murmur at or below the pulmonary area may be heard. This murmur may reflect obstruction to right ventricular (RV) outflow. Examining the jugular venous pulse frequently reveals a prominent a-wave that rises on inspiration, depending on the degree of RV diastolic dysfunction. Rarely, this is accompanied by an RV fourth heart sound.

Effect of ventriculomyectomy operation in subaortic obstructive HCM

Ventriculomyectomy

↓ Septal thickness

↑ LVOT size

Abolish SAM

Abolish obstruction — Abolish apical murmur — Abolish mitral regurgitation

↓ LA size

↓ LVEDP

↓ LAP

Abolish symptoms

FIGURE 5-7. Management of obstructive HCM that does not respond to medical therapy. When patients with obstructive HCM are unresponsive to medical therapy, or are dissatisfied by the disease-imposed limitations or the side effects of medication, atrioventricular sequential pacemaker therapy, alcohol septal ablation, or surgery may be considered. Ventricular pacing from the right ventricular apex may cause a rightward septal shift and alleviation of the subaortic obstruction with resultant symptomatic improvement in some patients. This form of therapy is not, however, effective in all patients. The obstruction in some patients is not completely relieved, and up to 25% of patients require atrioventricular nodal ablation to achieve ventricular capture [5,6]. Ventriculomy-ectomy surgery, on the other hand, has been performed for over 30 years, and a number of centers have had extensive experience (and good to excellent results) [7–10]. The mechanisms of benefit of this procedure are illustrated. Myectomy thins the ventricular septum and widens the left ventricular outflow tract (LVOT), which abolishes mitral leaflet systolic anterior motion (SAM). This in turn abolishes the obstruction and mitral regurgitation. These effects eliminate the apical murmur and decrease the left ventricular end-diastolic pressure (LVEDP) as well as left atrial pressure (LAP) and size. Symptoms are dramatically relieved by these mechanisms. Myectomy is also indicated in recurrent atrial fibrillation to decrease left atrial size and restore normal sinus rhythm. The procedure should be performed in patients with obstructive HCM with unexplained syncope or cardiac arrest.

Alcohol ablation attempts to reduce the subaortic gradient by creation of myocardial dysfunction. Alcohol is injected into the septal branch or branches of the left anterior descending artery that supply the hypertrophied septum. If successful, the myocardial infarction decreases septal contraction and reduces the outflow gradient.

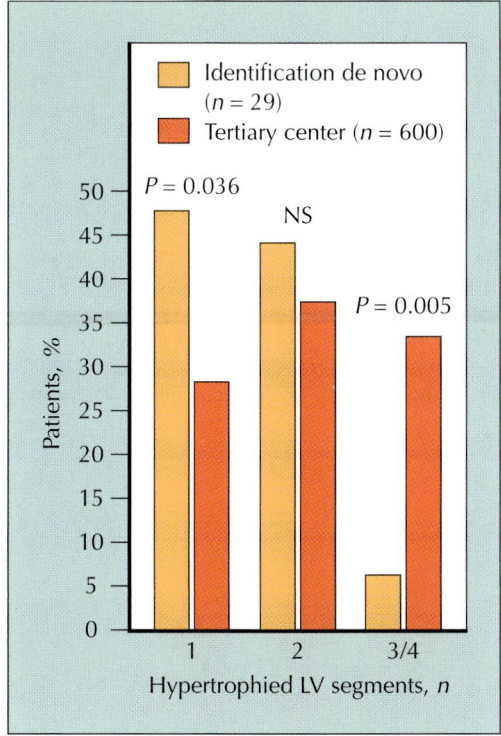

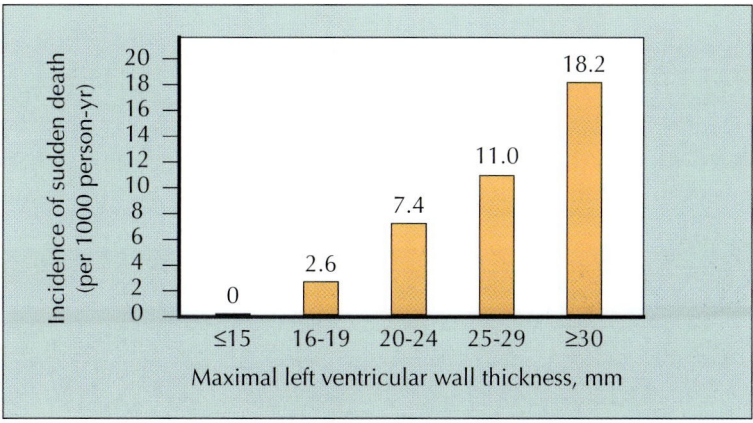

FIGURE 5-9. Patients with asymmetric septal hypertrophy die of progressive heart failure or sudden cardiac death. The risk of sudden death appears to correlate with the maximal left ventricular wall thickness. Severe hypertrophy may be present in young patients with mild or no symptoms [12]. (*Adapted from* Spirito *et al.* [12].)

FIGURE 5-8. Patients with hypertrophic cardiomyopathy may remain clinically unrecognized. On echocardiography, subjects screened in the community have fewer hypertrophied left ventricular segments than patients reported from tertiary centers [11]. (*Adapted from* Maron *et al.* [11].)

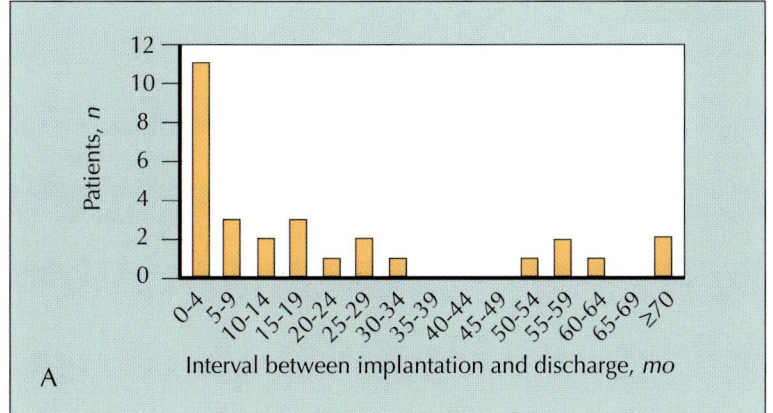

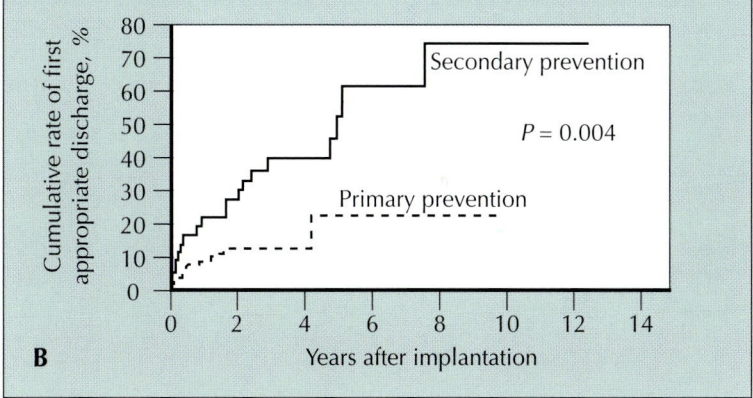

FIGURE 5-10. Implantable cardiovertor/defibrillators appear to prevent sudden cardiac death in some patients with hypertrophic cardiomyopathy. In patients who had defibrillators placed after sudden cardiac death or sustained ventricular tachycardia (secondary prevention), 11% received an appropriate AICD discharge per year. However, in patients where placement was used as primary prevention, 5% received appropriate discharges per year (**A**). Occasionally, the interval between implantation and discharge is long (**B**) [13]. (*Adapted from* Maron *et al.* [13].)

Idiopathic Dilated Cardiomyopathy

According to the World Health Organization, idiopathic dilated cardiomyopathy is characterized by dilatation of the left, right, or both ventricles with impaired systolic function and is of unknown cause.

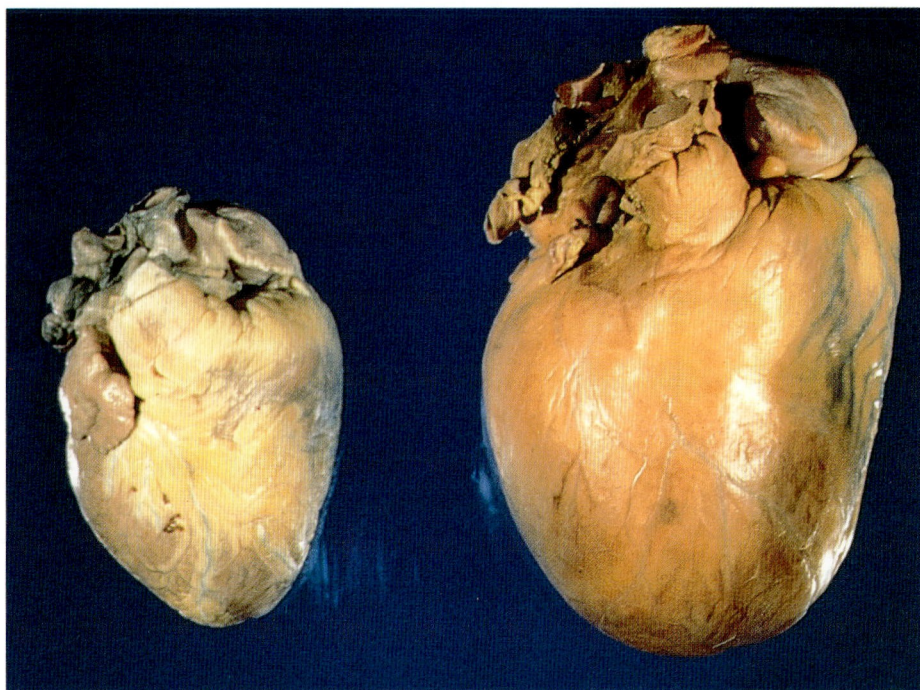

FIGURE 5-11. Gross pathology. In contrast to the normal heart (*left*), the heart in idiopathic dilated cardiomyopathy (*right*) is characterized by biventricular hypertrophy and four-chamber enlargement. The weight is often 25% to 50% above normal. Enlargement of the heart can be seen easily on chest radiography or cardiac echocardiography.

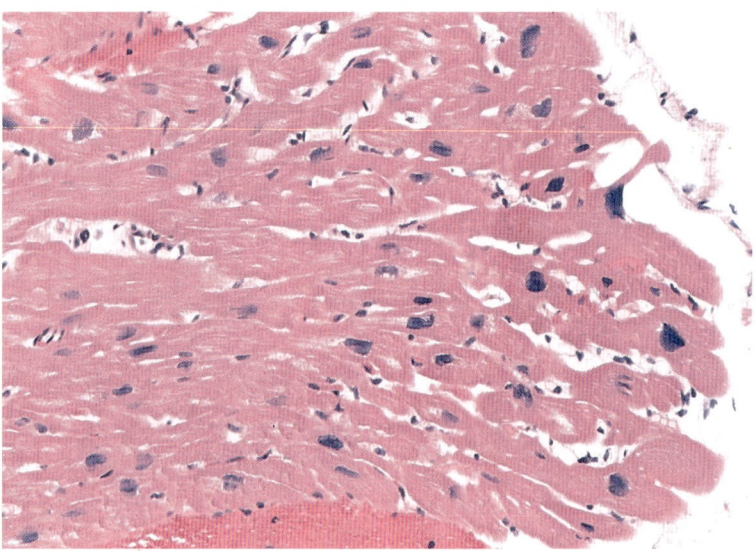

FIGURE 5-12. Endomyocardial biopsy from a patient with idiopathic cardiomyopathy. Large, irregularly shaped hyperchromatic nuclei are present, consistent with myocyte hypertrophy. The interstitium is cellular, but this should not be confused with myocarditis. These features, although nonspecific, support the diagnosis of idiopathic dilated cardiomyopathy. A completely normal endomyocardial biopsy does not support a diagnosis of idiopathic dilated cardiomyopathy and should suggest a focal cause, such as sarcoidosis, which requires further investigation [14].

SPECIFIC HEART-MUSCLE DISEASES

Heredofamilial	Sensitivities and toxic reactions
Familial cardiomyopathy	Ethanol
Muscular dystrophies	Anthracycline
Infectious	Cocaine
Bacterial	Cobalt
Viral	Catecholamines
Human immunodeficiency virus	Corticosteroids
Other	Lithium
Metabolic	Radiation
Endocrine	Heavy metal
Nutritional	Scorpion sting
Storage diseases	Other
Myocarditis	Uremia
Neoplastic	Anemia
Peripartum	Leukemia
Systemic	Obesity
Infiltrative	
Connective tissue disease	

FIGURE 5-13. Specific causes of dilated cardiomyopathy. These are also called secondary cardiomyopathies or specific heart-muscle diseases. Almost any disease process can involve cardiac muscle, as can be seen from this list. Multiple factors may actually play a causative role in any single patient. (*Adapted from* Abelmann [15].)

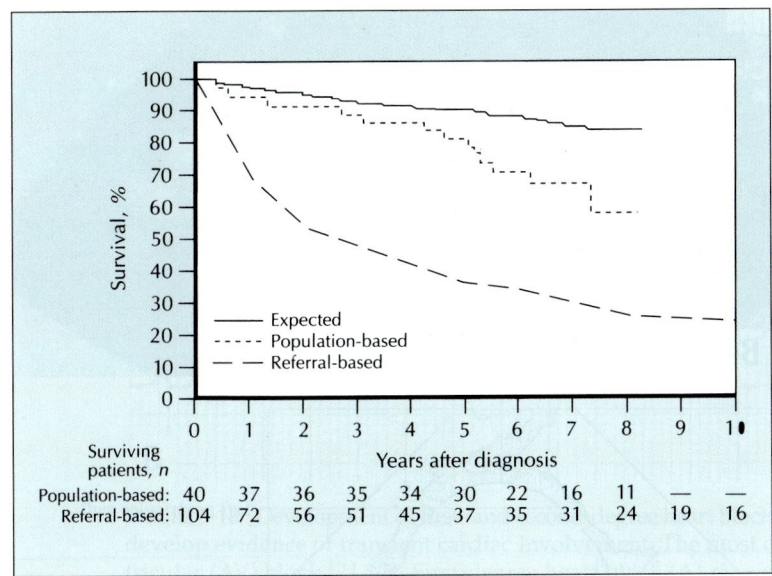

Surviving patients, n	0	1	2	3	4	5	6	7	8	9	10
Population-based:	40	37	36	35	34	30	22	16	11	—	—
Referral-based:	104	72	56	51	45	37	35	31	24	19	16

FIGURE 5-14. Survival after the initial diagnosis of idiopathic dilated cardiomyopathy. Survival among residents of Olmsted County, Minnesota, from 1975 to 1984 was poor [16]. Survival was better in a population-based rather than a referral-based cohort of patients. Not surprisingly, however, survival was still impaired compared with an age- and sex-matched cohort without idiopathic dilated cardiomyopathy (expected). (*Adapted from* Sugrue *et al.* [17].)

SIGNS AND SYMPTOMS

SYMPTOMS

Palpitation

Syncope

Dyspnea on exertion, paroxysmal
nocturnal dyspnea, orthopnea

Weakness and exercise intolerance

Peripheral edema, abdominal distension,
loss of appetite

Atypical chest pain

SECONDARY EFFECTS

Atrial tachyarrhythmias

High-degree atrioventricular block and
cerebral thromboembolism

Pulmonary congestion and pleural effusion

Low cardiac output

Right ventricular failure

Arrhythmias? pulmonary hypertension?
pulmonary embolism?

SIGNS

S_4 in patients with normal sinus rhythm

S_3 either from left or right ventricular origin

Moist rales in the lung fields

Jugular venous distension, hepatosplenomegaly,
ascites, pretibial edema, jaundice

FIGURE 5-29. Although there are no specific signs or symptoms of restrictive cardiomyopathy, this condition is manifested principally as congestive heart failure, pulmonary hypertension, thromboembolism, and arrhythmias.

HYPEREOSINOPHILIC HEART DISEASE (LÖFFLER'S SYNDROME)

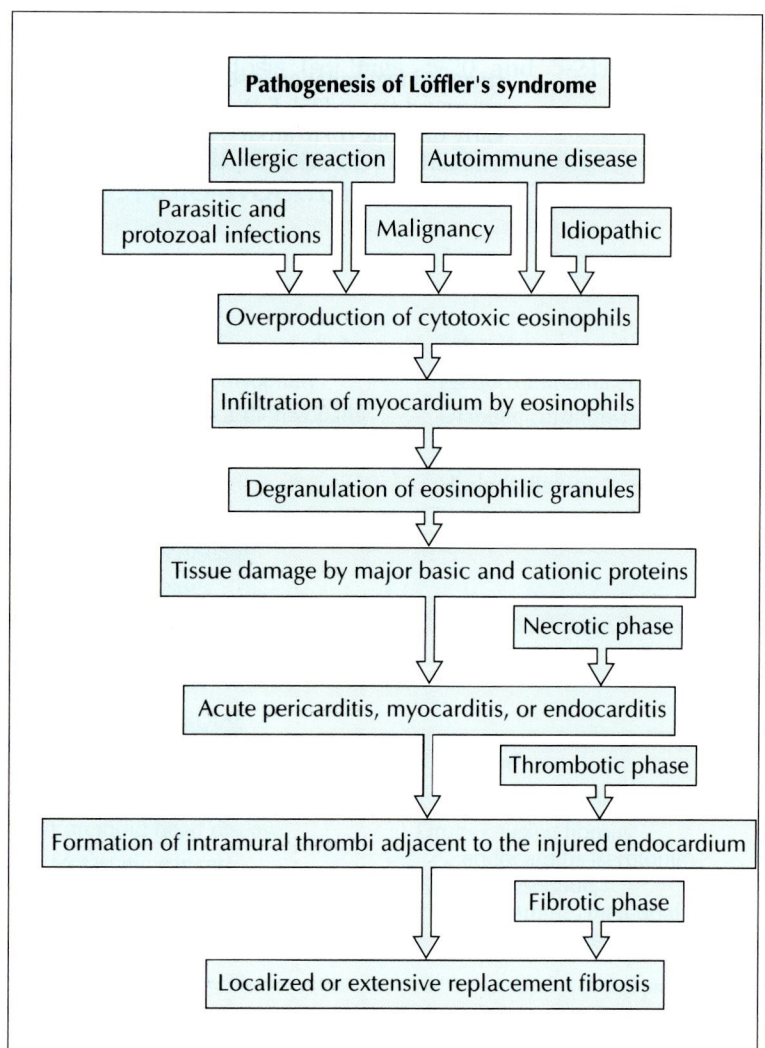

Pathogenesis of Löffler's syndrome

Allergic reaction · Autoimmune disease

Parasitic and protozoal infections · Malignancy · Idiopathic

↓

Overproduction of cytotoxic eosinophils

↓

Infiltration of myocardium by eosinophils

↓

Degranulation of eosinophilic granules

↓

Tissue damage by major basic and cationic proteins

→ Necrotic phase →

Acute pericarditis, myocarditis, or endocarditis

→ Thrombotic phase →

Formation of intramural thrombi adjacent to the injured endocardium

→ Fibrotic phase →

Localized or extensive replacement fibrosis

FIGURE 5-30. The pathogenesis of Löffler's syndrome. Tissue damage is caused by major basic and cationic proteins derived from cytotoxic eosinophils [36–40]. These cytotoxic proteins may stay in the myocardium for a prolonged period and produce continuous tissue damage. At the fibrotic phase, various types of heart diseases, such as endomyocardial fibrosis, dilated cardiomyopathy, atrioventricular block, or valvular regurgitation can be seen according to the difference of the most dominantly involved site.

Necrotic phase

Manifestations of acute endo-, myo-, or pericarditis with hypereosinophilia

Thrombotic phase

Cavity obliteration with intramural thrombi with or without hypereosinophilia (common in the tropics and rare in the temperate zone)

Fibrotic phase

Atrioventricular block

Valvular regurgitation

Heart failure with restrictive physiology (ranging from diastolic dysfunction to endomyocardial fibrosis) or systolic dysfunction

Absence of hypereosinophilia

FIGURE 5-31. The clinical manifestations of Löffler's syndrome and endomyocardial fibrosis [36,39]. The necrotic phase is acute, lasting for months. The thrombotic phase is subacute, lasting for months to 2 years. The fibrotic phase is chronic, and lasts for years.

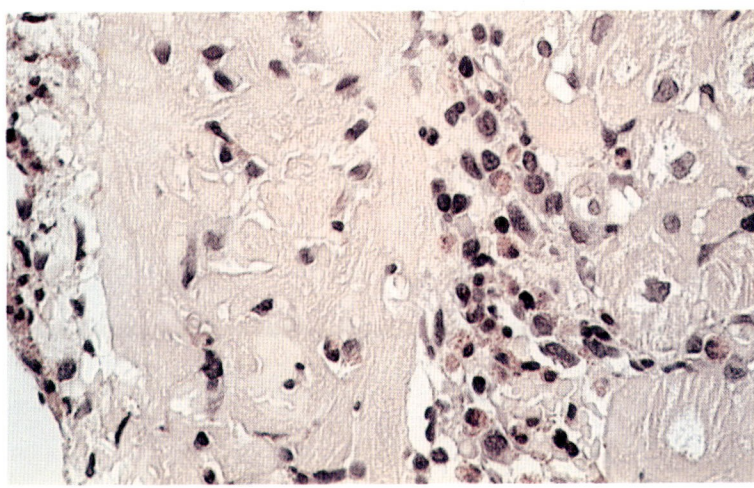

FIGURE 5-32. Histologic view of a biopsy specimen (same patient as in Fig. 5-39) showed massive infiltration of eosinophils in the myocardium as well as in the endocardium (hematoxylin and eosin).

CLINICAL MANIFESTATIONS WITH CARDIAC INVOLVEMENT

MUSCULAR DYSTROPHY

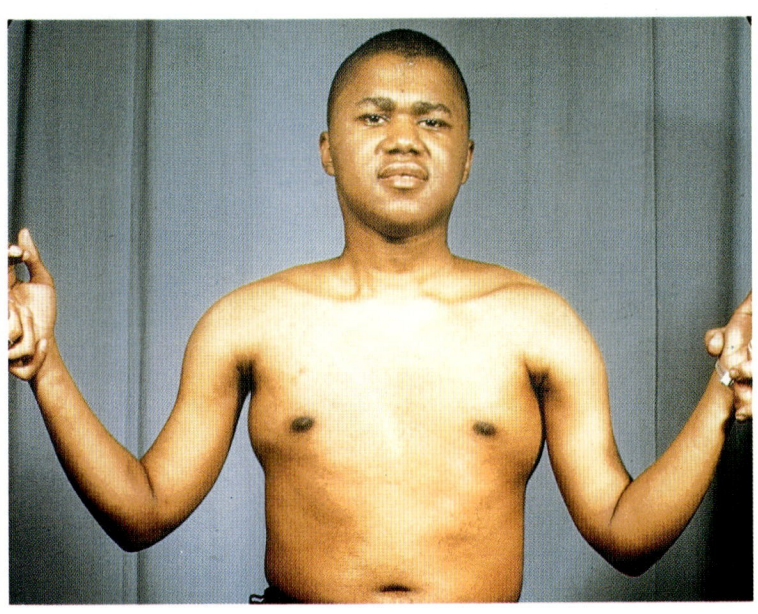

FIGURE 5-33. A 17-year-old boy with Duchenne muscular dystrophy demonstrating striking enlargement (hypertrophy-pseudohypertrophy) of the deltoid and pectoralis major muscles. There is also enlargement of the calves, which is the earliest clinical expression (phenotype) of human Duchenne dystrophy in skeletal muscle. Such calf enlargement has been called "pseudohypertrophy" because of extensive infiltration if not replacement by connective tissue and fat. However, before age 2 years, connective tissue and fat can be minimal, so calf enlargement is due to true hypertrophy rather than pseudohypertrophy. Exceptionally, regional muscle enlargement (hypertrophy-pseudohypertrophy) in Duchenne dystrophy can be striking in muscle groups other than the calves, as is illustrated here. Animal models shed further light on hypertrophy, at least in striated muscle. Dystrophin-deficient mice and cats do not experience overt clinical dystrophy but instead manifest hypertrophy of striated muscle in both the early and late stages of the disease. Especially striking is the systemic striated muscle hypertrophy in dystrophin-deficient cats that have a paucity of overt muscle necrosis but remarkable hypertrophy of individual muscle fibers. The hypertrophy-pseudohypertrophy distribution shown in this patient is rare in humans with Duchenne dystrophy, but is typical of the dystrophin-deficient cat.

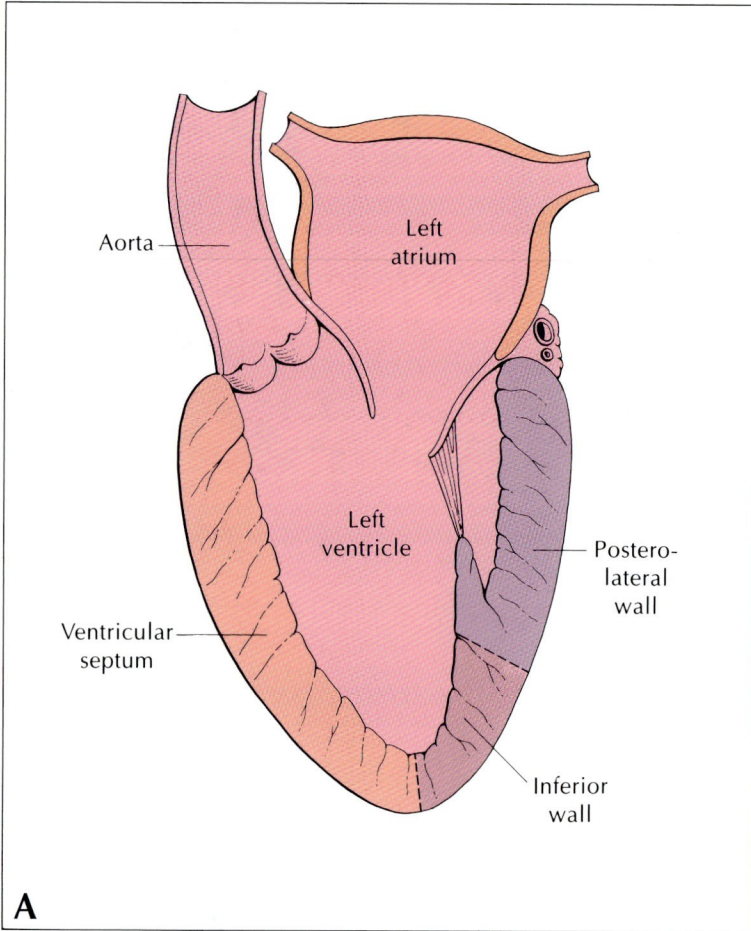

A

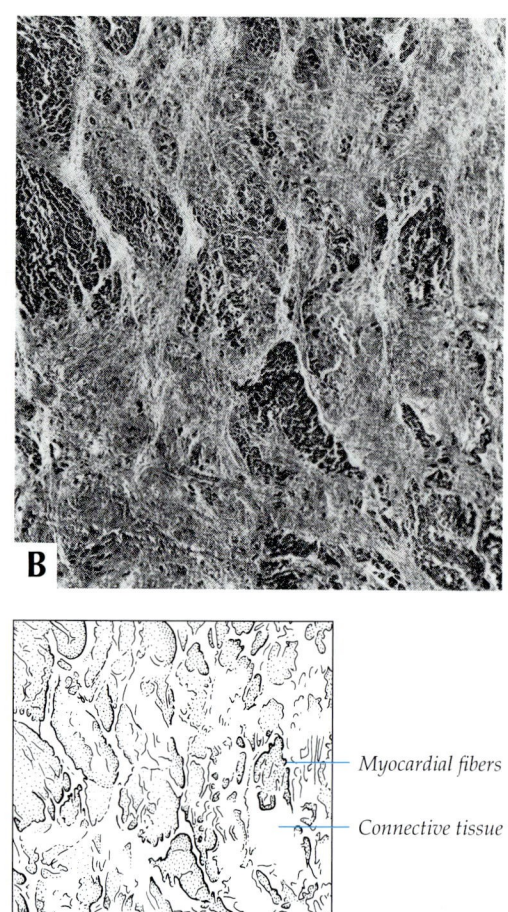

B

Myocardial fibers

Connective tissue

FIGURE 5-34. A, The posterolateral (infra-atrial) involvement of the left ventricle in Duchenne dystrophy. **B,** Posterobasal portion of the left ventricular wall. In contrast to the posterobasal wall, which shows extensive connective tissue proliferation with scattered islands of myocardial fibers, no fibrous scars are present in the ventricular septum (hematoxylin and eosin, × 25). A reduction in or loss of electromotive force caused by the location of myocardial dystrophy in the posterobasal and contiguous lateral left ventric-

ular walls is believed to be responsible for the characteristic scalar electrocardiogram, and is represented by tall right precordial R waves and deep but narrow Q waves in leads 1, aVL, and the left precordium. Duchenne dystrophy emerges as a unique form of heart disease characterized by a genetically determined predilection for specific regions of myocardium.

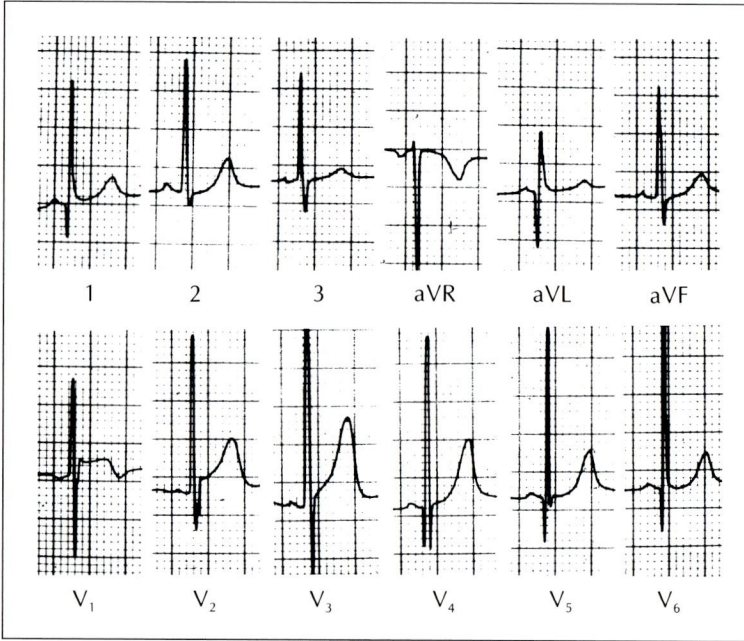

FIGURE 5-35. Typical electrocardiogram of Duchenne muscular dystrophy in a 10-year-old boy. The P-R interval is short (0.10 seconds in lead 2). The QRS complex shows an anterior shift in the right precordial leads (tall R waves) and deep but narrow Q waves in leads 1, aVL, and V_{4-6}. A reduction in or loss of electromotive force caused by myocardial dystrophy in the postero-basal and contiguous lateral left ventricular walls is believed to be responsible for the QRS pattern. The standard scalar electrocardiogram is the simplest and most reliable tool for detecting cardiac involvement in Duchenne dystrophy. Abnormal electrocardiograms are present even in early childhood. Tall right precordial R waves and increased R:S amplitude ratios, together with deep Q waves in leads 1, aVL, and V_{5-6}, are characteristic of classic, rapidly progressive X-linked Duchenne dystrophy.

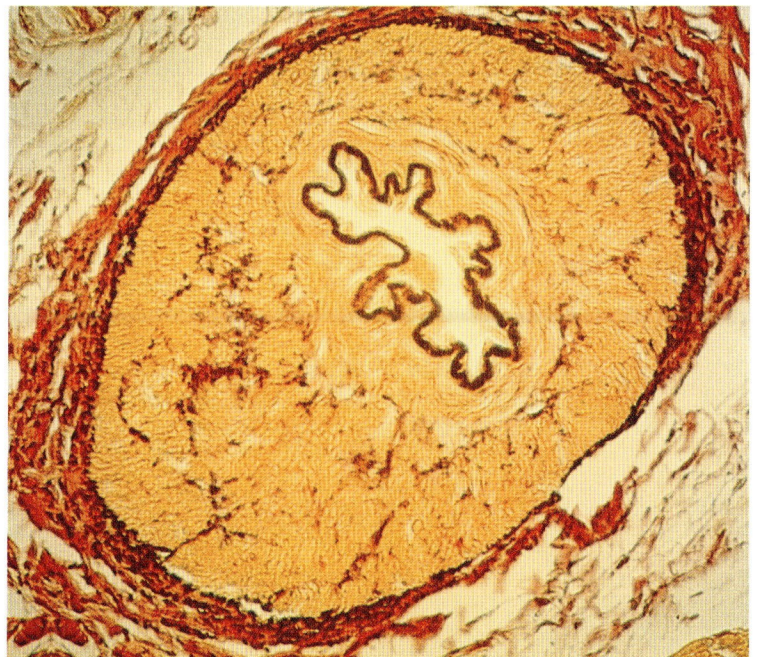

FIGURE 5-36. Histologic section of small intramural coronary arteries in the left atria of patient with Duchenne dystrophy. Striking hypertrophy of medial smooth muscle with luminal narrowing (Verhoeff-von Gieson elastic tissue stains, × 260). The coronary arteriopathy is characterized principally by striking hypertrophy of the media with luminal narrowing, and less commonly by coexisting cystic degeneration. The dystrophin content of vascular smooth muscle cells (shown here) is similar to that of striated myofibers. The smooth muscle form of dystrophin is believed to be slightly smaller than the predominant striated muscle dystrophin, implying that a smaller form might represent a vascular smooth muscle isoform. A fundamental question is why dystrophin deficiency in the vascular smooth muscle of Duchenne dystrophy (in contrast to striated muscle) expresses itself chiefly as hypertrophy rather than necrosis.

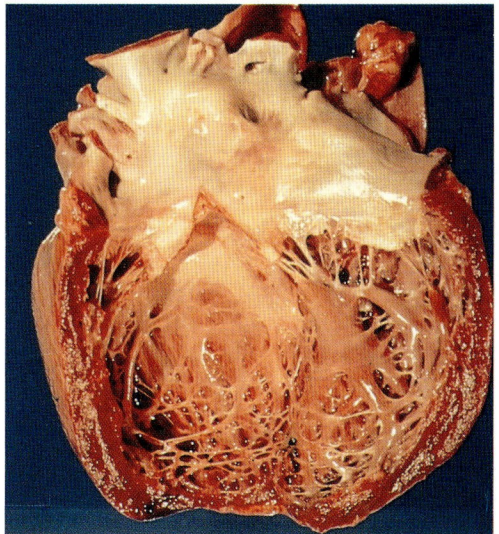 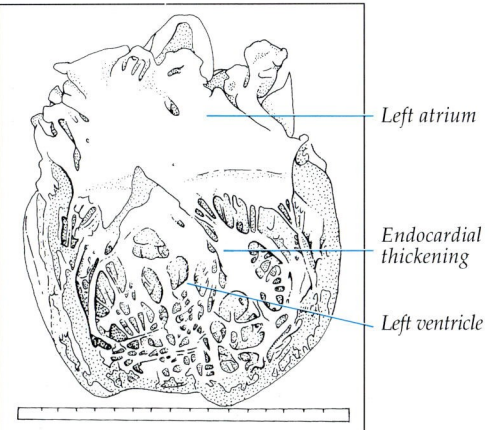

Left atrium

Endocardial thickening

Left ventricle

FIGURE 5-37. Gross and microscopic cardiac pathologic specimen from a 45-year-old man with late-onset, slowly progressive Becker muscular dystrophy. The left atrium was also dilated. No significant coronary artery disease was identified. In Becker dystrophy, the protein product of the gene is present but is abnormal in molecular weight, while in Duchenne dystrophy the protein product is absent or scanty but of normal molecular weight. In contrast to Duchenne dystrophy, cardiac involvement in Becker dystrophy involves all four chambers, with dilatation and failure of the ventricles in addition to abnormalities of the His bundle and infranodal conduction that express themselves as fascicular block and complete heart block.

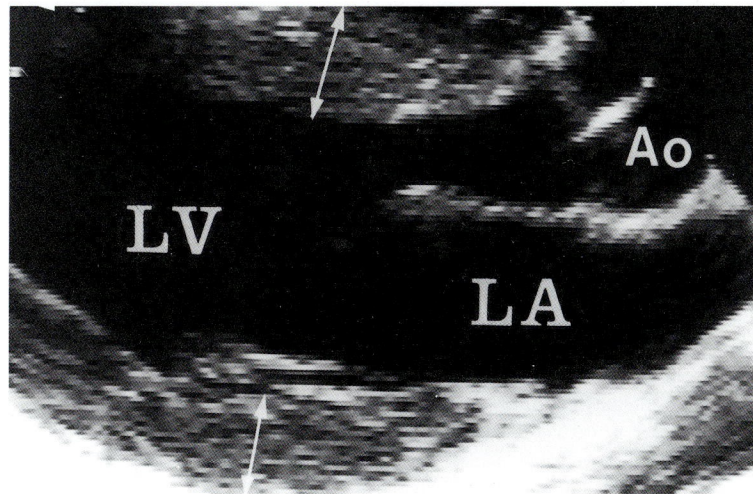

FIGURE 5-38. Two-dimensional echocardiogram (parasternal long axis diastolic frames) from a 14-year-old girl with Friedreich's ataxia and concentric hypertrophy (*arrows*) of the left ventricle (LV). The most common echocardiographic finding in Friedreich's ataxia is concentric (symmetric) left ventricular hypertrophy. Asymmetric septal hypertrophy occurs less frequently, and is occasionally accompanied by a left ventricular to aortic systolic gradient. Septal cellular disarray, which is the histologic hallmark of genetic hypertrophic cardiomyopathy, has not been identified in necropsy studies of Friedreich's ataxia—an observation that may in part explain why the potentially malignant ventricular arrhythmias that prevail in genetic hypertrophic cardiomyopathy are essentially unknown in Friedreich's ataxia. In hypertrophic cardiomyopathy of Friedreich's ataxia, systolic ventricular function is normal, not supernormal, and diastolic function is not deranged as in genetic hypertrophic cardiomyopathy. Ao—aorta; LA—left atrium.

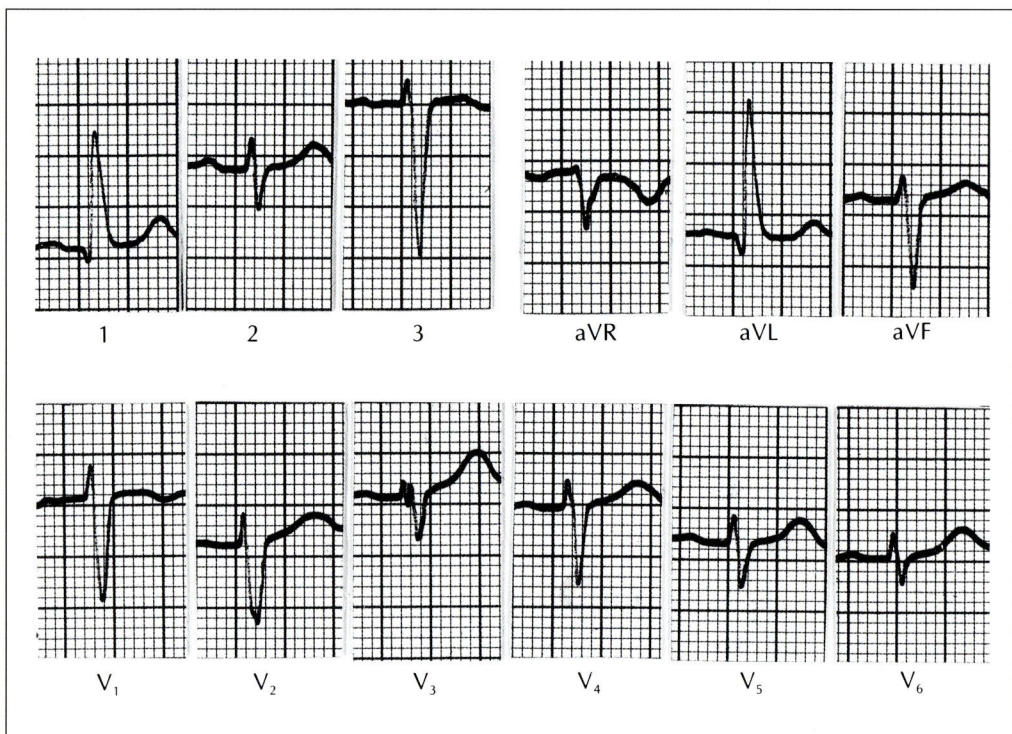

FIGURE 5-39. Typical electrocardiogram from an adult man with myotonic muscular dystrophy. There is P-R interval prolongation (0.20 seconds) and left anterior fascicular block. Cardiac involvement is relatively selective in myotonic dystrophy, primarily targeting specialized tissues, and more specifically the His-Purkinje system. The most common electrocardiographic abnormalities—prolongation of the P-R interval, left anterior fascicular block, and increased QRS duration—reflect the His-Purkinje disease that can progress rapidly, culminating in fatal Stokes-Adams episodes unless anticipated by pacemaker insertion.

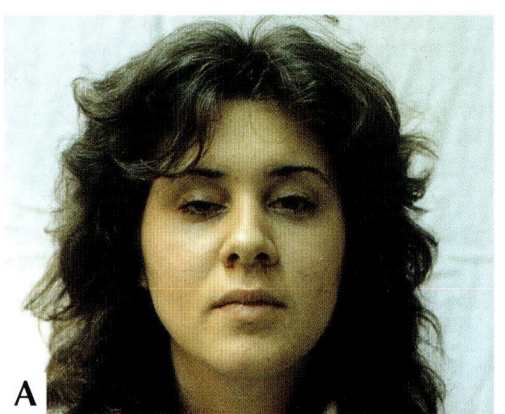
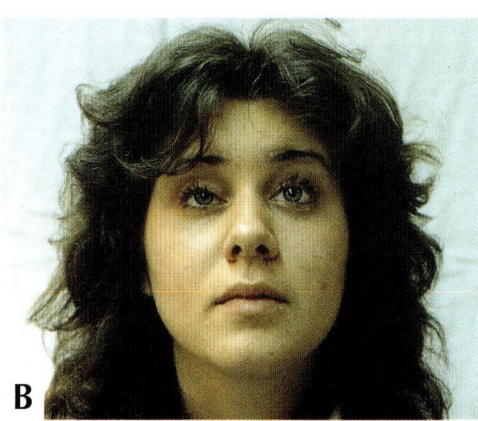

FIGURE 5-40. Kearns-Sayre syndrome is a mitochondrial myopathy expressed as external ophthalmoplegia, pigmentary retinopathy, and cardiac involvement that typically afflicts specialized conduction tissues culminating in complete heart block [41]. This 18-year-old girl with Kearns-Sayre syndrome and bilateral asymmetric ptosis had pigmentary retinopathy and an electrocardiogram that progressed from normal to bifascicular block. **A,** The asymmetric ptosis is present when the patient looks straight ahead. **B,** Ptosis of the right lid persists during upward gaze.

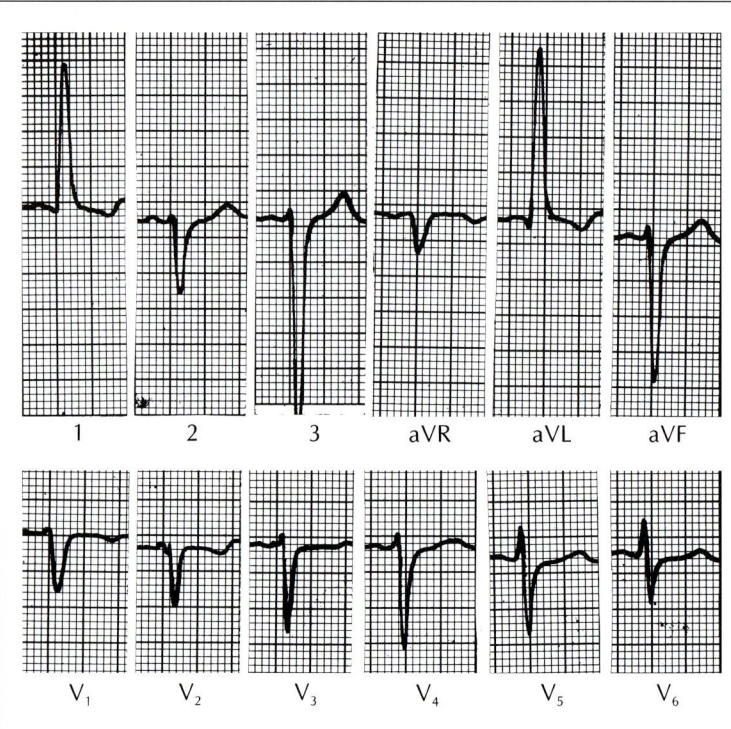

FIGURE 5-41. Twelve-lead scalar electrocardiogram from a 14-year-old girl with Kearns-Sayre syndrome. There is left anterior fascicular block and right bundle branch block (bifascicular block); 4 years earlier, the electrocardiogram showed isolated left anterior fascicular block. The patient had bilateral asymmetric ptosis that was especially apparent on upward gaze. Ophthalmologic examination disclosed pigmentary retinopathy. Skeletal muscle biopsy identified ragged red fibers in the trichrome stain. Clinically overt myocardial disease is exceptional in Kearns-Sayre syndrome, despite the fact that ultrastructural abnormalities, especially in mitochondria, are well established. Two derangements of the specialized conduction pathways generally coexist: 1) gradually progressive impairment of infranodal conduction (left anterior hemiblock, right bundle branch block, and complete heart block), and 2) enhancement of atrioventricular nodal conduction. The morphologic basis for impaired infranodal conduction lies in the extensive changes in distal portions of the His bundle extending to the origins of the bundle branches. Evidence of enhanced atrioventricular nodal conduction has been identified by His bundle electrograms.

GENE MUTATIONS CAUSING DILATED CARDIOMYOPATHY

CHROMOSOME	PROTEIN	DISEASE	INHERITANCE
1p1–q21	Lamins A and C	Dilated cardiomyopathy	Autosomal dominant
1q11–21	Unknown	Dilated cardiomyopathy*°	Autosomal dominant
1q11–23	Lamins A and C	Autosomal dominant Emery-Dreifuss muscular dystrophy	Autosomal dominant
1q32	Unknown	Dilated cardiomyopathy	Autosomal dominant
2q11–22	Unknown	Dilated cardiomyopathy	Autosomal dominant
2q31	Unknown	Dilated cardiomyopathy	Autosomal dominant
3p22–25	Unknown	Dilated cardiomyopathy	Autosomal dominant
6q23	Unknown	Dilated cardiomyopathy*	Autosomal dominant
9q13–22	Unknown	Dilated cardiomyopathy	Autosomal dominant
10q21–23	Unknown	Dilated cardiomyopathy	Autosomal dominant
10q22	Metavinculin	Dilated cardiomyopathy	Unknown
15q14	Actin	Dilated cardiomyopathy	Autosomal dominant
17q12–21.33	alpha-Sarcoglycan (adhalin)	Dilated cardiomyopathy*	Autosomal recessive
Xq28	Emerin	Emery-Dreifuss muscular dystrophy	X-linked
Xp21	Dystrophin	X-linked dilated cardiomyopathy	X-linked
Xp21	Dystrophin	Becker type muscular dystrophy	X-linked
Xp21	Dystrophin	Duchenne type muscular dystrophy	X-linked

*This form is associated with limb-girdle muscular dystrophy.
°Although the loci on chromosome 1q are similar to those for Emery-Dreifuss muscular dystrophy, the disease form is distinct.

FIGURE 5-42. Specific genetic mutations are increasingly being associated with both hypertrophic and dilated cardiomyopathy. Familial (genetic) dilated cardiomyopathy may account for 20% of all patients presenting with cardiomyopathy [42].

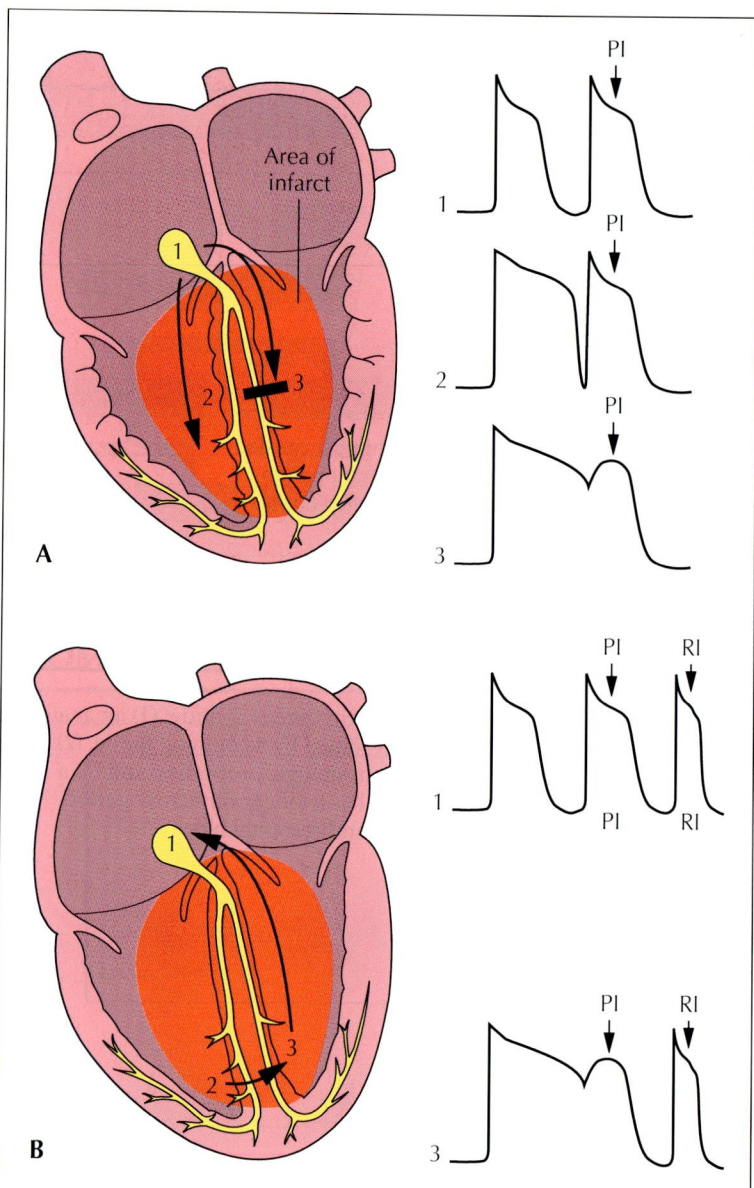

Figure 6-10. Mechanism for reentry resulting from dispersion of refractoriness in the subendocardial Purkinje fiber network over an area of extensive myocardial infarction. This figure shows the endocardial surface of the left ventricular anterior papillary muscle. The color area in each diagram is the scar resulting from the myocardial infarct that is covered by a blanket of the surviving Purkinje fibers. As depicted, Purkinje fibers in different regions have markedly different action potentials with respect to duration and refractory periods. Action potentials are recorded from normal tissue (site 1) and from subendocardial Purkinje fibers with prolonged repolarization phases (sites 2 and 3), surviving in the infarct. In **A**, premature impulse (PI) occurs at the infarct border (site 1) and conducts into the infarcted regions as indicated by the large arrows. Note that the action potentials are prolonged. The action potential at site 3 is longer than at site 2 in the infarcted area. Consequently, premature impulses can excite cells at site 2, but conduction blocks at site 3. **B,** The continuation of these events after the premature impulse conducts through site 2 and activates the cells at site 3. As a reentering impulse (RI), it then proceeds to its site of origin (site 1), which also re-excites as a reentry impulse (RI). (*Adapted from* Wit *et al.* [6].)

ANTIARRHYTHMIC DRUGS

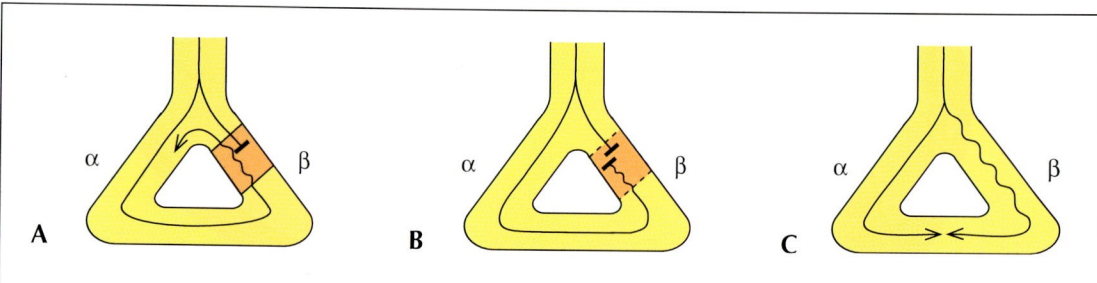

Figure 6-11. Effect of antiarrhythmic drugs on reentry. The question of how antiarrhythmic drugs suppress arrhythmias must be addressed by considering arrhythmia mechanisms. Most arrhythmias based on abnormal conduction involve reentry circuits, as illustrated in **A** (described in Figs. 6-8 and 6-9). The *shaded area* represents the depolarized tissue in which conduction block occurs, and retrograde conduction is slow enough to allow the cells in limb α to recover and propagate the reentrant impulse. Antiarrhythmic drugs can eliminate reentry tachyarrhythmias by impairing conduction sufficiently to cause interruption of conduction through the circuit (**B**) or by improving conduction in limb β, which prevents the development of conduction block (**C**). Class I drugs prevent reentry by causing a greater amount of slow conduction in depolarized tissue, thus producing conduction block in both the forward and reverse directions in limb β.

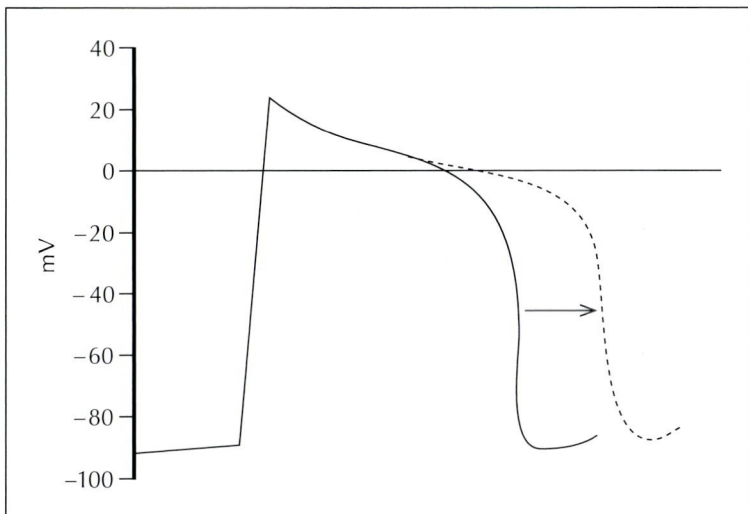

FIGURE 6-12. Class III antiarrhythmics. Class III action consists of prolongation of the action potential duration, which leads to a prolongation of refractoriness. The diagram represents a normal action potential of a Purkinje cell (*solid line*) and the effects of d-sotalol (*dotted line*) on the action potential duration.

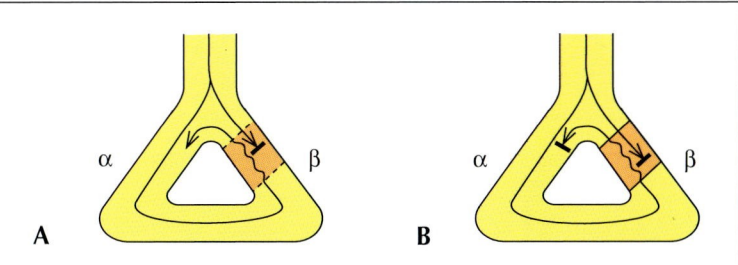

FIGURE 6-13. The probable effect of a drug with Class III antiarrhythmic action on a reentry circuit. Class III drugs can affect a prototypic reentry circuit (**A**; described in Figs. 6-8 and 6-9) by sufficiently prolonging the refractory period of path α, thus preventing reentry from occurring (**B**).

COMPARATIVE EFFICACY OF ORAL ANTIARRHYTHMIC DRUGS

DRUG	PREMATURE ATRIAL CONTRACTIONS	ATRIAL FIBRILLATION	ANTEGRADE SLOWING OF AV NODAL CONDUCTION	AV NODE RE-ENTRANT TACHYCARDIA	EFFECTS ON ACCESSORY PATHWAY CONDUCTION	WPW-PAROXYSMAL SUPRAVENTRICULAR TACHYCARDIA	SUSTAINED VENTRICULAR TACHYCARDIA/VENTRICULAR FIBRILLATION PES, %
Quinidine	++	++	+/-	+	+	+	20–25
Procainamide	++	++	+/-	+	+	+	20–25
Disopyramide	++	++	+/-	+	++	++	20–25
Tocainide	0	0	0	0	+/-	0	10–15
Mexiletine	0	0	0	0	+/-	0	10–20
Moricizine	+	NE	0	NE	+	NE	20
Flecainide	++	++	+	++	+++	+++	20–25
Encainide	++	++	++	++	+++	+++	20–25
Propafenone	++	++	++	++	++	++	20–25
Recainam	+	++	+	++	++	++	20
β blockers	+*	+	++	+	0	+	5
Amiodarone	++	+++	++	++	+	++	20–60
Sotalol	+	++	++	++	+	+	30
Digoxin	0	+*	++	+	+/-	+	NA
Verapamil	0	+*	++	+	+/-	+	NA
Diltiazem	0	+*	++	+	+/-	+	NA

*Rate control data

FIGURE 6-14. Efficacy of antiarrhythmic drugs. This table compares the efficacy of a number of antiarrhythmic drugs on some of the more common types of arrhythmias. NA—not applicable; NE—not established; PES—programmed electrical stimulation.

SINUS NODE DISORDERS

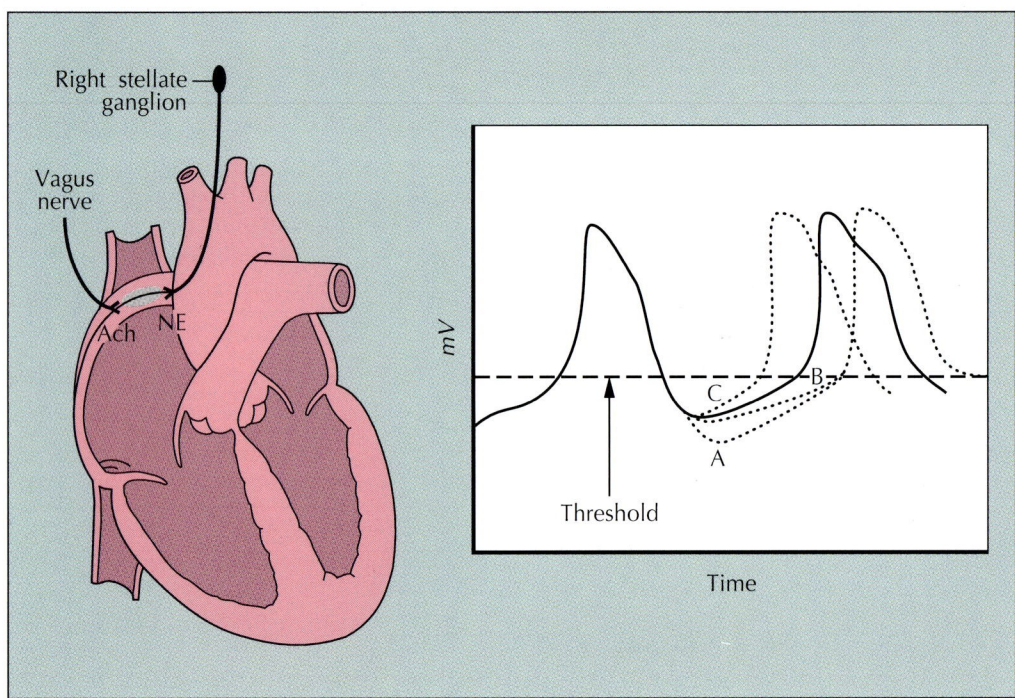

FIGURE 6-15. Autonomic nervous system inputs to the sinus node. Parasympathetic stimulation via the vagus nerve results in the release of acetylcholine (Ach). This produces a *negative* chronotropic response due to a decrease in the maximum diastolic potential (hyperpolarization) (A) and a decrease in the slope of phase and depolarization (B). Sympathetic stimulation via the right stellate ganglion results in norepinephrine (NE) release from the postsynaptic nerve terminals within the sinus node. This produces a *positive* chronotropic response mainly by an increase in the rate of phase 4 depolarization (C).

Modulation of the sinus rate is therefore due to the interactions of the two limbs of the autonomic nervous system (parasympathetic and sympathetic). During sleep and in response to some stimuli (nausea, and in some people, the sight of blood or pain, for example), parasympathetic stimulation predominates, and the heart rate slows. During exercise and in response to fright or to some kinds of pain, sympathetic stimulation predominates, and the heart races. (*Adapted from* Talano *et al.* [7].)

TYPES OF SINUS NODE DYSFUNCTION

CONDITIONS ASSOCIATED WITH SINUS NODE DYSFUNCTION

INTRINSIC	EXTRINSIC
Aging	Hypothermia
Hypertension	Electrolyte abnormalities
Coronary artery disease	Hypothyroidism
Rheumatic heart disease	Abnormalities of autonomic nervous system (carotid hypersensitivity)
Cardiomyopathies	Hyperbilirubinemia
Pericarditis	Drugs
Congenital heart abnormalities	Cardiac glycosides
Collagen vascular disease	β-Adrenergic receptor blockers
Amyloidosis	Calcium-channel blockers
Trauma	Methyldopa
Surgical	Reserpine
Closure of ASD (sinus venosus type)	Lithium carbonate
Mustard procedure	Cimetidine
Placement of caval cannula	Amitriptyline
Tumor	Phenothiazines
Irradiation	

FIGURE 6-16. Conditions associated with sinus node dysfunction. Sinus node dysfunction may be due to a pathologic process that directly involves the sinus node (intrinsic) or other processes and drugs that have secondary effects on the sinus node (extrinsic). ASD—atrial septal defect.

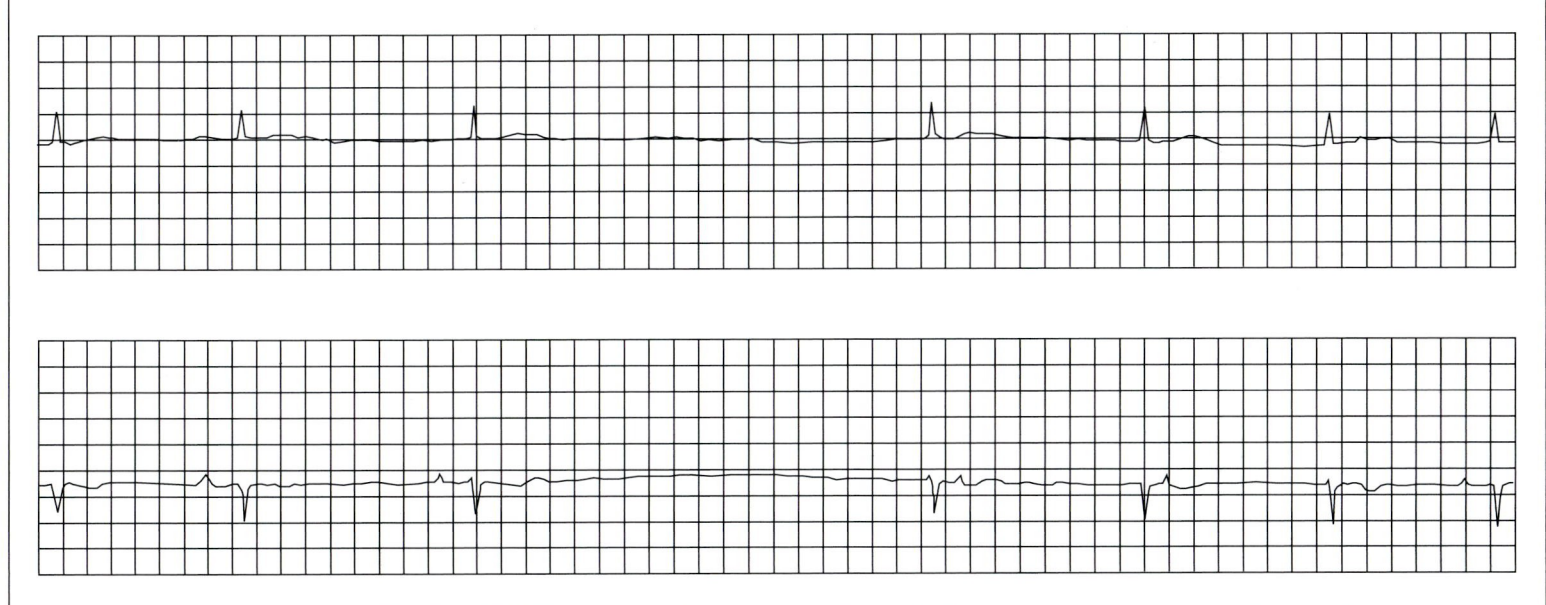

FIGURE 6-17. Failure of impulse generation. Sinus node dysfunction can be manifested as a failure of impulse generation. This can result in sinus bradycardia (defined as sinus rhythm <60 bpm) or sinus arrest. However, this rate is considered normal during sleep or in a trained person at rest. Sinus bradycardia is clinically significant only if it results in failure to meet the patient's metabolic demands. This may result in physical signs such as hypotension or congestive heart failure or symptoms of fatigue, shortness of breath, exercise intolerance, angina, lightheadedness, or even syncope.

Simultaneous leads V_5 (*top*) and V_1 (*bottom*) of a Holter recording from an 85-year-old woman with a history of syncope. Both sinus bradycardia (38 bpm) and sinus arrest (4.2-second pause) with a junctional escape rhythm are represented. (*Adapted from* Evans [8].)

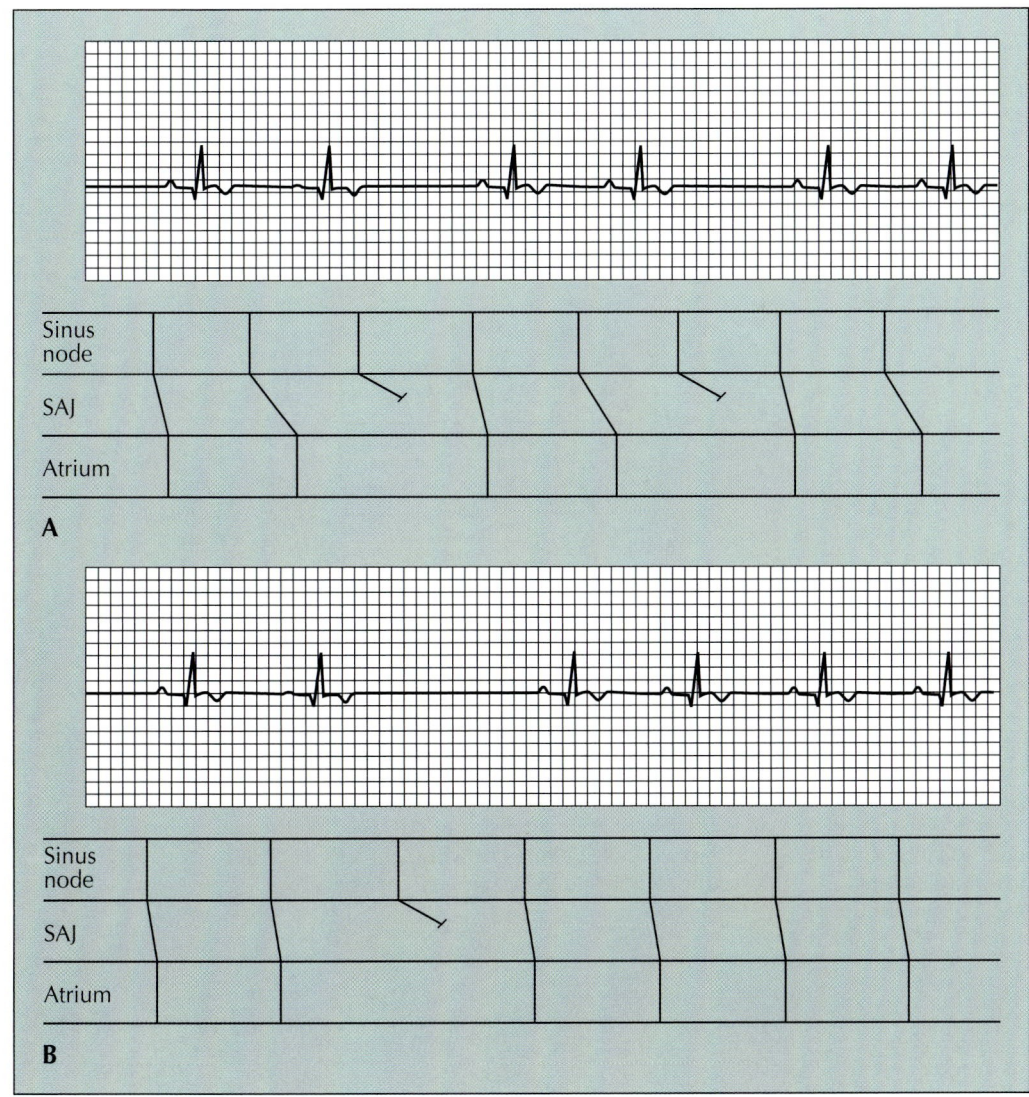

FIGURE 6-18. Abnormalities of impulse conduction. Sinus pauses can be due to sinoatrial exit block of the impulse generated from the primary pacemaker cells in the node itself or at the sinoatrial junction.

Block may be manifested in one of two forms. **A,** A typical Wenckebach pattern, with progressive slowing of conduction (in the sinoatrial junction [SAJ]), resulting in progressive shortening of the P-wave–P-wave interval, ending in a sinus pause (blocked impulse). The pause is less than twice the shortest atrial cycle length. **B,** Sudden block, with no prior evidence of conduction slowing, may be observed. In this setting the pause is equal to twice the atrial cycle length (Mobitz II SA block). In *A,* Wenckebach block in the SAJ can be seen. There is progressive slowing (represented by a deceased slope) of conduction in the SAJ prior to block (beats 3 and 6). In *B,* there is no change in conduction through the SAJ. Block (beat 3) occurs suddenly. (*continued*)

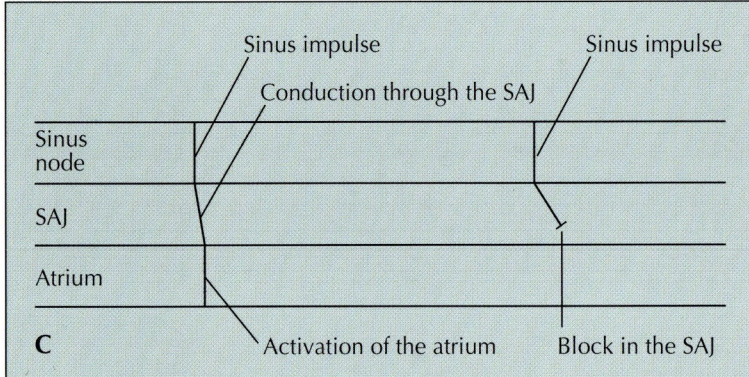

FIGURE 6-18. (*continued*) **C,** A ladder diagram with explanation. Throughout this chapter, ladder diagrams are used to demonstrate electrophysiologic phenomena. Each horizontal area represents a region within the heart. Impulse origin and conduction are represented by the vertical (or slanting) lines. Conduction block is represented by a vertical line with a perpendicular line at the end of it.

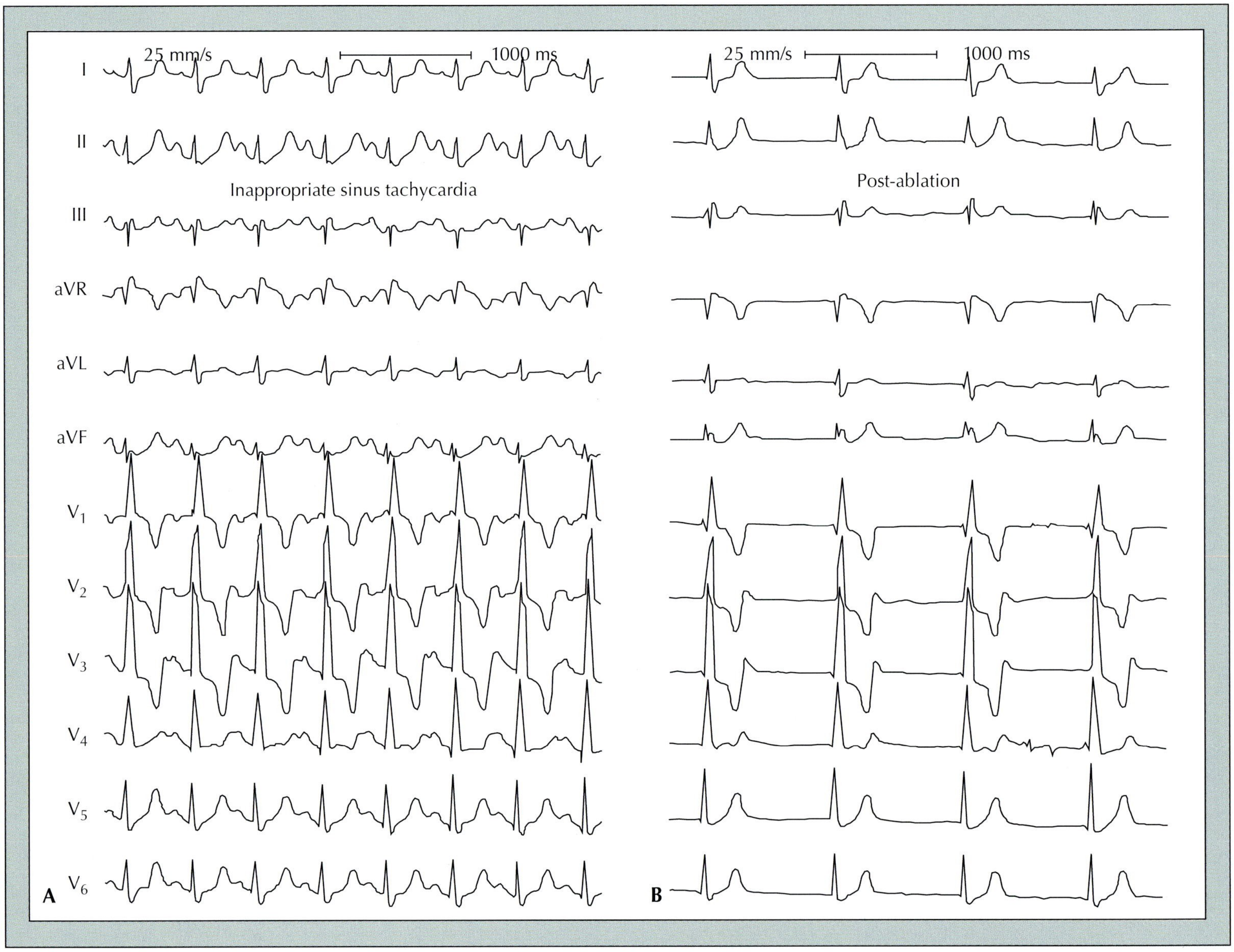

In the diagram (panel C): Sinus impulse · Sinus impulse · Conduction through the SAJ · Sinus node · SAJ · Atrium · Activation of the atrium · Block in the SAJ

Panel A: 25 mm/s · 1000 ms · Inappropriate sinus tachycardia · Leads I, II, III, aVR, aVL, aVF, V₁, V₂, V₃, V₄, V₅, V₆

Panel B: 25 mm/s · 1000 ms · Post-ablation

FIGURE 6-19. Inappropriate sinus tachycardia often can be difficult to treat, and in many cases even combination drug therapy fails to control this arrhythmia adequately [9]. Transcatheter sinus node ablation and/or modification using radiofrequency energy appears to be a treatment option in patients with this refractory arrhythmia. **A,** A 12-lead electrocardiogram from a patient with drug-resistant inappropriate sinus tachycardia. **B,** Following sinus node ablation the patient initially had a junctional rhythm, but within a week a stable atrial rhythm that appropriately responded to exercise was evident.

PHARMACOLOGIC INTERVENTIONS FOR ASSESSMENT OF SINUS NODE DISORDERS

DRUG	STUDY	DOSAGE	RESPONSE		COMMENTS
			NORMAL	ABNORMAL	
Atropine	Dauchot and Gravenstein [16]	1.0 mg	>17% decrease in cycle length	<25% increase in sinus rate	Relatively easy, safe; helpful only if positive
	Eckberg et al. [17]	0.04 mg/kg	>15% increase in HR		
	Lekieffre et al. [18]	0.03 mg/kg	HR >90 bpm		
	Medvedowsky and Barnay [19]	0.04 mg/kg	HR >85 bpm		
Isoproterenol	Mandel et al. [20]	3 mg/min	>25% increase in HR	<25% increase in sinus rate	Helpful if positive; may be dangerous in patients with ventricular arrhythmias or CAD
	Strauss et al. [21]	Variable	Based on dose required for 20% increase in HR		
Propranolol	Eckberg et al. [17]	0.2 mg/kg	≥12% decrease in HR	>20% decrease in sinus rate	May be dangerous in patients with marked bradycardia or decreased LV function
	Vasquez et al. [22]	0.1 mg/kg	≥12% decrease in HR		
Atropine + propranolol	Jose and Collison [23]	0.04 mg/kg + 0.2 mg/kg	IHR=118.1-(0.57 × age); SD depends on age	>10% decrease in age-predicted rate	Wide variability
	Tonkin and Heddle [24]	0.03 mg/kg + 0.15 mg/kg	IHR=118.1-(0.57 × age); SD depends on age		

FIGURE 6-20. Pharmacologic interventions for the assessment of sinus node disorders. A variety of pharmacologic interventions can be used to assess sinus node competence. Included in this table are agents that either enhance or block autonomic activity in the heart. Although abnormal responses may suggest sinus node dysfunction, these interventions are neither sensitive nor specific. CAD—coronary artery disease; HR—heart rate; IHR—intrinsic heart rate; LV—left ventricular; SD—standard deviation [7,10,11].

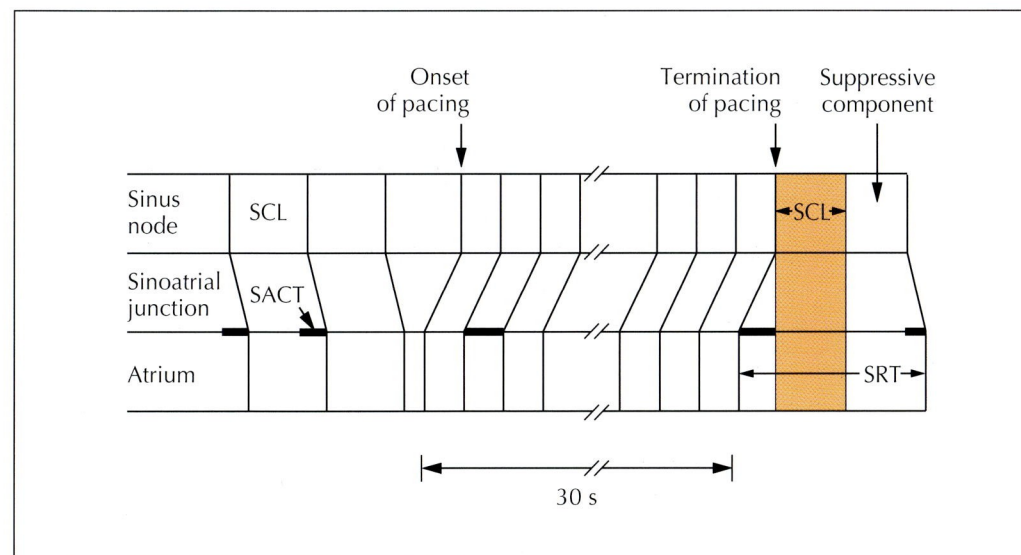

FIGURE 6-21. Sinus node recovery time (SRT). By pacing the atrium at rates progressively faster than the sinus rate (atrial decremental pacing), the SRT can be determined. Rapid stimulation of the sinus node may suppress intrinsic automaticity, resulting in a delay in the post-pacing response. This ladder diagram depicts events during decremental atrial pacing to assess sinus recovery time. At the termination of pacing, the SRT, as determined from recordings in the atria, actually consists of three elements: retrograde atriosinus conduction, the intranodal cycle length (which is an interval equal to the basic sinus cycle length [SCL] plus an interval resulting from overdrive suppression), and antegrade sinoatrial conduction. The length of sinoatrial conduction time (SACT) is emphasized periodically with a thickening of the rung between the sinoatrial junction and the atrium. (*Adapted from* Reiffel [12].)

THERAPEUTIC OPTIONS FOR SINUS NODE DISORDERS

DIAGNOSIS

Symptomatic sinus node dysfunction (bradycardia,
     chronotropic incompetence, sinus arrest, sinoatrial exit block)

Tachy-brady syndrome

Sinus node reentry

Inappropriate sinus tachycardia

Carotid sinus hypersensitivity

THERAPY

AAIR pacing when no evidence of AV conduction disease

DDDR pacing with evidence of AV conduction disease

Type I or III antiarrhythmics to treat atrial arrhythmias

β-Blockers, calcium-channel blockers, and/or digoxin to control
     ventricular response

VVI or DDD pacing for bradycardic episodes (drug used to treat atrial
     arrhythmia may worsen bradyarrhythmias and precipitate the need for
     cardiac pacing)

AV junction ablation with DDDR or VVIR pacing in patients whose
     ventricular response is difficult to control

β-Blockers, calcium-channel blockers

Type I and III antiarrhythmics

Catheter ablation (sinus node modification)

β-Blockers, calcium-channel blockers

Catheter ablation (sinus node ablation/modification)

Pindolol, Norpace

Cardiac pacing

Avoidance of tight collars

FIGURE 6-22. Therapeutic options for sinus node disorders. Pacing nodes are standard. AAIR—rate-responsive atrial pacing; AV—atrioventricular; DDD—dual chamber pacing; DDDR—rate-responsive dual chamber pacing; VVI—ventricular pacing; VVIR—rate-responsive ventricular pacing.

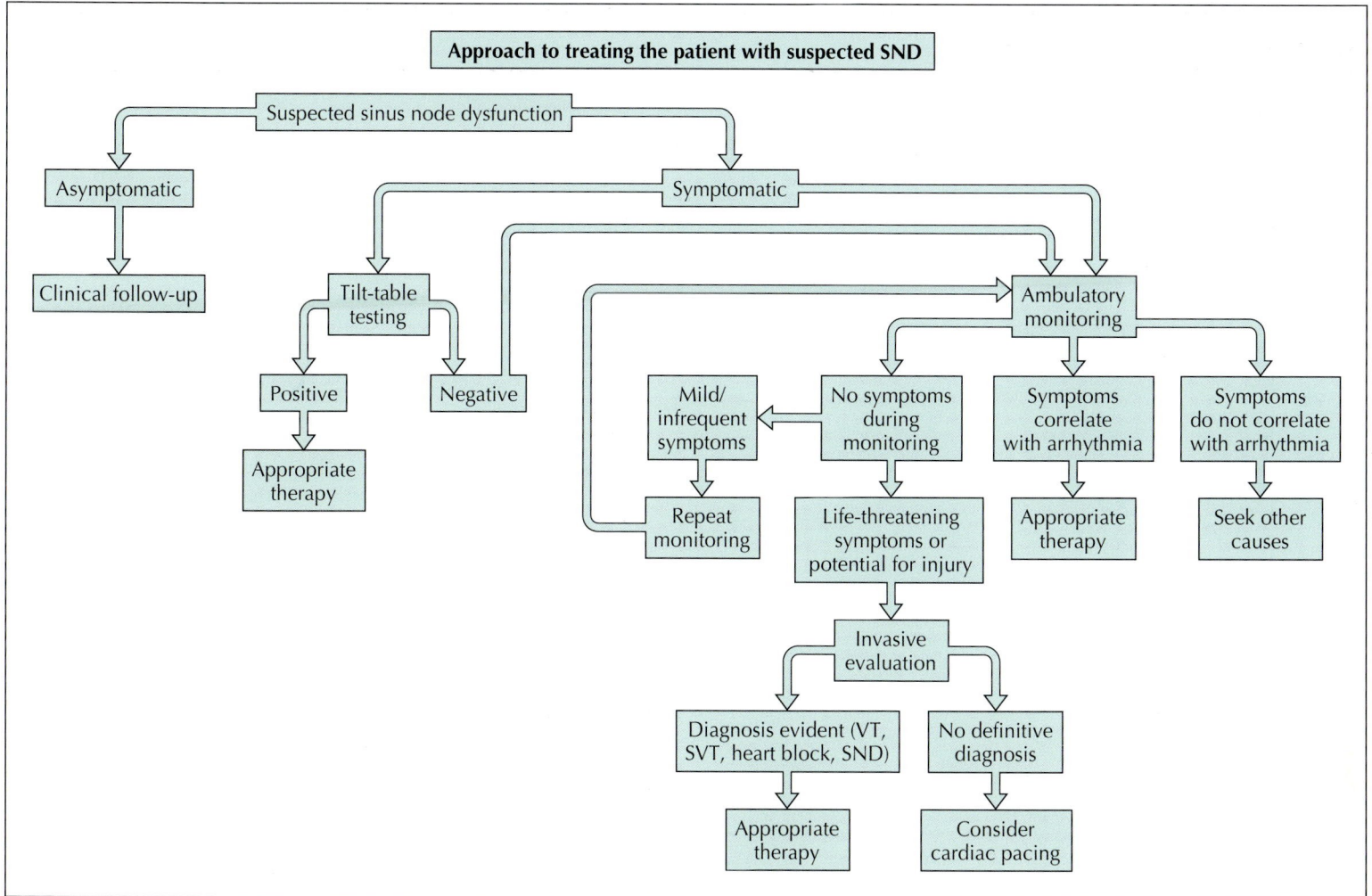

FIGURE 6-23. The approach to diagnosing and treating sinus node dysfunction (SND). In patients with suspected SND, the correlation with symptoms is crucial. The presence of bradycardia alone is not an indication for treatment. In symptomatic patients, a careful history may reveal diagnostic clues. In patients with syncope or syncope associated with standing, a tilt-table test may be in order. In patients with frequent symptoms, 24-hour monitoring is often diagnostic. When symptoms are less frequent, an event-type recorder may be more useful. If symptoms do not correlate with cardiac arrhythmias, other causes (ie, neurologic) should be sought. If no symptoms occur during monitoring but the patient has recurrent syncope or has been injured during episodes, a more invasive evaluation is indicated. SVT—supraventricular tachycardia; VT—ventricular tachycardia. (*Adapted from* Gomes [13].)

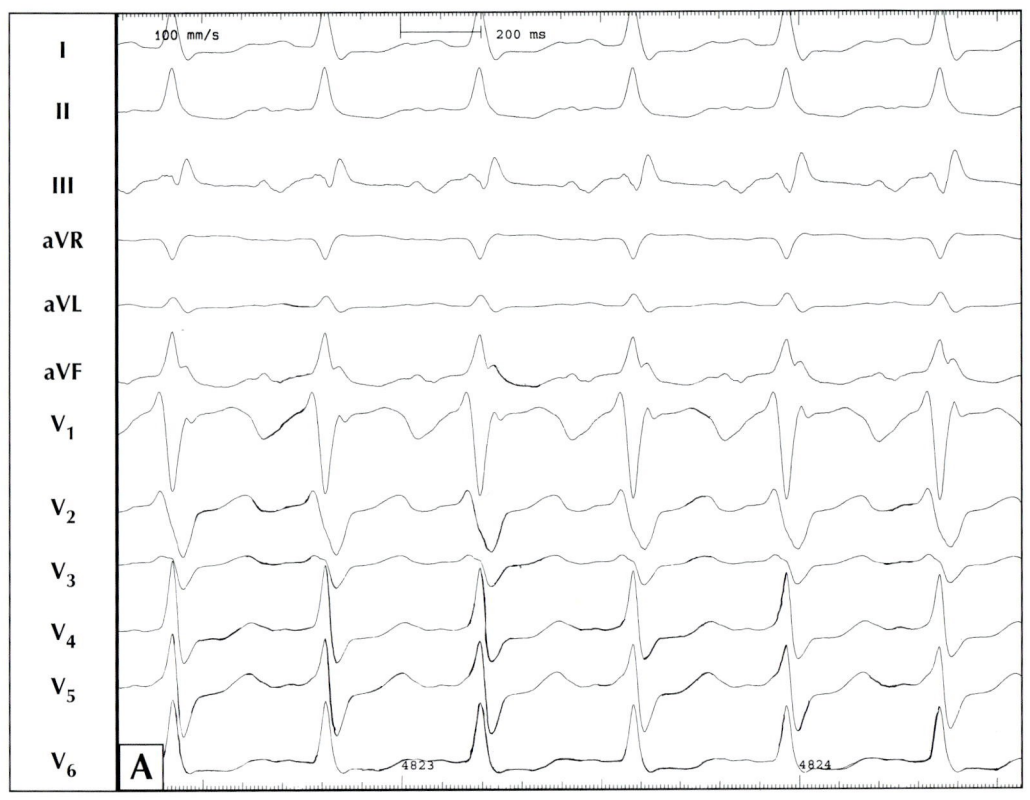

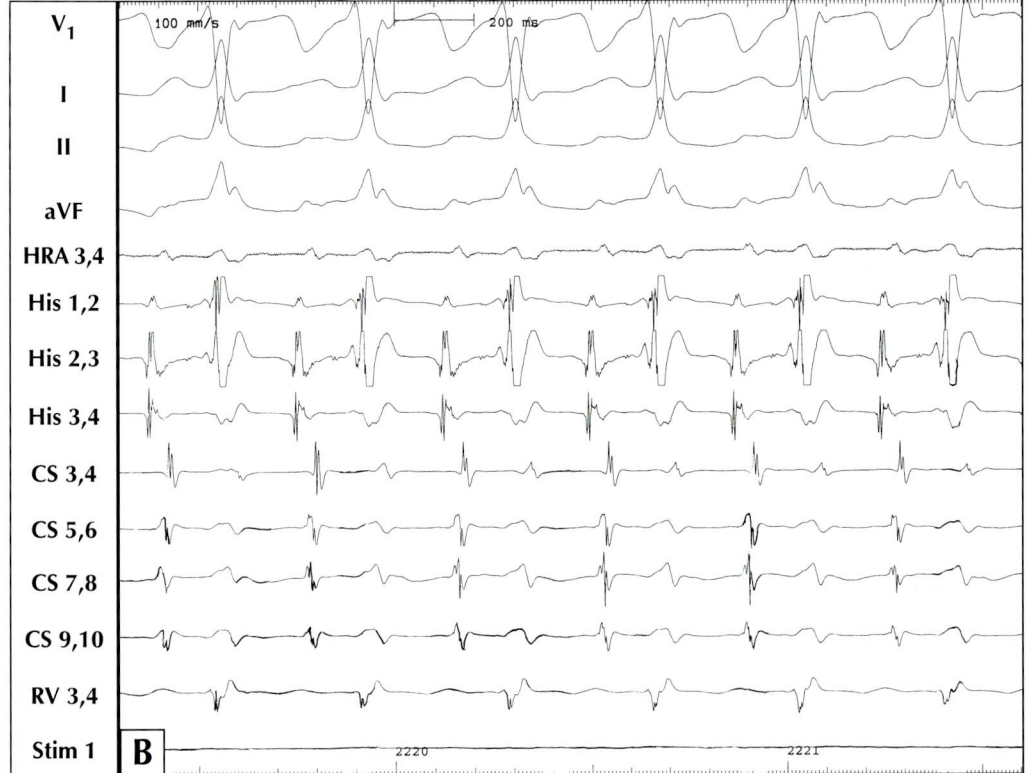

Figure 6-24. Atrial tachycardia. **A,** 12-lead electrocardiogram (ECG) of an atrial tachycardia. This ECG shows a narrow complex tachycardia with a rate of 130 beats per minute. Note the upright P waves in leads II, III, aVL, and aVF, and negative P wave in lead V_1. The relationship between the P wave and the QRS complex is consistent with a long RP tachycardia. The differential diagnosis of a long RP tachycardia includes atypical atrioventricular (AV) node reentry, a slowly conducting bypass tract, or an atrial tachycardia. From the intracardiac recordings in **B** we clearly see the atrial and ventricular ECG relationship. Atrial intracardiac electrograms from the coronary sinus (CS) catheter, along the left atrioventricular groove, come after the right septal (His bundle) electrograms. Tachycardia initiation required isoproterenol and was induced with programmed stimulation. Surface leads are V_1, I, II, and aVF. Intracardiac leads include high right atrium (HRA 3,4), His bundle recording (His 1,2–His 3,4), CS recordings (CS 3,4–CS 9,10), and right ventricular apex. (*continued*)

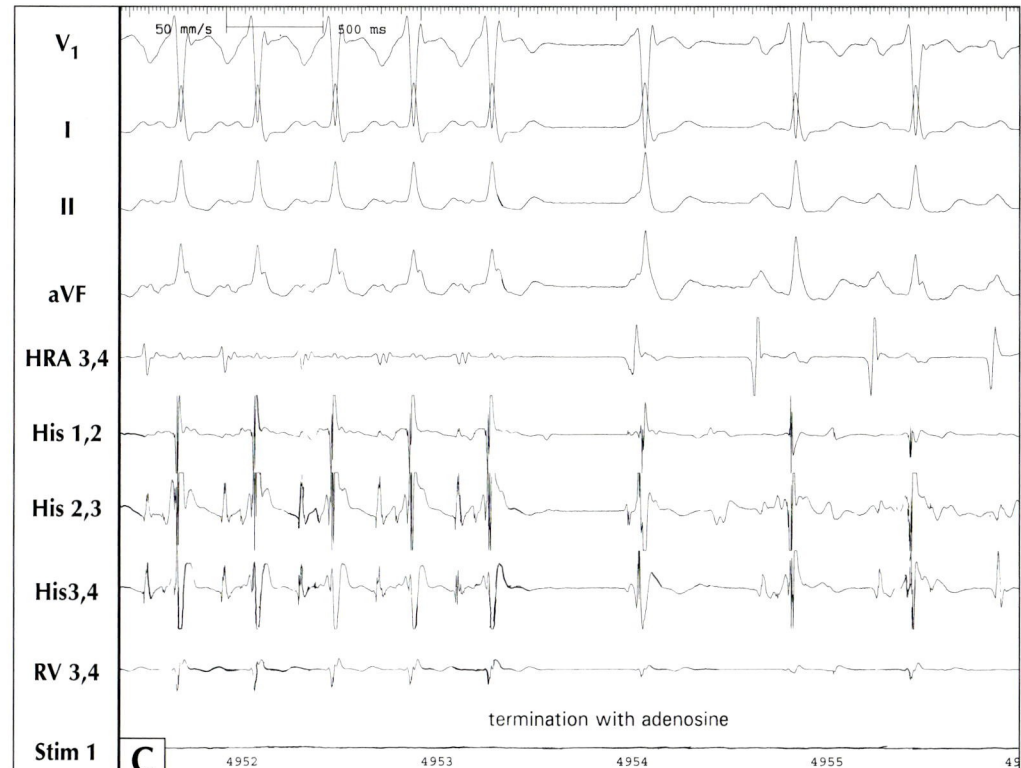

FIGURE 6-24. (*continued*) In **C** the tachycardia was terminated with adenosine. There was no evidence for an accessory pathway or dual AV nodes. These findings are consistent with an adenosine-sensitive atrial tachycardia. Note, the first beat after the tachycardia is terminated in a junctional beat [14].

MECHANISMS

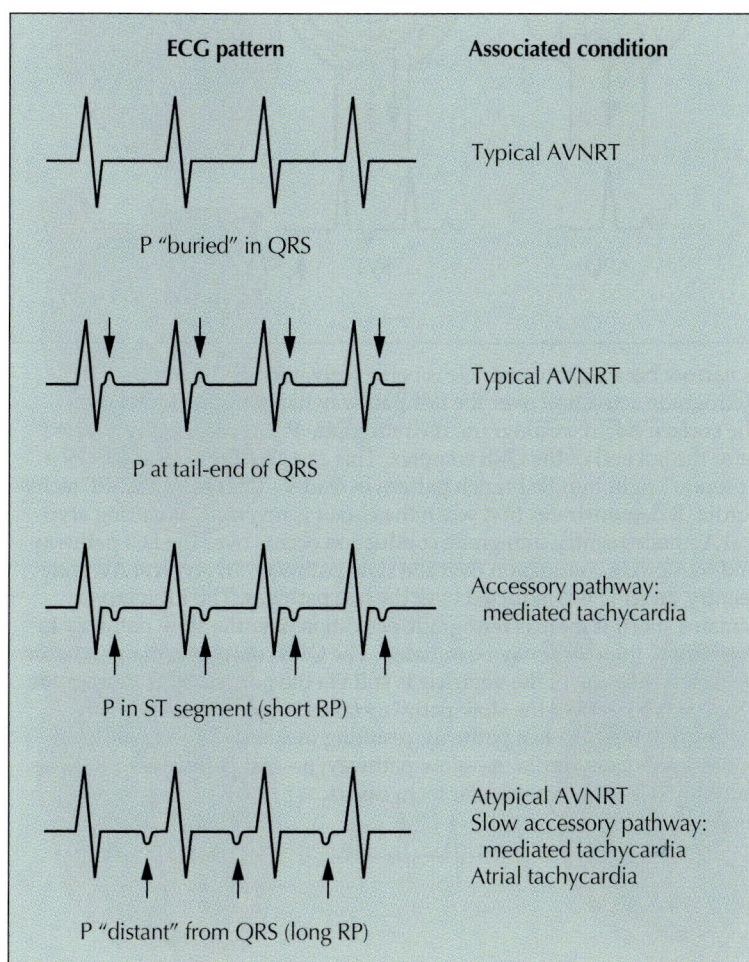

FIGURE 6-25. Electrocardiographic patterns of narrow complex tachycardias. The most important clue to the mechanism of a narrow complex tachycardia is the relationship of the P wave to the QRS complex. No visible P wave often means that the P wave is buried in the QRS complex. This is usually due to typical atrioventricular (AV) nodal reentry. With typical AV nodal reentry, the P wave may also be located just at the start or end of the QRS complex, giving a qRs or Rsr' pattern. When the P wave is located close to the previous QRS complex, it is identified as a short-RP tachycardia. This is often seen with accessory pathway–mediated tachycardia and is due to retrograde atrial activation over the accessory pathway. The P wave may also be far from the previous QRS complex and classified as a long-RP tachycardia. If the P wave is inverted, it may be the result of atypical AV node reentry, or it may be using a slowly conducting accessory pathway in the retrograde direction. AVNRT—atrioventricular nodal reentry tachycardia; ECG—electrocardiogram [15].

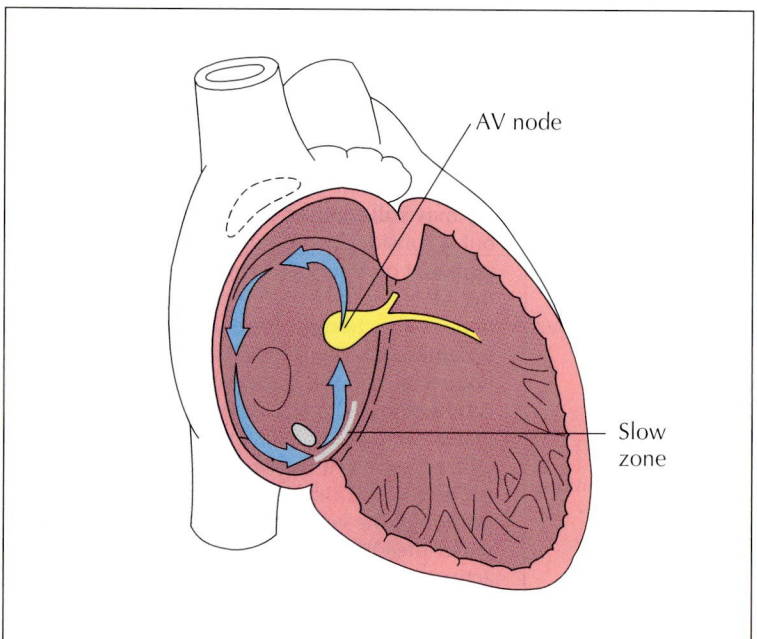

Figure 6-29. Atrial flutter circuit. With atrioventricular (AV) nodal reentry, AV reentry utilizing an accessory pathway, and a reentrant atrial tachycardia, there is usually a defined circuit which, if interrupted, can terminate the tachycardia. We now have learned that atrial flutter is a macro reentrant circuit in the right atrium. The circuit involves conduction in a counterclockwise (or clockwise) direction from the low posterior right atrium near the tricuspid valve annulus (TA), the posteroseptal region near the coronary sinus os, the interatrial septum, the high lateral right atrium, and down the crista terminalis to the isthmus between the inferior vena cava and the TA. The region of the posterior right atrium is thought to be the slow zone of conduction in the circuit. Evidence that supports this theory consists of data showing that atrial flutter can be entrained with atrial pacing. This has led to the development of techniques allowing electrophysiologists to ablate the critical regions of the circuit causing atrial flutter, thus, rendering the circuit inoperable [16].

ATRIAL FIBRILLATION

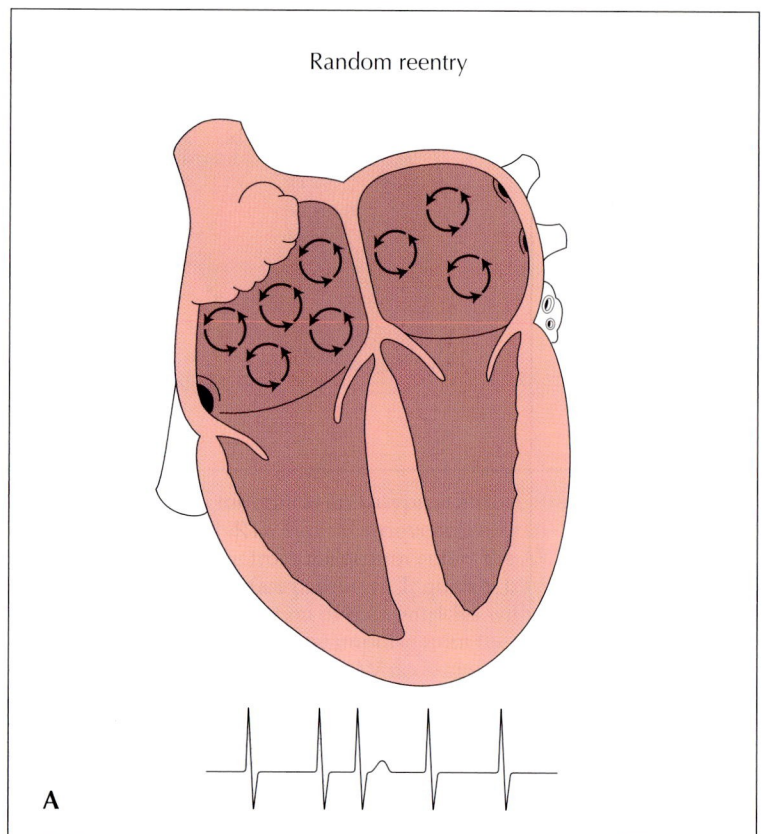

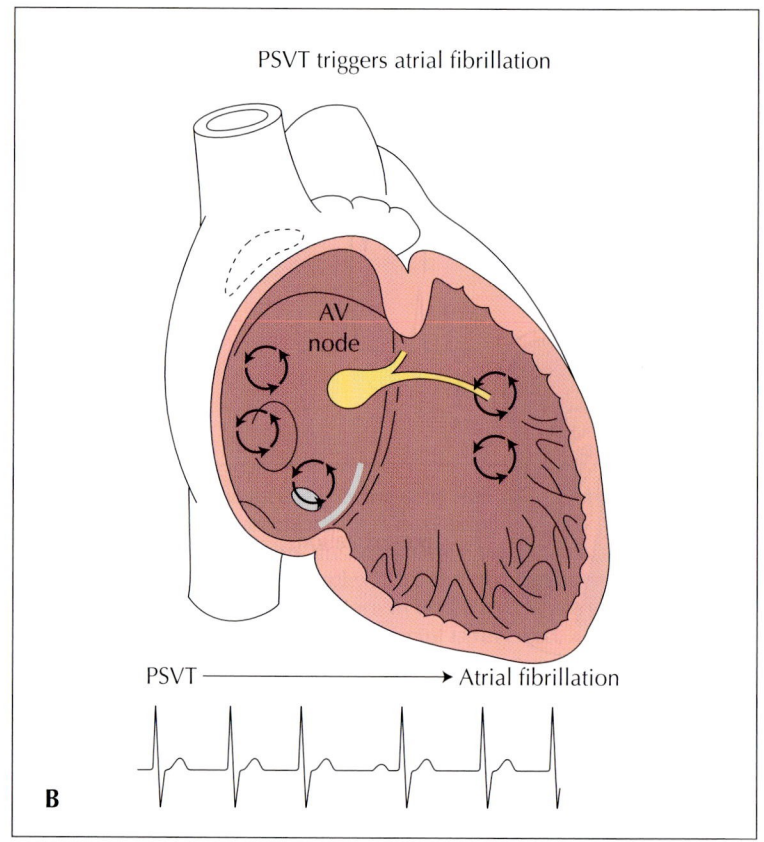

Figure 6-30. Mechanisms of atrial fibrillation (AF). AF is the most common sustained arrhythmia and is particularly prevalent in the elderly. While atrial flutter has one reentrant circuit, AF demonstrates multiple random reentrant circuits. This leads to clot formation and systemic embolic events. Thus, most patients with persistent or permanent AF require anticoagulation. Patients with "lone AF" (no structural heart disease or hypertension under age 60) are considered to have a lower risk of stroke and do not generally require anticoagulation. **A,** Random reentry. AF is thought to be due to multiple wavelets produced by functional or anatomic reentry [17]. **B,** Paroxysmal supraventricular tachycardia (PSVT) can trigger AF. Ablation of the PSVT may, in some cases, prevent AF recurrence [18]. (*continued*)

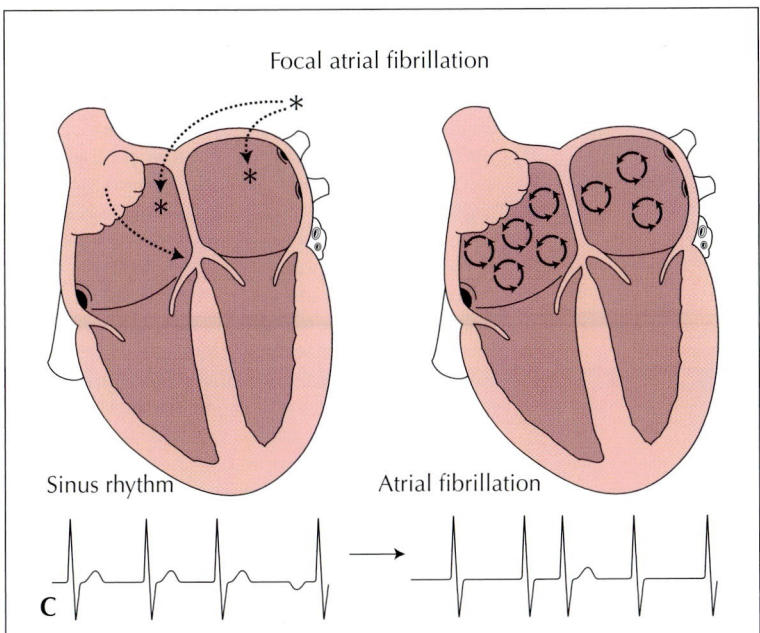

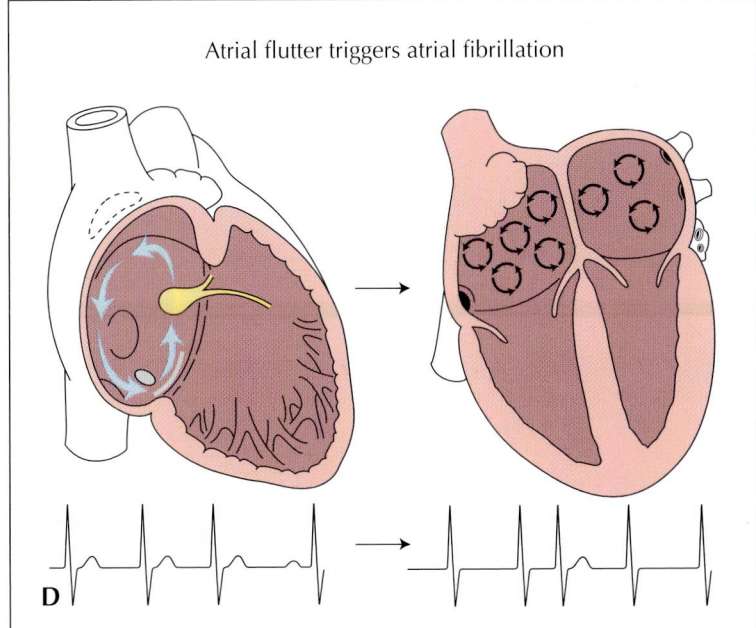

FIGURE 6-30. (*continued*) **C,** Focal atrial premature complexes usually originating from pulmonary veins can initiate AF [19,20]. Ablation of these arrhythmogenic focal triggers can restore rhythm. This finding opens an exciting era in electrophysiology with the possibility of curing

AF by ablation. **D,** Atrial flutter (AFL) triggers AF. There is a relationship between the more organized reentrant AFL arrhythmia and AF [21,22]. Certain class IC drugs (such as propafenone) can convert AF to AFL. Additionally, the two rhythms often coexist in the same patient.

TREATMENT MODALITIES FOR ATRIAL FIBRILLATION

Pharmacologic therapy: goal is to restore sinus rhythm or rate control
    AV nodal blocking agents: β-blockers, calcium channel blockers, digoxin
    Class IA: procainamide, disopyramide
    Class IC: flecainide, propafenone
    Class III: amiodarone, sotalol, dofetilide
Acute cardioversion
    Electrical
    Chemical: ibutilide or ibutilide + chronic amiodarone
Catheter ablation
    Complete AV node ablation + pacemaker
    Focal pulmonary vein ablation
    Catheter maze procedure (right and/or left atria)
Surgery
    Maze procedure

FIGURE 6-31. Treatment of atrial fibrillation (AF). Many drugs are available for rate control of AF. Acute cardioversion can be attempted by electrical means (monophasic or biphasic shocking waveforms) [23] or by chemical means with ibutilide (class III drug) [24,25] or ibutilide and amiodarone [26]. Dofetilide is a new class III drug that can be used for cardioversion in patients with congestive heart failure [27]. Using ibutilide or dofetilide in patients with renal failure increases the incidence of torsade de pointes. Anticoagulation should be maintained for one month after cardioversion. Complete atrial ventricular (AV) node ablation and placement of a permanent pacemaker can be performed for rate control. Other catheter ablation techniques include ablation of atrial premature beats from pulmonary veins that trigger focal AF [19,20]. The catheter Maze procedure places drag lesions in the right and/or left atria to restore sinus rhythm.

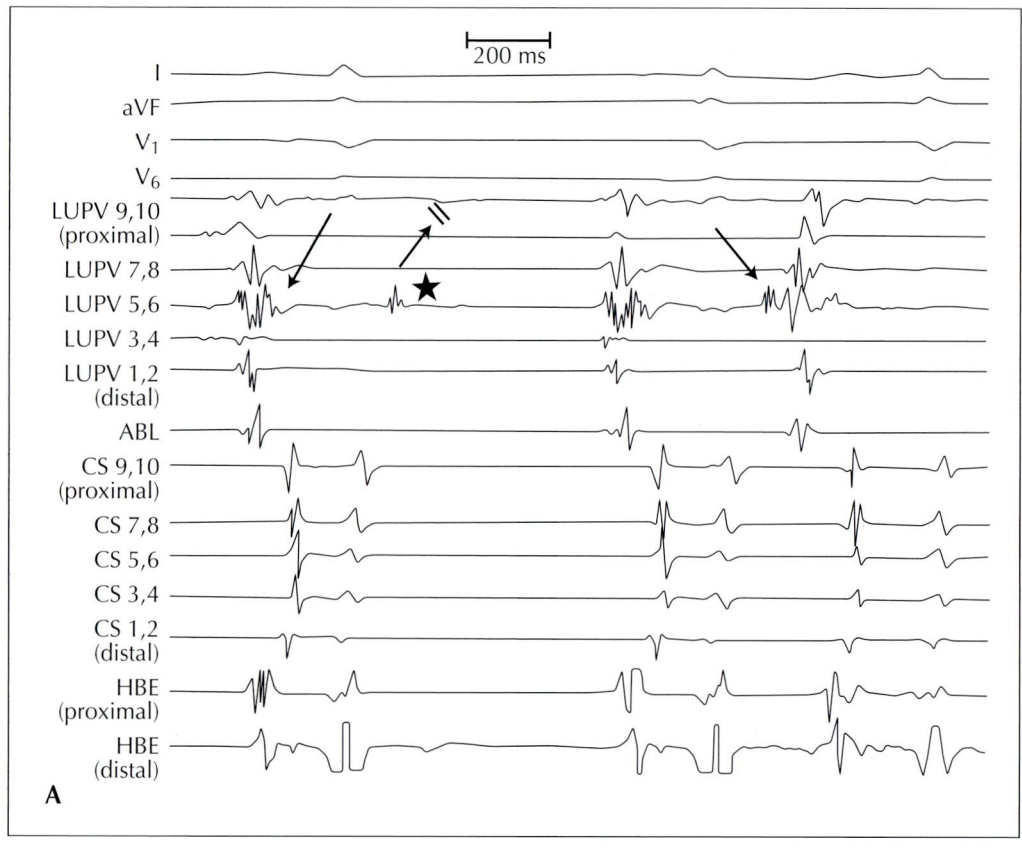

A

Figure 6-32. Focal origin of atrial fibrillation (AF). **A,** Intracardiac electrocardiograms demonstrating pulmonary vein potentials. A 38-year-old man with paroxysmal AF underwent an ablation procedure for focal AF. *Arrows,* a pulmonary vein potential that follows the left atrial activation in the first (sinus) beat but precedes left atrial activation in the premature beat; *star,* a blocked premature beat originating in the left upper pulmonary vein (LUPV). The pulmonary veins are wrapped in atrial myocardium that extends for several centimeters into the pulmonary veins. Such atrial tissue can become arrhythmogenic foci that fire rapidly and initiate AF. The upper pulmonary veins are common origins for these foci. **B,** Intracardiac electrocardiograms during an ablation procedure for focal AF in a 35-year-old man with paroxysmal AF. Note that an atrial premature complex (*star*) originating from the LUPV initiates sustained AF. Elimination of this focal trigger by radiofrequency ablation appears to restore sinus rhythm in the patient over long-term follow-up. The finding of focal triggers to AF has heralded an exciting new era in arrhythmia management. Potential complications of focal AF ablations include tamponade (due to transseptal puncture), pulmonary vein stenosis, and stroke. ABL—ablating catheter; CS—coronary sinus; CT—crista terminalis (in lateral right atrium); HBE—His bundle electrogram; LUPV—left upper pulmonary vein.

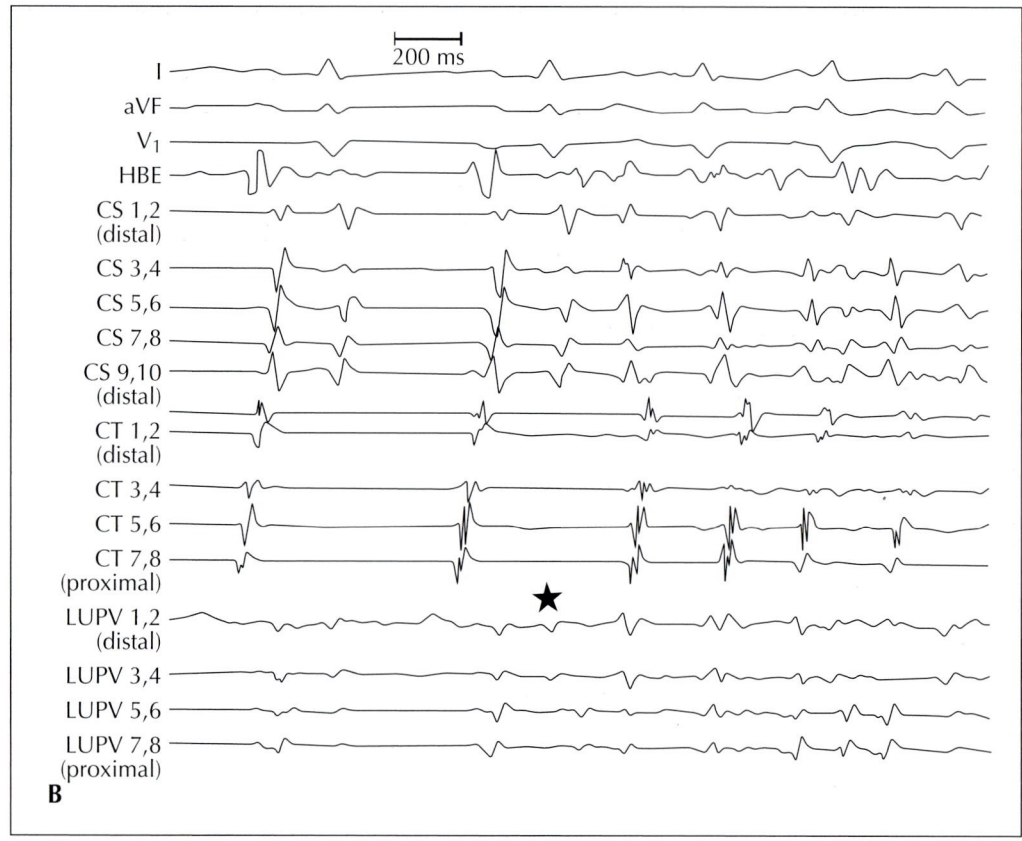

B

CLASS III ANTIARRHYTHMIC DRUGS

<u>IBUTILIDE</u>

Inhibits I_{Kr} channels (outward repolarizing current)

Enhances slow inward sodium current

Prolongs QT interval

Intravenous formulation only

Useful for terminating acute onset atrial fibrillation or flutter

Post-cardiac surgery atrial arrhythmias

Facilitates transthoracic electrical cardioversion

Can be used to treat rapid atrial fibrillation with Wolff-Parkinson-White syndrome

Causes torsades de pointes

<u>DOFETILIDE</u>

Inhibits I_{Kr} channels

Intravenous and oral formulation

Prolongs QT interval

Useful for conversion of atrial arrhythmias and maintenance of sinus rhythm

Can be used in high-risk patients with heart failure or post-myocardial infarction

Causes torsades de pointes—narrow therapeutic window

<u>AZIMILIDE</u>

Inhibits both I_{Kr} and I_{Ks} channels

Intravenous and oral formulation

Prolongs QT interval

Useful for atrial arrhythmias

Causes torsades de pointes

FIGURE 6-33. New class III antiarrhythmic drugs. Ibutilide, dofetilide, and azimilide represent potassium-channel blocking agents useful for cardioversion of atrial fibrillation and flutter [24,25,27,28]. All three drugs increase the atrial refractory period and exhibit reverse-use dependence, or greater drug effect at slow heart rates. As a general class effect, they prolong the QT interval and can exhibit proarrhythmic effects including torsades de pointes. Risk factors for torsades de pointes with these drugs include hypokalemia, female gender, the presence of heart failure, and renal failure.

DIAGNOSIS

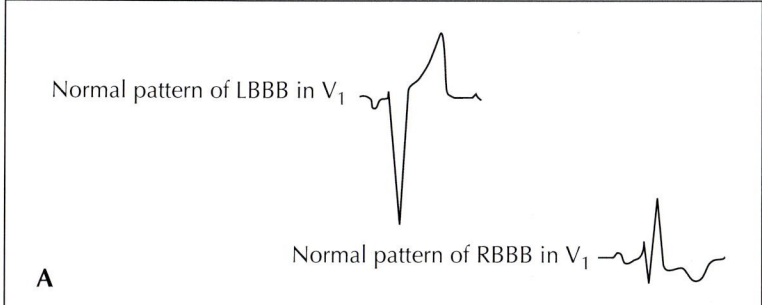

Normal pattern of LBBB in V_1

Normal pattern of RBBB in V_1

A

FIGURE 6-34. The 12-lead electrocardiogram in the differential diagnosis of wide complex tachycardia. Brugada *el al.* [29] analyzed 384 cases of ventricular tachycardia (VT) and 170 cases of supraventricular tachycardia (SVT) with aberrancy, representing 554 patients with tachycardia (those taking antiarrhythmic medications were excluded). They then devised a systematic approach for diagnosing wide QRS complex tachycardia with regular rhythmicity. **A,** The first step is to exclude sinus tachycardia or atrial tachycardia with right bundle branch block (RBBB) or left bundle branch block (LBBB). This can usually be done by finding P waves in lead V_1: the ST segment and T wave are always smooth, unless distorted by a P wave. However, missing this diagnosis should not affect the ability to diagnose VT or SVT, unless the patient is taking QRS-lengthening drugs. **B,** Steps in diagnosis of SVT with aberration. A *yes* answer at any point indicates that no further steps need to be taken. When the answer is *no*, proceed to the next step. The cumulative sensitivity using this method is 97% and specificity is 99%. (*continued*)

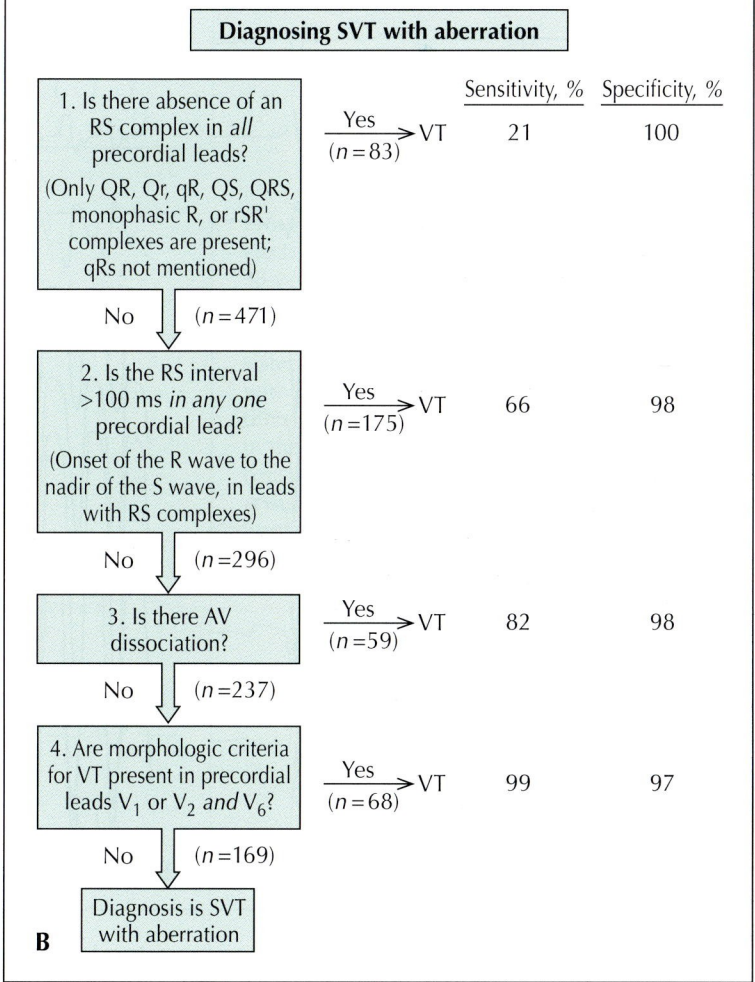

Diagnosing SVT with aberration

		Sensitivity, %	Specificity, %
1. Is there absence of an RS complex in *all* precordial leads? (Only QR, Qr, qR, QS, QRS, monophasic R, or rSR' complexes are present; qRs not mentioned)	$\xrightarrow[(n=83)]{\text{Yes}}$ VT	21	100
No $(n=471)$			
2. Is the RS interval >100 ms *in any one* precordial lead? (Onset of the R wave to the nadir of the S wave, in leads with RS complexes)	$\xrightarrow[(n=175)]{\text{Yes}}$ VT	66	98
No $(n=296)$			
3. Is there AV dissociation?	$\xrightarrow[(n=59)]{\text{Yes}}$ VT	82	98
No $(n=237)$			
4. Are morphologic criteria for VT present in precordial leads V_1 or V_2 *and* V_6?	$\xrightarrow[(n=68)]{\text{Yes}}$ VT	99	97
No $(n=169)$			
Diagnosis is SVT with aberration			

B

B

TYPE	ION CHANNEL MUTATION/ CHROMOSOME LOCATION	ARRHYTHMIA TRIGGER	INCIDENCE OF KNOWN GENOTYPES
LQT1	I_{Ks}/chromosome 11	Exercise, swimming, strong emotion, rarely auditory stimuli	≈50%
LQT2	I_{Kr} ("HERG")/chromosome 7	Auditory stimuli, abrupt arousal from sleep	≈45%
LQT3	SCN5A (sodium)/chromosome 3	Usually not related to exercise; may occur during sleep	≈5%
LQT4	?/chromosome 4	?	?
LQT5	minK/chromosome 21 Interacts to form I_{Ks}	Exercise, swimming, strong emotion, rarely auditory stimuli	?
LQT6	MiRP1/chromosome 21 Interacts to form I_{Kr}	Auditory stimuli, abrupt arousal from sleep	?

FIGURE 6-37. (*continued*) **B,** Only half of all patients with LQTS can be currently genotyped because their mutations have not yet been identified. LQTS is an autosomal dominant genetic disorder (Romano-Ward syndrome) with incomplete penetrance [31,32]. Up to 30% of patients with LQTS have normal or only borderline prolonged QT intervals, which can make diagnosis difficult. If both parents carry the defective gene for the I_{Ks} channel and pass it on, the child will have a severe form of LQTS associated with congenital hearing loss (Jervell-Lange-Nielsen syndrome). Treatment options include beta-blocker therapy, dual-chamber pacemaker, and/or dual-chamber pacemaker-defibrillator therapy [33].

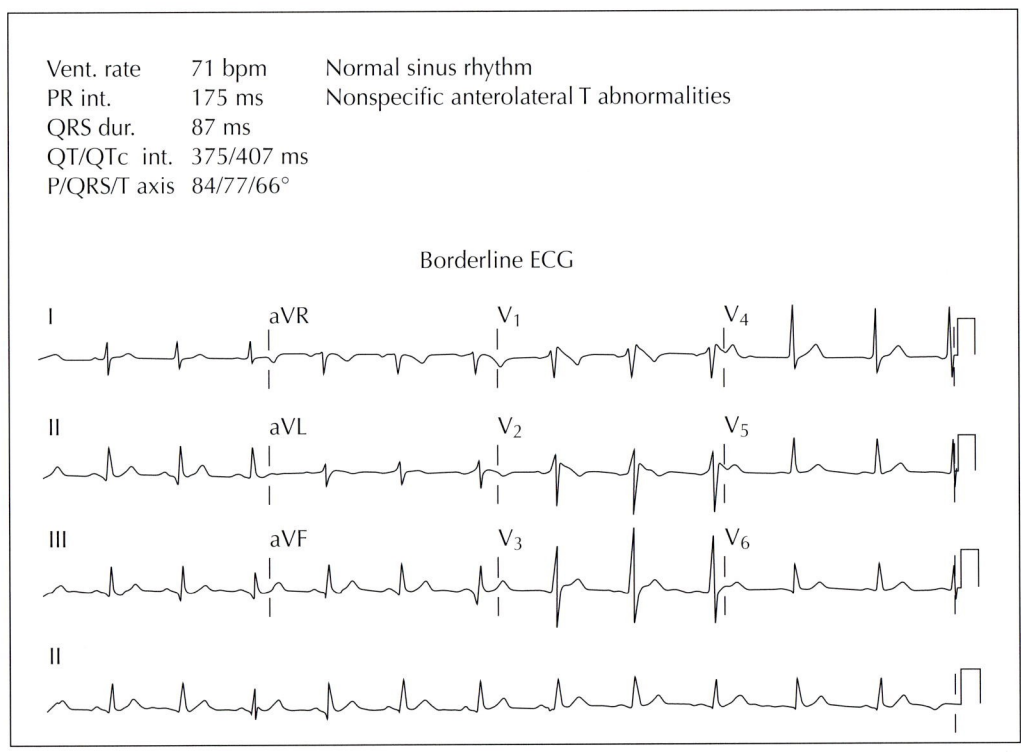

Vent. rate	71 bpm	Normal sinus rhythm
PR int.	175 ms	Nonspecific anterolateral T abnormalities
QRS dur.	87 ms	
QT/QTc int.	375/407 ms	
P/QRS/T axis	84/77/66°	

Borderline ECG

FIGURE 6-38. A 12-lead electrocardiogram (ECG) obtained from a 57-year-old man without structural heart disease who survived a cardiac arrest. The ECG has features that suggest Brugada's syndrome, including persistent ST elevation in leads V_1–V_3, right bundle branch block-type pattern, prominent J wave (positive deflection at the end of the QRS complex), and inverted T waves. The prevalence of primary ventricular fibrillation in symptomatic individuals is 40%–60%, and defibrillator implantation is often recommended for these patients. Brugada's syndrome appears to be a genetic disorder caused by mutations in SCN5A, the cardiac sodium channel [34,35]. Flecainide or other sodium channel blocker drugs can unmask the typical ECG phenotype in these patients.

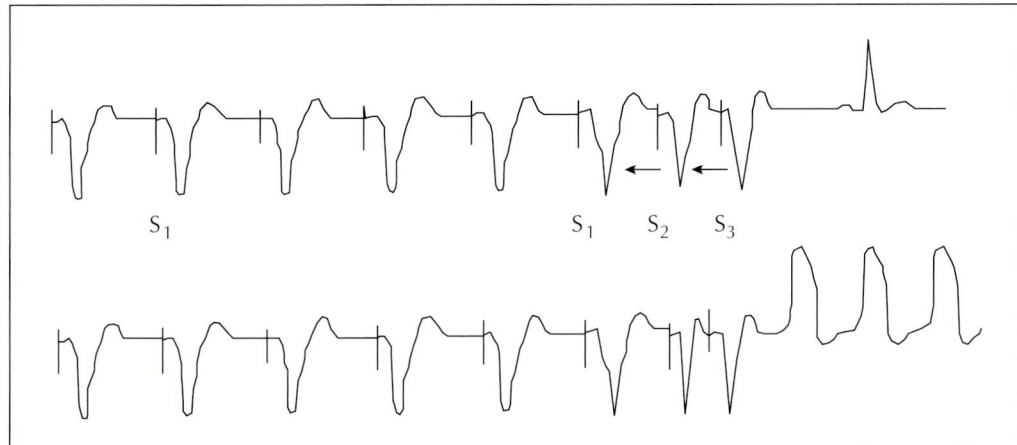

FIGURE 6-39. Programmed electrical stimulation (PES). PES can be used in the diagnosis and management of ventricular tachycardia (VT) by inserting a catheter into the right ventricle. Although this is the typical application, the left ventricle can also be used. Eight or more beats at a basic drive rate (S_1) are introduced, followed by one, two, or three premature extra beats (S_2, S_3, S_4). These extra beats are placed at programmed intervals, and the intervals are shortened by scanning diastole until refractoriness. This technique has a sensitivity and specificity of over 90% for the induction of reentrant sustained monomorphic VT in patients with healed myocardial infarction (MI). However, it is not sensitive in patients whose VT is due to acute MI, reversible ischemia, electrolyte disturbances, or other etiologies. The induction of nonsustained VT, polymorphic VT, or ventricular fibrillation has reduced specificity, especially if induced with aggressive stimulation with very early premature beats. Repeat PES following drug administration in patients with inducible sustained VT may be used to help predict drug efficacy.

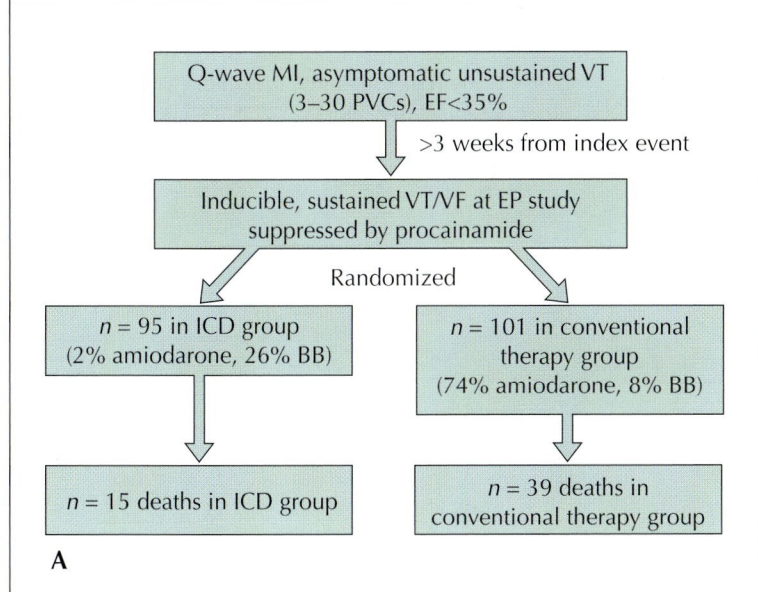

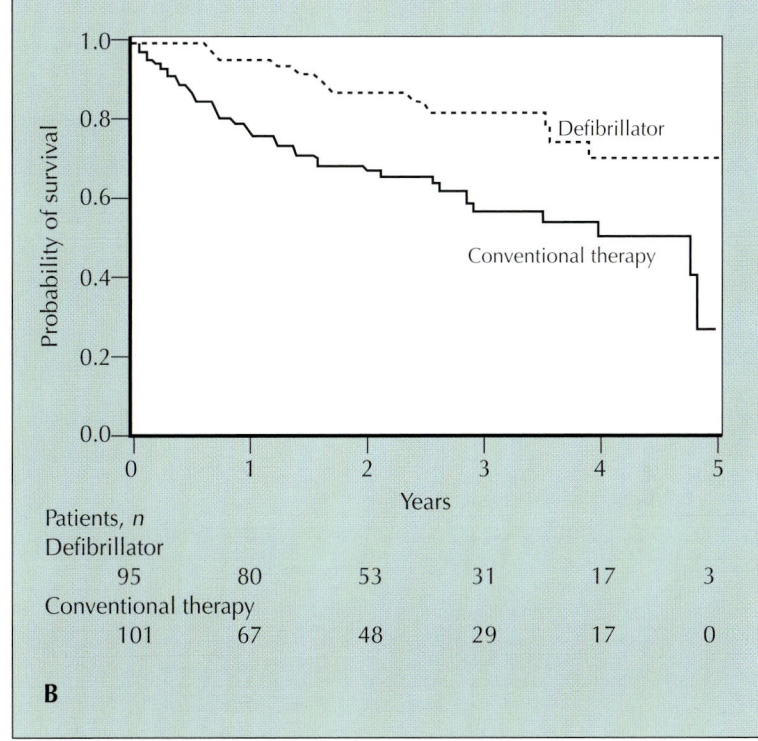

FIGURE 6-40. Multicenter Automatic Defibrillator Implantation Trial (MADIT). **A**, MADIT was a primary prevention study where high-risk patients with known coronary artery disease and asymptomatic unsustained ventricular tachycardia (VT) not suppressible by procainamide were randomly assigned to receive an implantable cardioverter/defibrillator (ICD) or conventional medical therapy, which consisted mainly of amiodarone therapy. **B**, There was a significant difference in survival between the two treatment groups ($P = 0.009$), with fewer deaths reported in the ICD group at follow-up after 27 months. BB—beta-blocker; EP— electrophysiology; EF—ejection fraction; MI—myocardial infarction; PVC—premature ventricular complexes; VF—ventricular fibrillation. (*Adapted from* Moss *et al.* [36].)

TREATMENT OPTIONS FOR SYMPTOMATIC SUSTAINED VT OR VF NOT DUE TO A REVERSIBLE CAUSE

NO STRUCTURAL HEART DISEASE

Calcium-channel blockers

β-blockers

Class I or III agents (propafenone, sotalol, amidarone)

RF catheter ablation

IDIOPATHIC CARDIOMYOPATHY

Drugs (especially amiodarone)

Implanted defibrillator with ATP

Catheter ablation for bundle branch reentrant VT, if present

PRIOR MYOCARDIAL INFARCTION

Class III agents (sotalol if preserved EF; amiodarone)

Catheter ablation

Implanted defibrillator with ATP

LONG QT SYNDROME

β-blockers and dual-chamber pacing to shorten QT interval

Implanted defibrillator with atrial pacing

FIGURE 6-41. Treatment options for patients with ventricular tachycardia (VT) or ventricular fibrillation (VF). The therapy recommended depends on presentation and substrate. ATP—antitachycardia pacing; EF—ejection fraction; RF—radiofrequency.

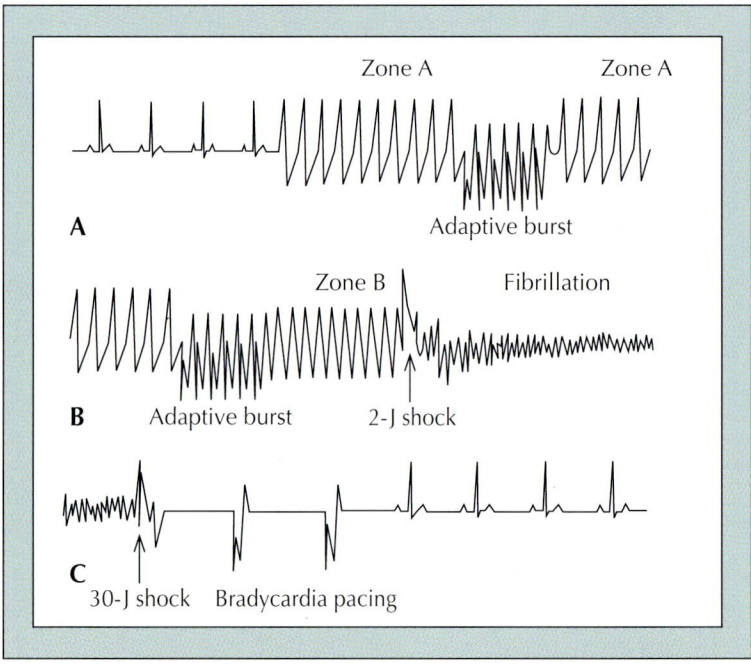

FIGURE 6-42. Incorporation of tiered or *zone* therapy in newer implantable devices for selective antitachycardia pacing, lower energy cardioversion, or high-energy defibrillation. Recordings show idealized tiered anti-tachycardia therapy. **A,** Onset of ventricular tachycardia (VT) with slower rate (zone A). Overdrive pacing is initiated with an adaptive burst, but tachycardia resumes with the same rate. **B,** Repeat burst pacing leads to acceleration of VT rate (zone B), and a low-energy (2 J) cardio-version shock leads to ventricular fibrillation (VF). **C,** VF is effectively terminated with 30-J shock delivery. (*Adapted from* Akhtar *et al.* [37].)

DEVICES FOR TACHYCARDIA: INDICATIONS FOR AICD

Failure of diagnosis

 Sudden death, noninducible, negative Holter monitor
  recording

Failure of therapy

 Clinical recurrence on a drug predicted effective by
  electrophysiologic testing

 Clinical recurrence on amiodarone

 Clinical recurrence after surgery or ablation

Predicted failure of therapy

 Still inducible on type I drug

 Amiodarone with multiple risk factors

 Inducible after surgery or ablation

FIGURE 6-43. Indications for using automatic implantable cardioverter/defibrillator (AICD).

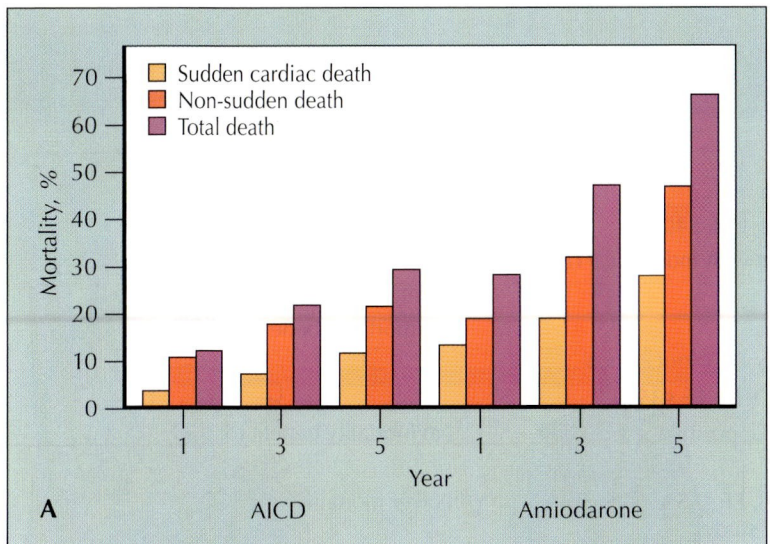
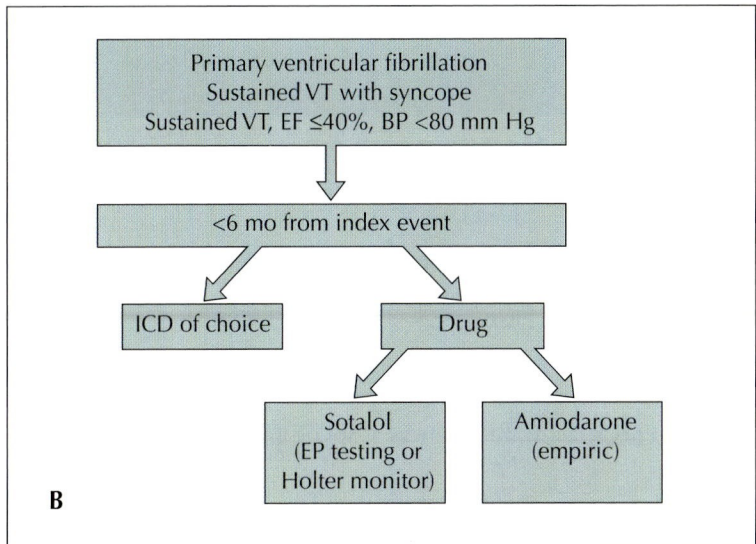

FIGURE 6-44. Automatic implantable cardioverter/defibrillator (AICD) versus drug therapy. The results of studies shown in **A** indicate that AICD therapy is associated with a lower incidence of sudden and nonsudden death compared with treatment with amiodarone, which is probably the most effective antiarrhythmic drug available. Caution must be exercised, however, in comparing studies that probably did not enroll comparable patient groups. It is still unknown whether amiodarone (or sotalol, another effective class III drug) or AICD is best in a matched cohort of patients with sustained ventricular tachycardia (VT) or ventricular fibrillation (VF). **B**, The Antiarrhythmic Drug Versus Implanted Defibrillator (AVID) Trial, sponsored by the National Institutes of Health, was an important secondary prevention trial studying implantable cardioverter/defibrillator (ICD) versus drug therapy for patients with hemodynamically unstable VT or VF. A total of 1016 high-risk patients were randomized to an ICD versus drug therapy (amiodarone or sotalol). At two years' follow-up, 82% of the patients in the drug therapy group were taking amiodarone; only 9% were using sotalol. ICD therapy conferred a survival benefit comparable to the drug therapy group. BP—blood pressure; EF—ejection fraction; EP—electrophysiology. (Panel A *adapted from* Winkle *et al.* [38].)

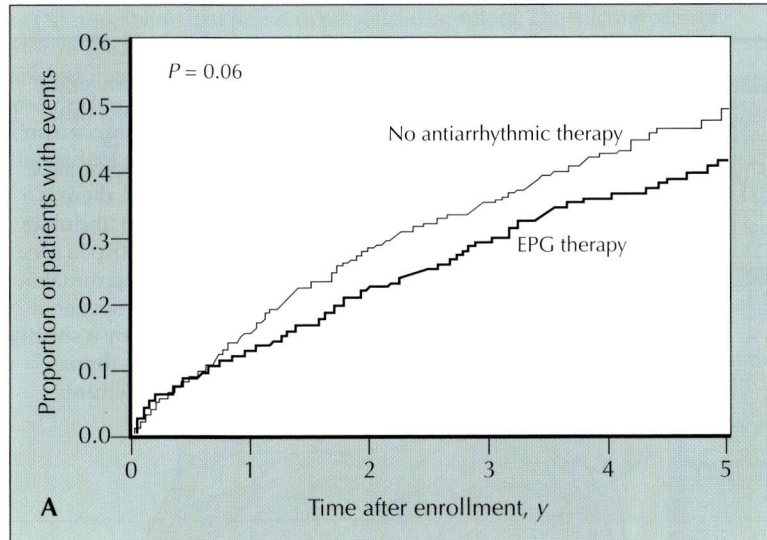
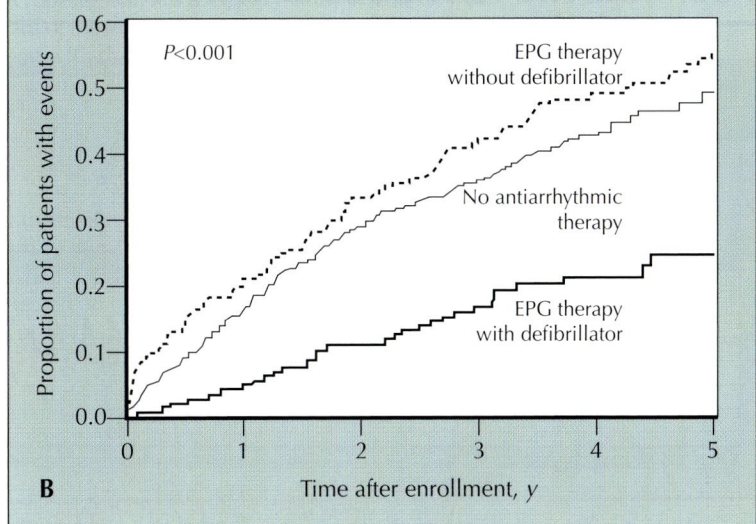

FIGURE 6-45. Use of electrophysiology (EP)-guided therapy. **A, B**, The Multicenter Unsustained Tachycardia Trial (MUSTT) study examined the hypothesis that EP-guided therapy would decrease the risk of sudden cardiac death in high-risk patients [39]. Study participants had a history of coronary artery disease, EF <40%, and asymptomatic unsustained ventricular tachycardia (VT). Those patients with inducible monomorphic VT, polymorphic VT, or ventricular fibrillation at EP study were randomized to EP-guided therapy (which included anti-arrhythmic drug or implantable cardioverter/defibrillator therapy) or to no anti-arrhythmic drug therapy. *Panel A* demonstrates that EP-guided therapy was not superior to the no-therapy group in long-term follow-up. *Panel B* shows that therapy with defibrillator conferred the greatest survival benefit in this study. EF—ejection fraction. (*Adapted from* Buxton *et al.* [39].)

CARDIAC PACING AND SURVIVAL

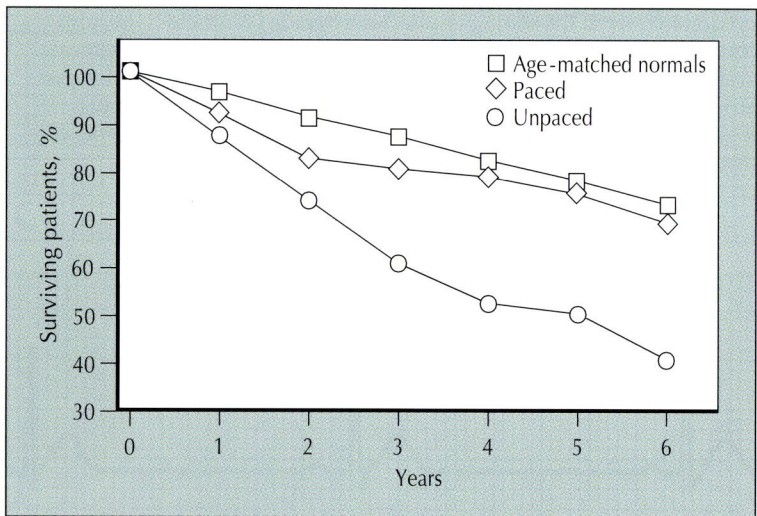

FIGURE 6-56. Heart block. Prior to the availability of pacemakers, survival among patients with third-degree heart block was dismal, approaching only 50% at 1 year and only 10% to 25% survival by 5 years [47]. Survival among patients with second-degree heart block is about 50% at 5 years compared with over 75% survival among patients receiving pacemakers [48].

RATE-ADAPTIVE PACING

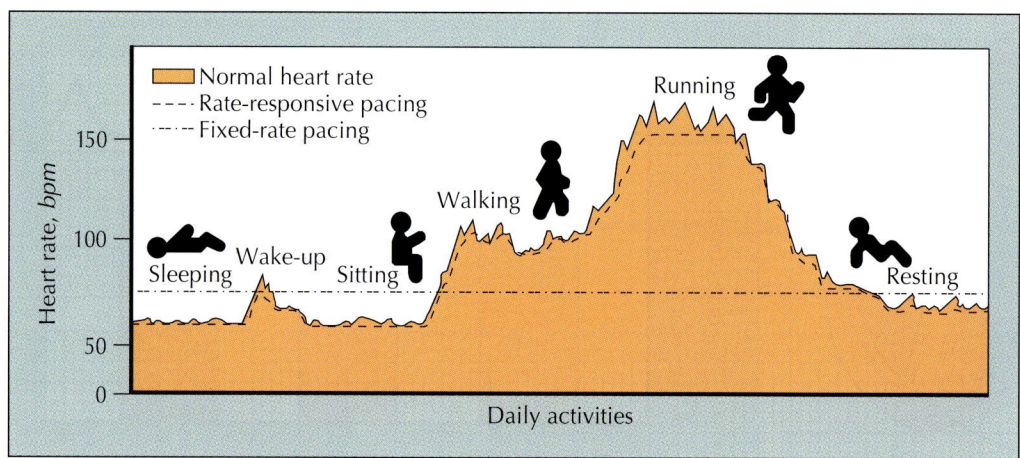

FIGURE 6-57. Adjusting heart rate to activity. Since the landmark achievement 35 years ago of restoring a stable cardiac rhythm with fixed-rate ventricular pacing (*straight dotted line*), efforts have focused on attempts to faithfully duplicate the rate responsiveness and physiologic characteristics of the native cardiac electrical pacemaking system. In the normal heart, rate (chronotropic) response accounts for a significant amount of the total cardiac reserve output in response to metabolic requirements with exercise (*shaded area*). A significant number, perhaps 50%, of patients receiving pacemakers today show variable amounts of chronotropic incompetence and may potentially benefit from pacing systems that offer chronotropic, rate-adaptive support. In addition, a significant number (estimated at 5% per year) of patients receiving pacing systems initially for heart block, develop rate-incompetence during follow-up and would benefit from such capability as well. The ideal pacemaker would duplicate the impressive responsiveness of the autonomic and cardiac nervous system, sinus node, and specialized interventricular conduction system to meet the full array of physiologic requirements (dotted line). (*Adapted from* Medtronic, Inc., Minneapolis, MN.)

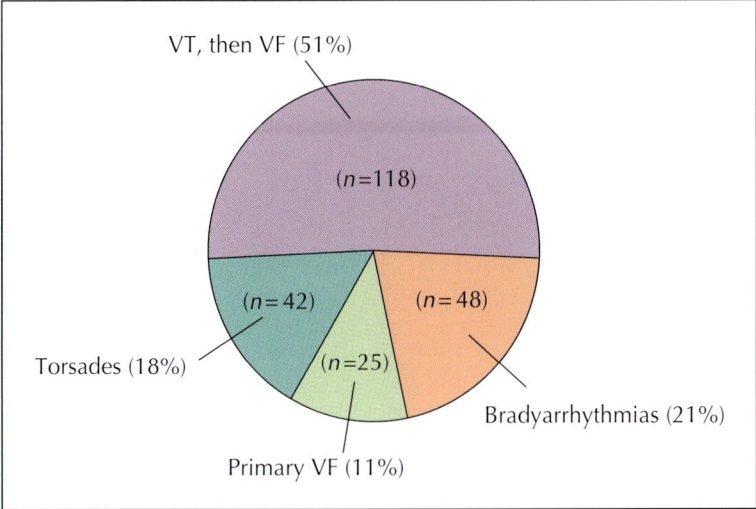

FIGURE 6-58. Cardiac arrhythmia at the time of sudden death. The cardiac rhythm present at the time of sudden death is usually ventricular tachycardia (VT) or fibrillation (VF) [31] as detected by ambulatory monitoring. The cardiac arrhythmogenic substrate is generally chronic, with various degrees of myocardial fibrosis such as that following myocardial infarction. This predisposes to lethal events following otherwise benign triggering events. (*Adapted from* Bayes de Luna *et al.* [49].)

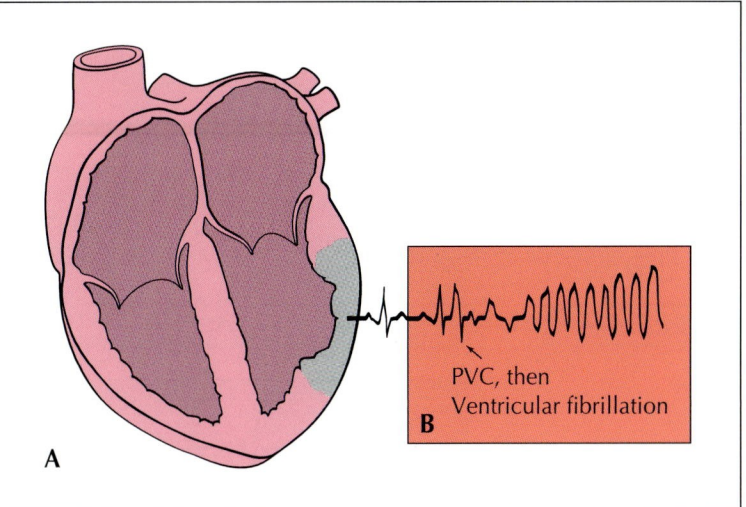

FIGURE 6-59. Substrate for malignant arrhythmias. **A,** Evidence of healed or recent myocardial infarction (shaded area) and significant coronary artery atherosclerosis [50], even in the absence of a suggestive clinical history [51], have been frequent findings at autopsy following sudden death. **B** shows premature ventricular contraction (PVC), resulting in ventricular fibrillation.

PREVENTION

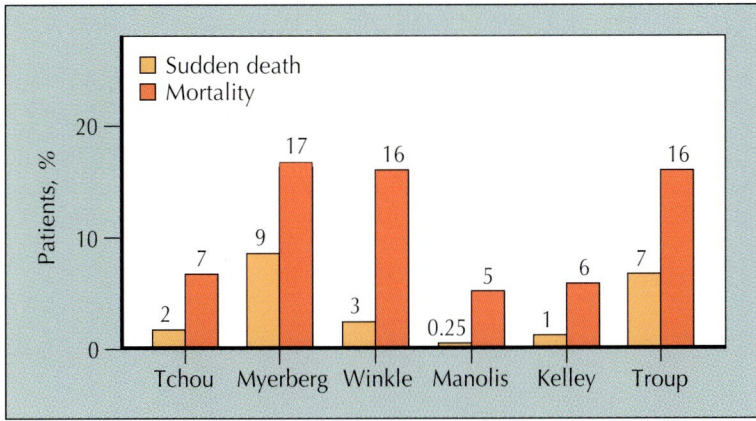

FIGURE 6-60. Improved survival after implantable cardioverter defibrillator therapy. The implantable defibrillator has had a remarkable impact on improving the freedom from recurrent sudden death relative to historical experiences, ranging from 91% at 1 year to 96% at 5 years, in a number of clinical studies. Overall survival has been reported to range from 95% at 1 year to 60% at 3 years. Most deaths are due to congestive heart failure and a much smaller proportion are due to bradyarrhythmias, electromechanical dissociation, or device failure [52–54]. (*Adapted from* Moss *et al.* [54].)

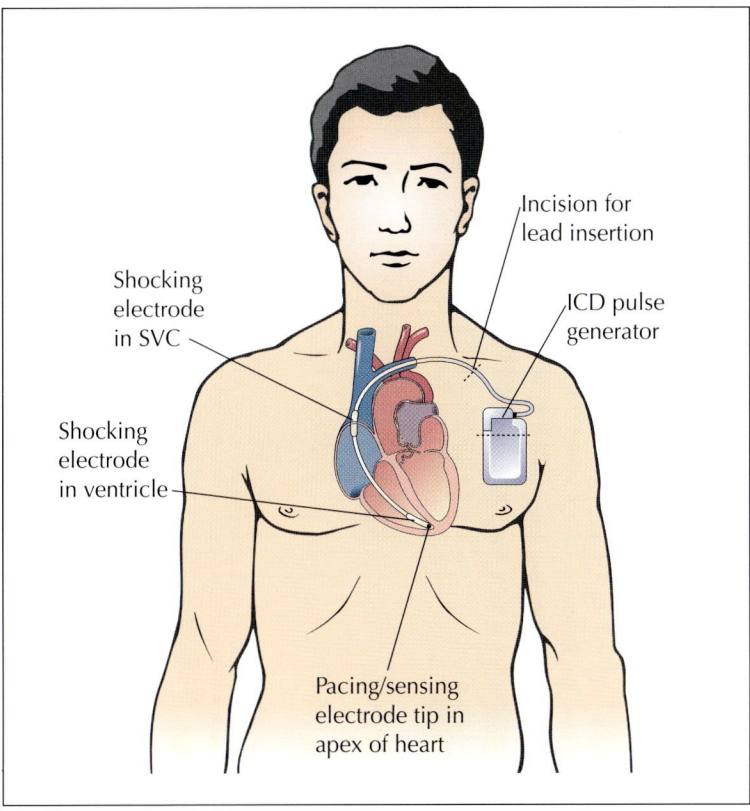

FIGURE 6-61. Pectoral implantable cardioverter/defibrillator (ICD). The ICD uses the defibrillation coils placed in the right ventricle apex and superior vena cava (SVC) with the titanium case of the pulse generator. Vascular access for the ICD leads is usually obtained via the left subclavian or cephalic vein. Typical volume for an ICD is 40 mL; typical weight is 80 g.

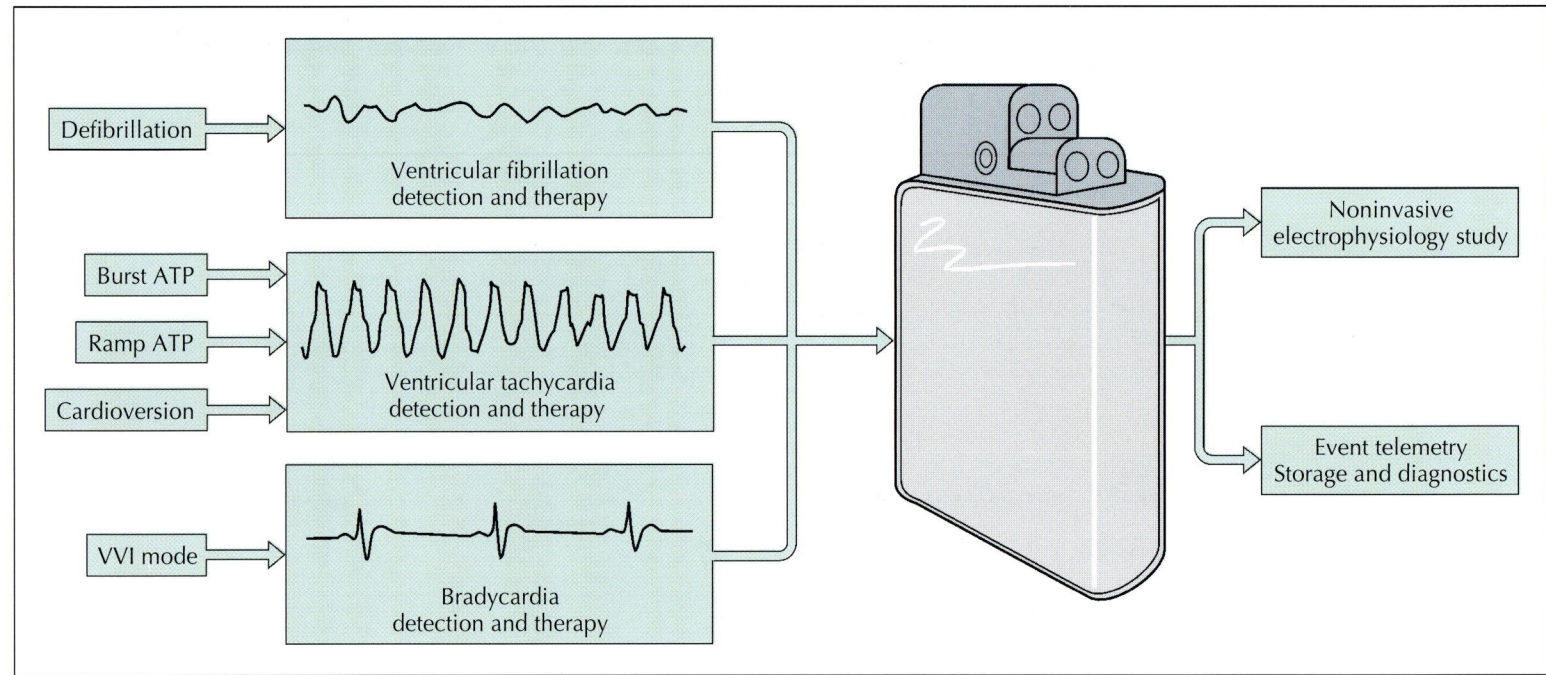

FIGURE 6-62. Tiered-therapy defibrillators. In addition to defibrillation, the implantable defibrillator has the capacity for several "tiered" functions including bradycardia pacing, antitachycardia pacing, and cardioversion. Therapy may be specifically programmed for individual patient needs and may include one or more "heart rate zones" based on both electrophysiologic testing and device-based testing after implantation. ATP—antitachycardia pacing; VVI—ventricular pacing, sensing, inhibiting. (*Adapted from* Medtronic, Inc., Minneapolis, MN.)

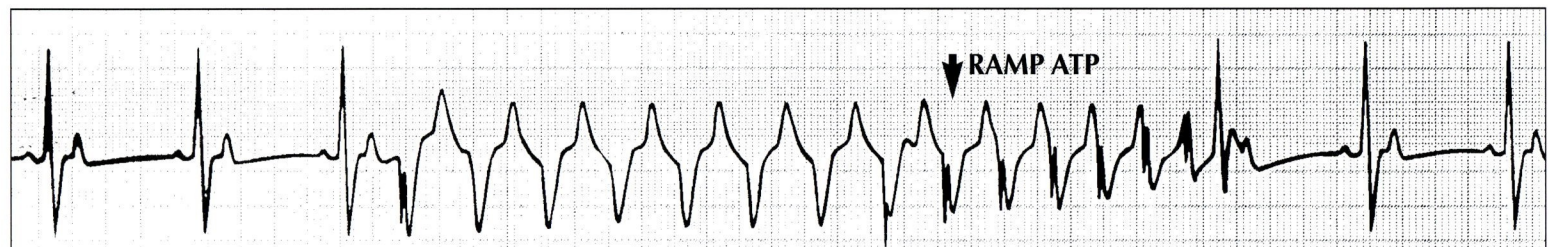

FIGURE 6-63. Antitachycardia pacing. Effective antitachycardia pacing burst patterns include those with between-burst decrement (SCAN) with or without an additional within-burst decrement (RAMP) pattern. In a randomized, controlled trial reported by Newman and colleagues [55], laboratory administration of adaptive SCAN or RAMP antitachycardia pacing patterns had a similar efficacy of 85% and 90% successful conversion among 29 patients with 65 inducible ventricular tachycardias. Acceleration due to antitachycardia pacing was observed in 7 (5 SCAN, 2 RAMP) of 65 (11%) tachycardias. Failure to convert tachycardia was associated with a shorter tachycardia cycle length. Basic cycle length=240–340 ms; delay= 36 ms. ATP—antitachycardia pacing.

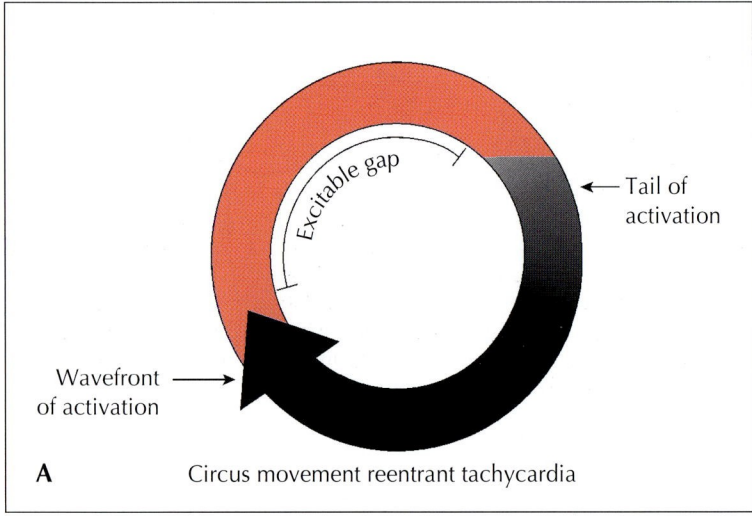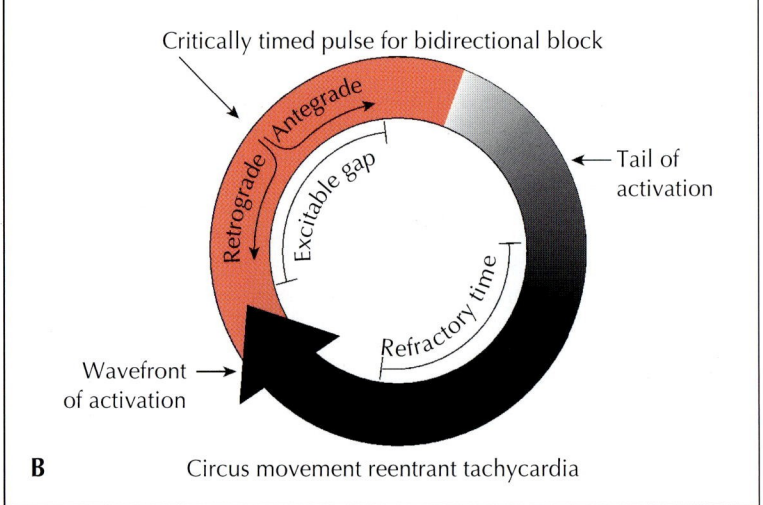

FIGURE 6-64. Reentrant tachycardia (**A**) may be terminated with critically timed stimulation resulting in twin propagated wavefronts (**B**) of depolarization in both antegrade and retrograde directions along the excitable reentrant pathway, resulting in bidirectional block to terminate the reentrant arrhythmia.

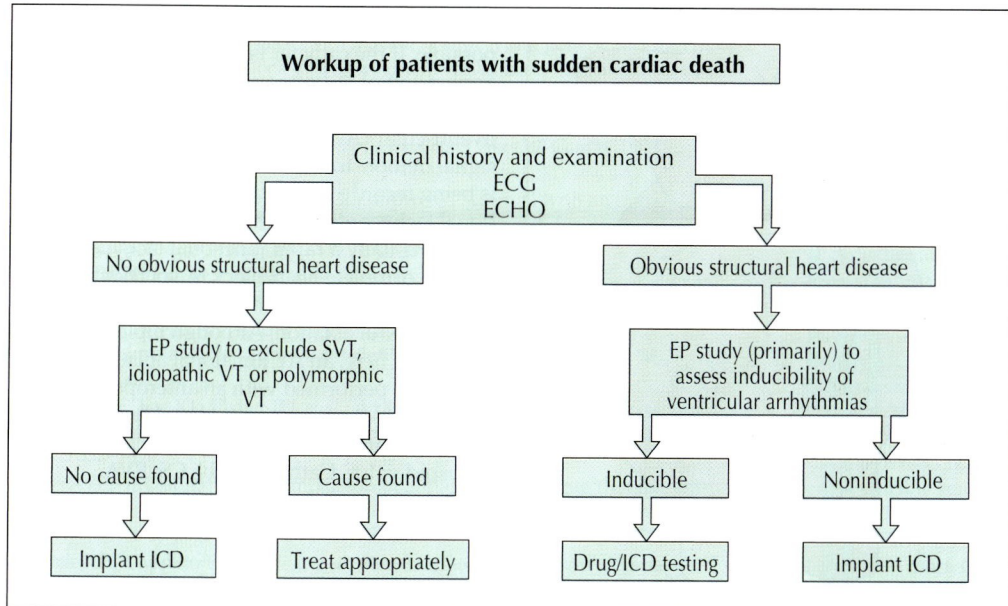

Workup of patients with sudden cardiac death

Clinical history and examination
ECG
ECHO

No obvious structural heart disease

Obvious structural heart disease

EP study to exclude SVT, idiopathic VT or polymorphic VT

EP study (primarily) to assess inducibility of ventricular arrhythmias

No cause found

Cause found

Inducible

Noninducible

Implant ICD

Treat appropriately

Drug/ICD testing

Implant ICD

FIGURE 6-65. Diagnostic work-up in patients with aborted sudden cardiac death. ECG— electrocardiogram; ECHO—echocardiogram; EP—electrophysiology; ICD—implantable cardioverter defibrillator; SVT; supraventricular tachycardia; VT—ventricular tachycardia.

CATHETER ABLATION

OVERVIEW OF CATHETER ABLATION

TYPE OF ARRHYTHMIA	SUCCESS RATE FOR CATHETER ABLATION (%)	ACCESS
WPW	85–95 (Right-sided) 95+ (Left-sided)	Transseptal or retrograde aortic approach for left-sided accessory pathways. Femoral right internal jugular or right subclavian for right-sided pathways.
AV node reentry	95+	Femoral
Atrial fibrillation: AV junction	95+	Femoral
Atrial flutter	80–90 for "typical atrial flutter"; 50–60 for "atypical atrial flutter"	Femoral
Atrial tachycardia	70–80	Femoral for right-sided atrial tachycardia; transseptal for left-sided atrial tachycardia

FIGURE 6-66. Summary of catheter ablation outcomes. In a number of large series [56], catheter ablation was used for treatment of the Wolff-Parkinson-White (WPW) syndrome. Approaches for left-sided accessory pathways have been highly successful. Transseptal approaches are highly useful in patients with aortic valve replacements, disease of the aortic arch, or congenital heart disease (associated with atrial septal defect). Patients with right-sided accessory pathways and Ebstein's anomaly may benefit from coronary artery mapping [57]. With atrioventricular (AV) node modification, the preferred approach is ablation of the slow AV nodal pathway rather than the fast pathway. With slow pathway modification, there is a less than 1% risk of requiring a permanent pacemaker [48]. Complete AV junction ablation requires the placement of a perma-

nent pacemaker and anticoagulation for chronic atrial fibrillation. The His bundle may need to be ablated from the left ventricular septum if necessary. AV modification is a means of altering AV node conduction without causing complete AV node block, thus making a permanent pacemaker unnecessary [58]. There is now investigation into reproducing the surgical Maze procedure with catheter techniques for cure of atrial fibrillation. Up to one third of patients may have a recurrence of their atrial flutter after an ablation and require a second ablation. A subset of patients may have recurrent (more stable) atrial fibrillation but not atrial flutter. The complications of an invasive procedure include bleeding, infection, emboli, and blood clots. The risk of tamponade (from catheter perforation), stroke, or death is less than 1%.

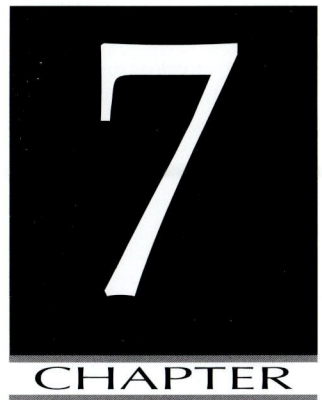

7

CHAPTER

HYPERTENSION

Edited by Norman K. Hollenberg

R. Wayne Alexander, John Amerena, Henry R. Black,
Emmanuel L. Bravo, Hans R. Brunner, Robert M. Carey,
William J. Elliott, Kathy K. Griendling, Randolph A. Hennigar,
Stevo Julius, Barry J. Materson, James A. Schoenberger,
Helmy M. Siragy, Bernard Waeber, Alan B. Weder, Matthew R. Weir

PATHOGENESIS OF HYPERTENSION

GENETIC AND ENVIRONMENTAL FACTORS

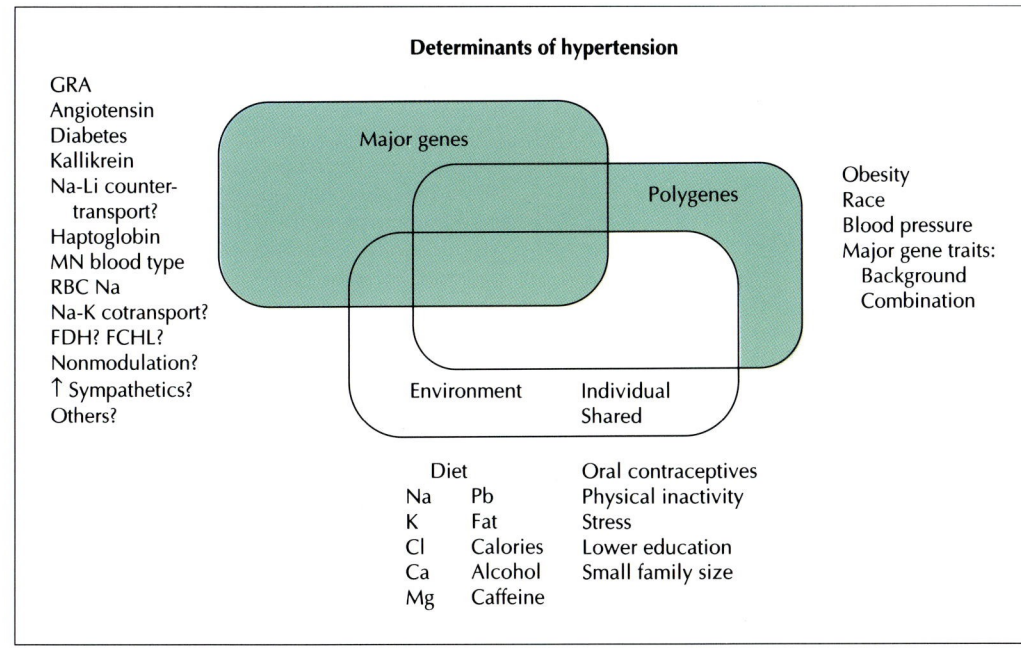

FIGURE 7-1. A model indicating the mechanisms by which essential hypertension could result from the combined effects of individual major genes that have a large impact on blood pressure, blended polygenes with small individual contributions, and environmental effects operating on individuals or within families. FCHL—familial combined hyperlipidemia; FDH—familial dyslipidemic hypertension; GRA— glucocorticoid-remediable aldosteronism. (*Courtesy of* Roger R. Williams, MD.)

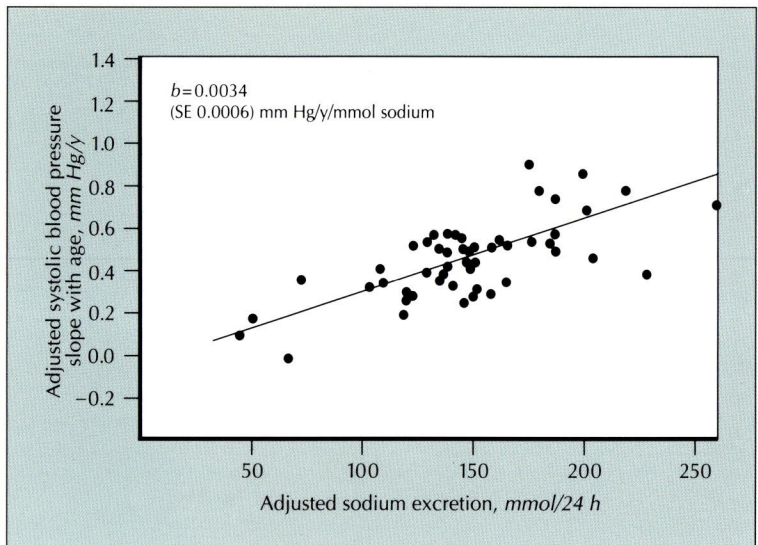

FIGURE 7-2. The INTERSALT Study [1] was undertaken to determine the relationship between urinary sodium excretion (which reflects dietary sodium intake) and blood pressure. Two hundred individuals were studied at each of 52 centers throughout the world. Averages for urinary sodium excretion (adjusted for age, sex, body mass index, and alcohol consumption) and blood pressure rise with age are shown. Each point represents one center. From the slope of the regression line (0.0034± mm Hg/y/mmoL Na$^+$) the magnitude of the effect of urinary sodium excretion can be estimated; reduction of sodium intake by 100 mmoL/d could reduce the rise in systolic blood pressure by 3.4 mm Hg for a period of 10 years [1].

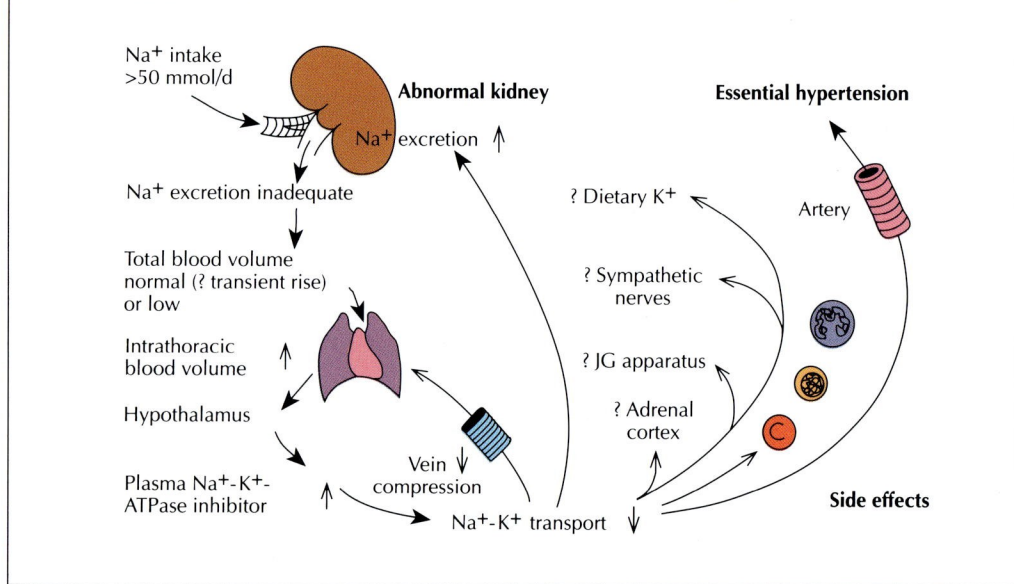

FIGURE 7-3. Hypothetical sequence of events demonstrating the role of sodium retention in cases of hypertension. An underlying genetic lesion may be expressed as a deficiency of sodium excretion, which becomes more apparent as sodium intake increases. The reduction in sodium excretion may initially cause a transient increase in total blood volume and a rise in intrathoracic blood volume. This change stimulates the hypothalamus to secrete a circulating sodium transport inhibitor, which adjusts renal sodium excretion, returning the sodium balance to normal. This balance is sustained only by a continuously high circulating sodium transport inhibitor, which raises the tone and reactivity of vascular smooth muscle. As a result, arterial pressure rises and venous compliance diminishes. Increased venous tone shifts blood from the periphery to the central vascular bed and thus raises intrathoracic pressure and perpetuates the stimulus for greater secretion of the sodium transport inhibitor. Total blood volume may be normal or low. (*Adapted from* de Wardener and MacGregor [2].)

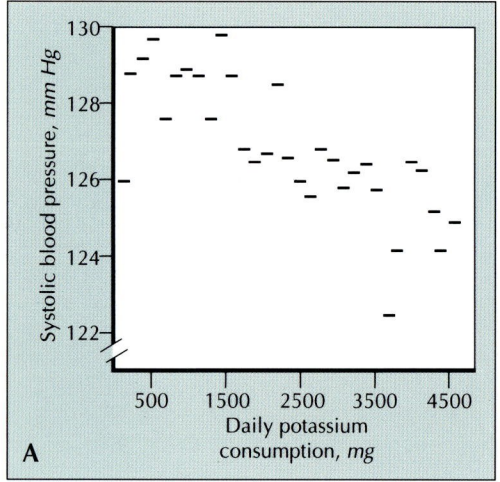

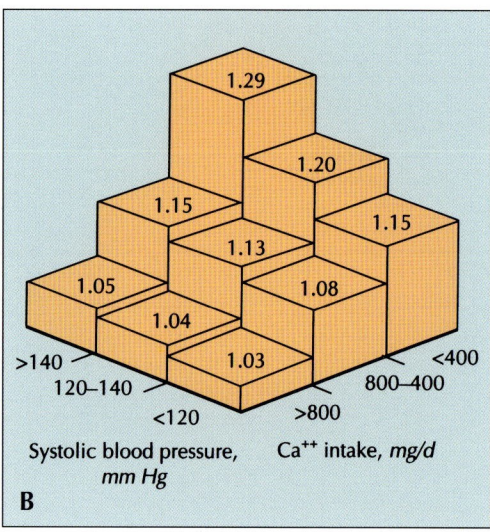

FIGURE 7-4. A, Dietary potassium intake is inversely related to systolic blood pressure. Displayed are values for systolic blood pressure and daily intake of potassium, as determined from dietary recall by participants in the NHANES-I cohort (a national population-based sample) [3]. **B,** Several dietary factors may interact to promote hypertension. The effect of dietary sodium and potassium on blood pressure may be conditioned by the contemporaneous intake of calcium. In this survey, continuous and graded relationships between blood pressure, dietary calcium, and the ratio of dietary sodium to potassium intake (numbers inside each bar) were found. Low calcium intake and an increased ratio of sodium to potassium intake were both associated with higher systolic blood pressure; the combination of both dietary habits was associated with the highest systolic blood pressure. (Part B *adapted from* Gruchow *et al.* [4].)

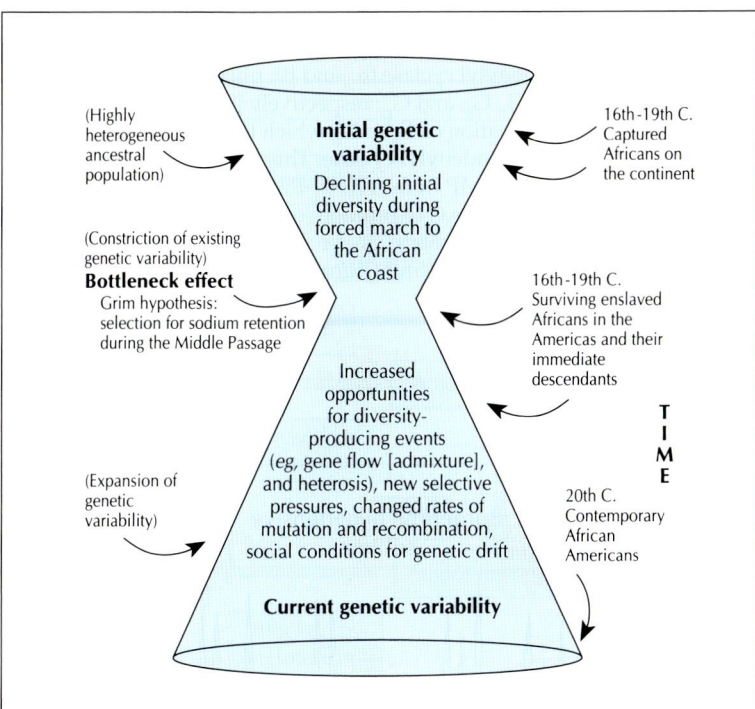

FIGURE 7-5. Blacks of the Western Hemisphere have a high prevalence of hypertension and a tendency toward salt sensitivity. One possible explanation of these observations is the slavery hypothesis [5]. Intense selection pressure mediated by the stresses of restricted availability of dietary salt and excessive salt wasting from heat and diarrhea is hypothesized to have resulted in a complement of genes optimized to conserve salt. As selection pressure waned and the salt-conserving genotype was exposed to a high-salt environment, excessive salt conservation is thought to have resulted in a tendency toward salt-sensitive hypertension. It is not clear that such genotypic homogeneity could have persisted during subsequent outbreeding [6].

ADRENERGIC NERVOUS SYSTEM

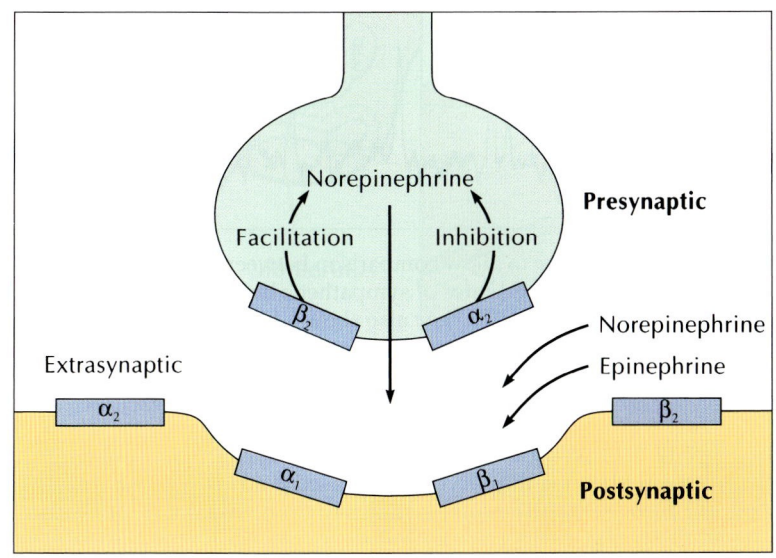

FIGURE 7-6. The pharmacologic and morphologic characteristics of peripheral adrenoreceptors. Nerve terminals within the autonomic nervous system are composed of several distinct receptor subtypes within and outside the synaptic cleft. These receptor subtypes have distinct and often opposing functional effects as well as different sensitivity to circulating catecholamines depending on their site and affinity. Stimulation of vascular postsynaptic α_1-receptors is predominantly by norepinephrine released locally (from the nerve terminal) and causes vasoconstriction. Extrasynaptic α_2-receptors, which are abundant in blood vessels, also cause vasoconstriction but are more responsive to circulating catecholamines (epinephrine > norepinephrine) because of their extrasynaptic location. Presynaptic α_2-receptors are more sensitive to locally released norepinephrine but decrease vasoconstriction by inhibiting further release of norepinephrine from the nerve terminal. Postsynaptic β_1-receptors are abundant in the heart and control heart rate and contractility while extrasynaptic β_2-receptors are predominantly located in resistance vessels in skeletal muscle and induce vasodilatation [7]. The overall physiologic effect of adrenergic receptor stimulation is determined by the degree of activation of the receptor subtypes and the balance between their opposing functional effects. (*Adapted from* Struyker Boudier [7].)

DISTRIBUTION AND PHYSIOLOGIC EFFECTS OF DIFFERENT ADRENERGIC RECEPTORS

TISSUE	RECEPTOR TYPE	EFFECT
Blood vessels	α_1 and α_2	Constriction
	β_2	Dilatation
Heart	β_1	Tachycardia; increased contractility
	α_1	Increased contractility
Bronchi	β_2	Relaxation
Thrombocytes	α_2	Aggregation
Kidneys	α_1 and α_2	Vasoconstriction
	β_1 and β_2	Renin release; inhibition tubular sodium reabsorption
Adipocytes	α_2	Inhibition lipolysis
	β_1, β_2, and β_3 (?)	Lipolysis

FIGURE 7-7. Adrenergic receptor subtype characterization by distribution and physiologic function. Subtypes of adrenergic receptors can be characterized by their distribution and physiologic function [7]. Along with variation in the distribution between organs there is variation in patterns of distribution within organs. For example, postsynaptic α_2-receptors are numerous in the peripheral vasculature but are present in greater numbers on the venous side of the circulation than on the arterial side. α- and β-receptors generally have opposite physiologic effects but in some organs, *eg*, the heart, the effects are complementary. β_3-receptors have been described recently in adipose tissue but their physiologic role is uncertain, although a role in lipolysis has been postulated [8].

MAJOR MECHANISMS OF RENIN RELEASE

Individual nephron signals
   Low macula densa sodium chloride (stimulates)
   Decreased afferent arteriolar pressure (stimulates)
Whole kidney modulating signals
   Angiotensin II negative feedback (inhibits)
   β-1 receptor stimulation (stimulates)
   Other humoral factors
     Vasopressin (inhibits)
     Atrial natriuretic peptide (inhibits)
     Dopamine DA-1 receptor (stimulates)
Local effectors
   Prostaglandins (stimulate)
   Nitric oxide (inhibits)
   Adenosine (inhibits)
   Kinins (stimulate)

FIGURE 7-13. Three major mechanisms are thought to govern renin release: 1) signals at the individual nephron, 2) signals involving the entire kidney, and 3) local effectors. Individual nephron signals include decreased sodium chloride load at the macula densa, which is the specialized group of distal tubular cells in approximation to the juxtaglomerular apparatus, and decreased afferent arteriolar pressure, which is probably mediated by a cellular stretch mechanism. Whole kidney signals include negative-feedback inhibition by angiotensin II at the juxtaglomerular cell, β_1-adrenergic receptor stimulation at the juxtaglomerular cell, and other hormonal factors. Local effectors include the prostaglandins E_2 and I_2, nitric oxide, adenosine, dopamine, and arginine vasopressin. The angiotensin II inhibitory feedback loop is thought to be the predominant and overriding mechanism that controls renin release in humans.

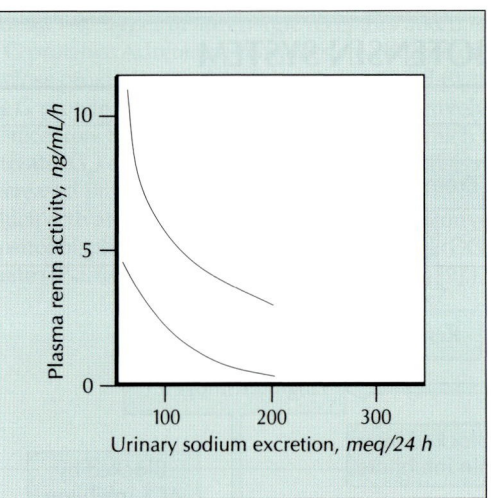

FIGURE 7-14. Relationship of plasma renin activity in ambulatory human subjects to the concurrent daily rate of urinary sodium excretion. The hyperbolic curves define the normal range. Approximately 25% of patients with untreated essential hypertension have low renin profiles, whereas approximately 15% have high renin profiles. Only 50% to 80% of patients with renovascular hypertension have elevated plasma renin activity. (*Adapted from* Brunner *et al.* [11].)

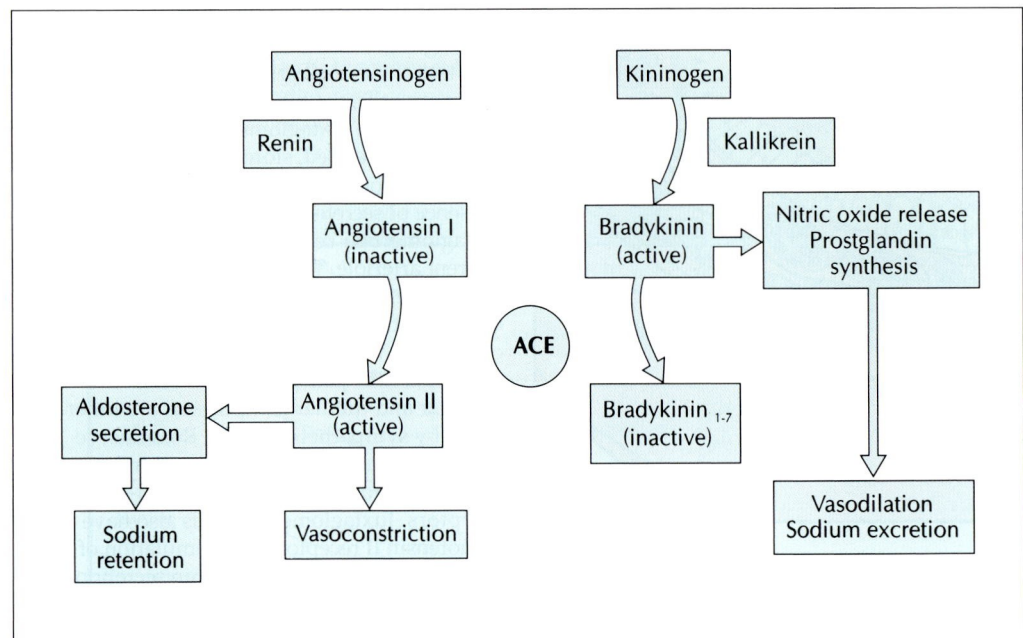

FIGURE 7-15. The actions of ACE. The left side of the figure demonstrates how the enzyme converts inactive angiotensin I to active angiotensin II. The right side depicts how ACE metabolizes bradykinin, an active vasodilator and natriuretic substance, to bradykinin$_{1-7}$, an inactive metabolite. ACE therefore increases production of a potent vasoconstrictor, angiotensin II, while promoting the degradation of a vasodilator, bradykinin. Both actions of ACE increase vasoconstriction, and inhibition of ACE leads to vasodilation and natriuresis. Bradykinin is formed by the action of the enzyme kallikrein on substrate kininogen. Bradykinin acts as a vasodilator and natriuretic substance by releasing nitric oxide (an endothelium-derived relaxing factor) and stimulating formation of prostaglandins E_2 and I_2.

CLASSIFICATION CRITERIA OF ANGIOTENSIN RECEPTOR SUBTYPES

	AT_1	AT_2
Potency order	Angiotensin II > angiotensin III	Angiotensin II = angiotensin III
Selective antagonists	Losartan (DuPont-Merck, Wilmington, DE)	PD 123177 (Morris Plains, NJ)
	EXP 3174 (DuPont-Merck)	PD 123319 (Morris Plains, NJ)
	DuP 532 (DuPont-Merck)	CGP 42112A (Basel, Switzerland)
	L-158,809 (Merck, West Point, PA)	
	SKF 108566 (Philadelphia, PA)	
	GR 117289 (Galaxo, Research Triangle Park, NC)	
	SR 47436 (Sanofi, Montpelier, France)	
Effector pathways	↑ Phospholipase C	↓ Guanylate cyclase
	↑ Phospholipase D	
	↓ Adenylate cyclase	
Sensitivity to dithiothreitol (sulfhydryl reducing agents)	↓ Binding	↑ Binding
Effect of GppNHp	↓ Affinity	No change
	↑ Hill coefficient to no change ~1	

FIGURE 7-16 Pharmacologic and biologic evidence suggests the existence of heterogeneity in the angiotensin (AT) II receptor population. AT_1 receptors are those selectively blocked by biphenylimidazoles, such as the compound Losartan (DUP 753), whereas AT_2 binding sites are blocked by tetrahydroimidazopyridines, typified by PD 123177. AT_1 receptors are more responsive to angiotensin II than to angiotensin III, are positively coupled to phospholipase C, and may be negatively coupled to adenylyl cyclase. AT_2 binding sites may be involved in modulation of the intracellular content of cGMP. Angiotensin II and angiotensin III are equally potent in binding to AT_2 receptors. AT_1 receptors mediate vascular smooth muscle contraction, aldosterone secretion, pressor and tachycardic responses, angiotensin II–induced water consumption, and hypertension in cases of renal artery stenosis. The physiologic effects of AT_2 receptor activation are unknown. GppNH—guanylyl-imidodiphosphate. (*Adapted from* Griendling *et al.* [12].)

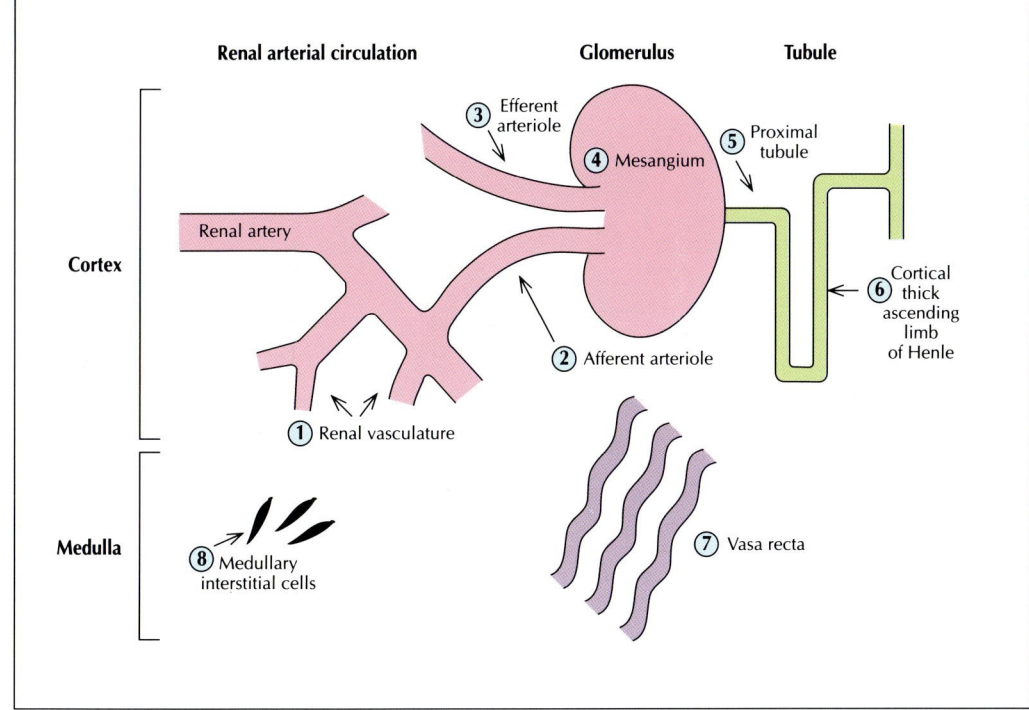

FIGURE 7-17. The renal tissue localization of angiotensin II receptors and the physiologic action stimulated by these receptors. Vasoconstriction occurs when angiotensin II acts at receptors in the arcuate and interlobular arteries, the afferent and efferent arterioles, and the medullary vasa recta. Angiotensin II preferentially constricts the efferent arteriole, thereby increasing glomerular filtration pressure; however, angiotensin II also acts on mesangial cell receptors to produce cellular contraction and reduce glomerular filtration. Angiotensin II receptors also are localized to the proximal tubule and the cortical thick ascending loop of Henle cells, which cause sodium resorption. Angiotensin II receptors recently have been found on renomedullary interstitial cell membranes, but the physiologic significance of these receptors is still unknown. 1—vasoconstriction; 2—limited vasoconstriction, and inhibition of renin synthesis and release; 3—preferential vasoconstriction; 4—contraction; 5 and 6—sodium reabsorption; 7—vasoconstriction; 8—unknown action.

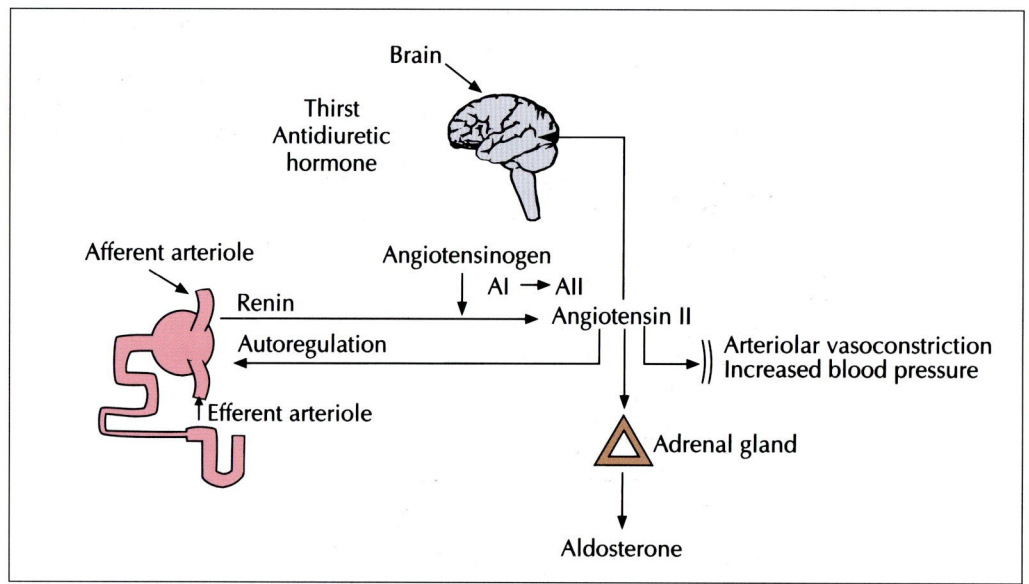

FIGURE 7-18. Angiotensin II has three major effects: 1) arteriolar vasoconstriction; 2) renal sodium retention; and 3) increased aldosterone biosynthesis, all of which result in sodium retention. These effects work together to maintain arterial blood pressure as well as blood volume. Angiotensin II also stimulates the sympathetic nervous system, particularly the thirst center in the hypothalamus.

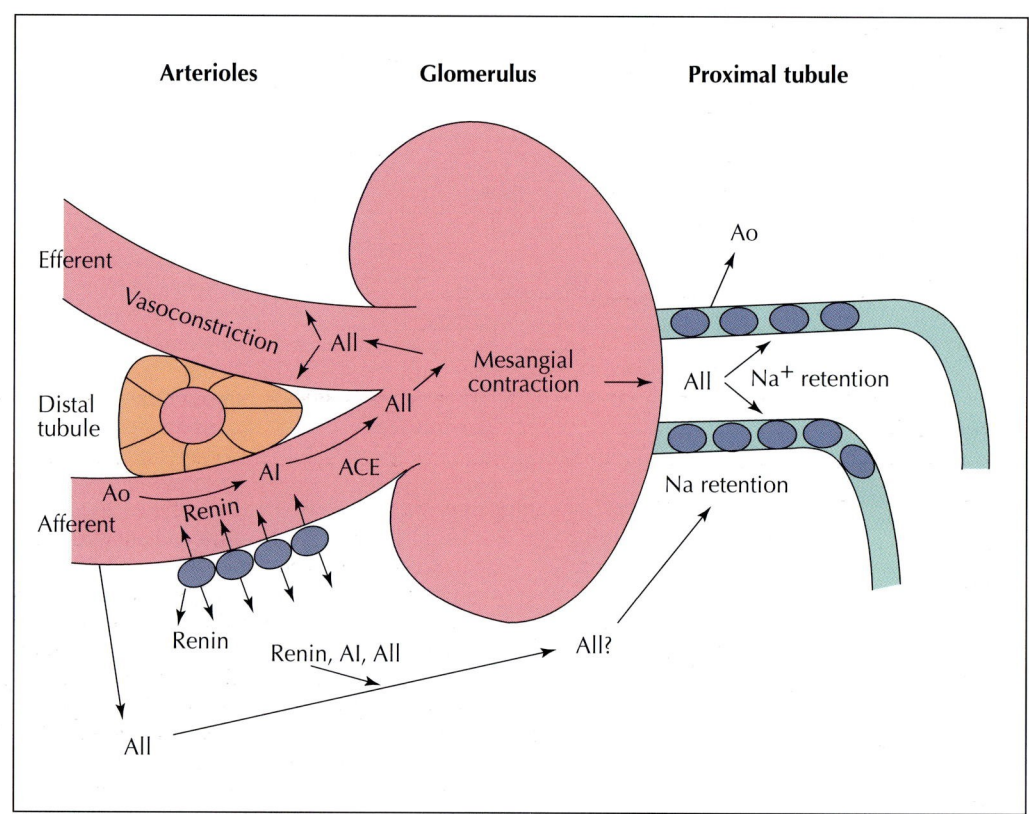

FIGURE 7-19. The cell-to-cell (*ie*, paracrine) effects of angiotensin II in the kidney. Angiotensinogen (Ao) either circulates to the kidney from the site of production in the liver or is synthesized in proximal tubular cells in the kidney. It is likely that renal interstitial angiotensinogen is derived predominantly from proximal tubular synthesis. Renin is synthesized and released from the juxtaglomerular cells into the afferent arteriolar lumen or into the renal interstitium. Angiotensin I (AI) is generated in the afferent arteriole and is converted to angiotensin II (AII) by angiotensin-converting enzyme (ACE). AII can cause mesangial cell contraction or efferent arteriolar constriction. AII can also be filtered at the glomerulus and may subsequently act at the proximal tubular cells to increase sodium reabsorption. In the renal interstitium, renin can cleave angiotensinogen to produce angiotensin peptides; these peptides may act at vascular and tubular structures. Angiotensin peptides may also be synthesized in and released from renal juxtaglomerular cells. Alternatively, the peptides may be taken up by renal cells from either interstitial fluid or the renal circulation.

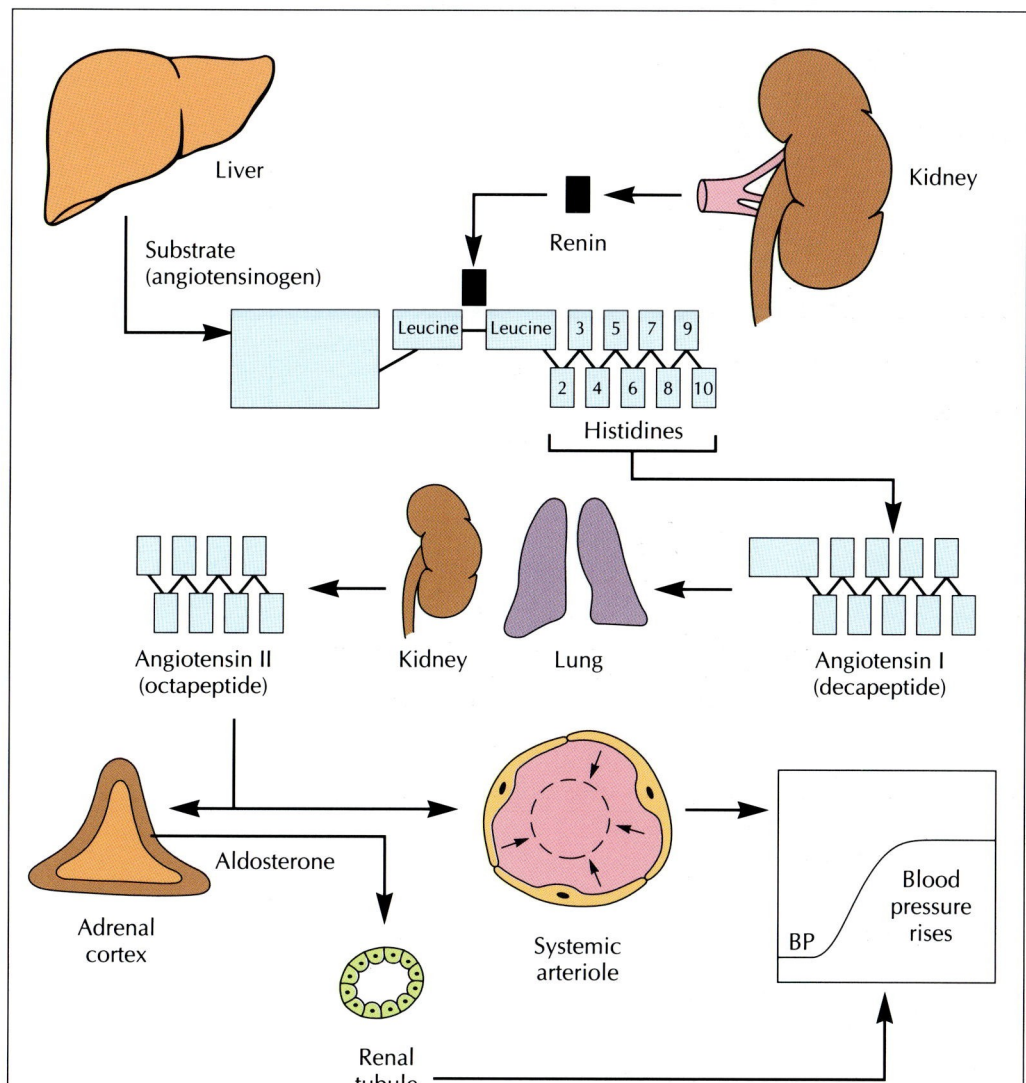

FIGURE 7-20. The circulating components of the renin-angiotensin system [13]. The circulating renin-angiotensin system plays a role in body fluid regulation, electrolyte homeostasis, and blood pressure control.

Liver

Substrate (angiotensinogen)

Renin

Kidney

Leucine Leucine 3 5 7 9

2 4 6 8 10

Histidines

Angiotensin II (octapeptide)

Kidney

Lung

Angiotensin I (decapeptide)

Adrenal cortex

Aldosterone

Systemic arteriole

BP Blood pressure rises

Renal tubule

VASCULAR MECHANISMS

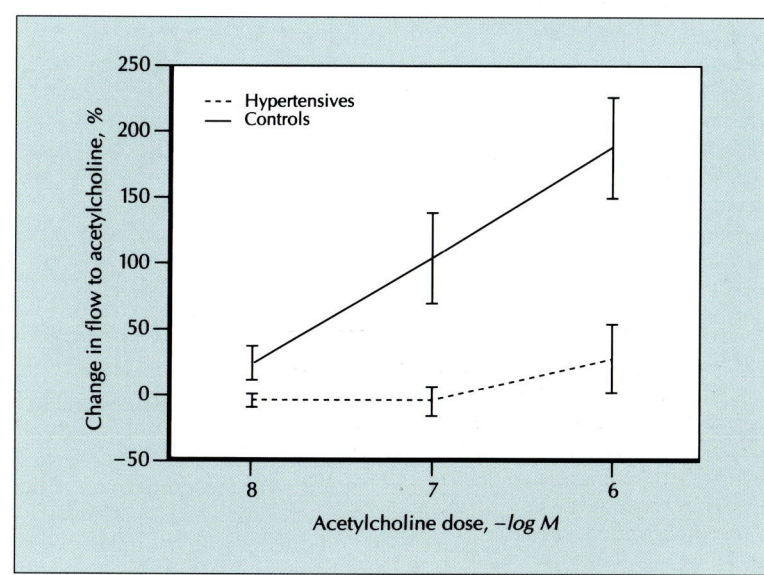

Change in flow to acetylcholine, %

- - - Hypertensives
— Controls

Acetylcholine dose, −*log M*

FIGURE 7-21. Evidence for defective endothelium-dependent relaxation in the coronary arteries of hypertensive subjects. Infusion of acetylcholine into the left anterior descending coronary artery of normal subjects leads to a dose-related increase in flow. The mechanism is presumably through the increased release of nitric oxide in the resistance circulation. In contrast, the increase in flow in response to acetylcholine infusion is markedly impaired in hypertensive subjects with ventricular hypertrophy. Maximal dilator capacity in response to nonendothelium-dependent dilators is not different between the two groups. The loss of this endothelial vasodilator mechanism probably contributes to disordered coronary flow regulation. Loss of endothelial-dependent vasodilator mechanisms could be associated more generally with the increase in vascular resistance in hypertension. M—molar. (*Adapted from* Treasure *et al.* [14].)

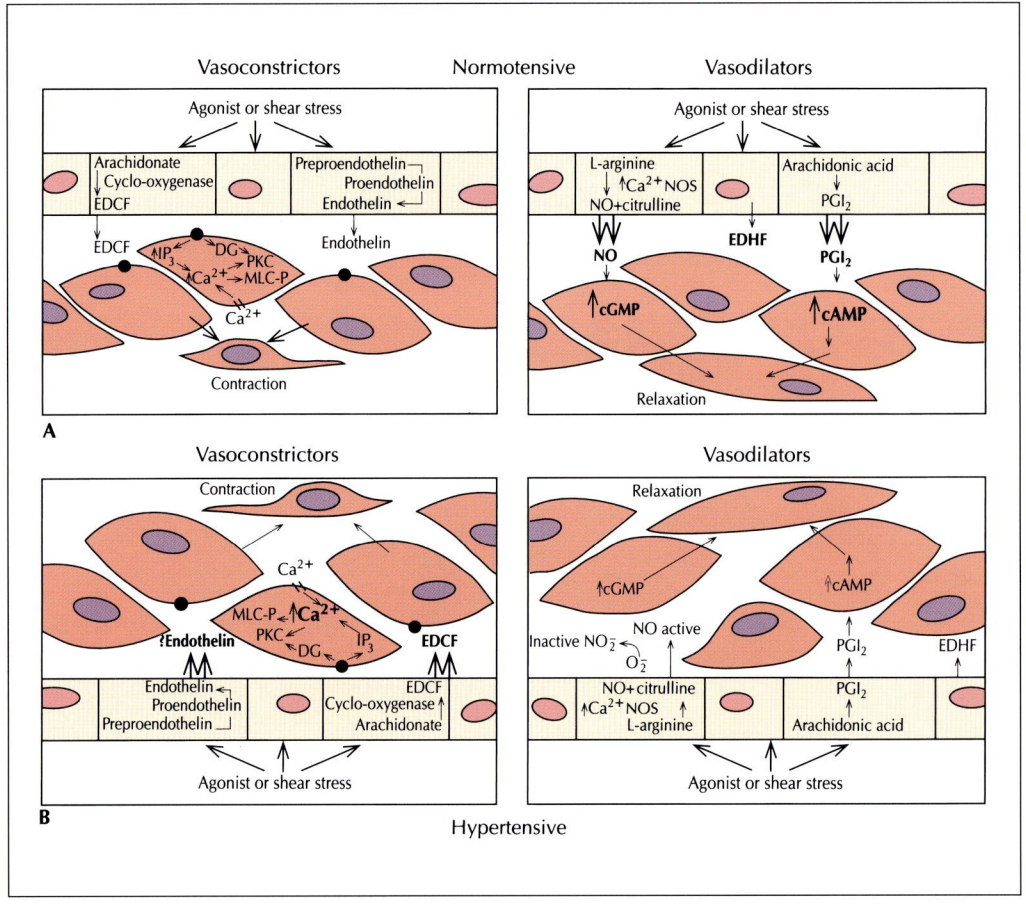

FIGURE 7-22. Endothelium-dependent vasodilator and vasoconstrictor mechanisms: modification in hypertension. Normal endothelial cells secrete both vasodilators, the most prominent of which are nitric oxide (NO), prostacyclin (PGI_2), and endothelium-derived hyperpolarizing factor (EDHF), and vasoconstrictors, including endothelin and endothelium-derived contracting factor (EDCF) [15]. Vessel tone is dependent on the balance between these factors and on the ability of the smooth muscle cell to respond to them.

A, In normotensive vessels there is a predominance of vasodilator secretion. These substances may also contribute to the inhibition of smooth muscle cell growth or hypertrophy. The relative concentrations of the vasoconstricting/vasodilating agents are indicated by the relative sizes of the arrows and bold type in the illustration.

B, In hypertension, release of vasoconstrictor substances may predominate [16]. In addition, vasodilator release may be decreased or, alternatively, the vasodilator itself may be inactivated by superoxide anion. Under certain circumstances, endothelin can also be growth-promoting, thereby contributing to smooth muscle cell hypertrophy or hyperplasia and intimal thickening. The biochemical pathways activated by endothelial agonists and by contracting and relaxing factors acting on smooth muscle can also be affected in hypertension. NO, produced by the conversion of L-arginine to citrulline, traverses the endothelial cell membrane, and activates the smooth muscle cell guanylate cyclase to generate intracellular cGMP. PGI_2 and EDCF are produced via cyclo-oxygenase action on arachidonic acid. PGI_2 relaxes vessels by increasing smooth muscle cell cAMP; the mechanism of action of EDCF is unknown. Endothelin is made and modified by endothelium. It then stimulates the phospholipase C pathway in smooth muscle to produce the second messengers inositol trisphosphate (IP_3) and diacylglycerol (DG), which in turn activate the Ca^{2+} and protein kinase C (PKC) signaling pathways. This leads to phosphorylation of the myosin light chain (MLC-P), causing contraction. Alterations of any of these signals could easily augment contraction or decrease the ability of the vessel to dilate.

<table>
<tr><td>

POTENTIAL MECHANISMS OF DEFECTIVE ENDOTHELIAL-DEPENDENT VASODILATION IN HYPERTENSION

Decreased production of nitric oxide

Increased degradation of nitric oxide by free radicals

Defective responsiveness of vascular smooth muscle to endothelial-dependent vasodilators

Increased production of endothelial-derived vasoconstrictors

</td></tr>
</table>

FIGURE 7-23. Possible mechanisms responsible for defective endothelium-dependent vasodilatation in hypertension. As described earlier, nitric oxide is perhaps the most important of the endothelium-derived relaxing factors. Therefore, decreased production of nitric oxide or increased degradation by free radicals markedly impairs vasodilatation [17]. The smooth muscle itself may exhibit decreased responsiveness to ambient endothelium-derived vasodilators. Finally, an imbalance in the production of endothelium-derived relaxing and contracting factors to favor excess production of the latter may also contribute to defective vasodilatation.

MEMBRANE ION TRANSPORT AND/OR CONTENT ABNORMALITIES THAT HAVE BEEN REPORTED IN HUMAN ESSENTIAL HYPERTENSION

Increased Ca^{2+} concentration in platelets

Decreased Na^+-Ca^+ exchange

Decreased Ca^{2+}-ATPase activity

Decreased activity of the Na^+/K^+-ATPase leading to increased intracellular Na^+ concentration

Increased Na^+ content in red and white blood cells

Low Na^+/K^+/(^+2Cl-) cotransport activity

Increased Na^+-Li^+ countertransport

Increased Na^+-H^+ exchange

Figure 7-24. Membrane ion transport or content abnormalities that have been reported in human essential hypertension. Studies of ion transport and content in cells from hypertensive patients are numerous. Many ion transporters have been examined, and many have been found to be altered in platelets or erythrocytes of subsets of hypertensive patients. This table summarizes the abnormalities identified in various cell types in human essential hypertension. In the following figures, each will be considered separately.

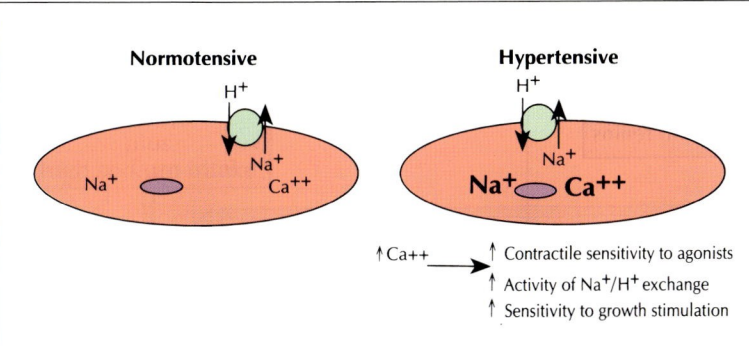

Figure 7-25. Unifying concept linking increased growth and contractility with ion abnormalities in vascular smooth muscle in hypertension. It has become apparent that human hypertension is associated with abnormalities of ion transport in vascular smooth muscle that result in an increase in intracellular Na^+ and Ca^{2+}. The increase in intracellular Ca^{2+} could enhance contractile sensitivity to agonists and increase activity of Na^+/H^+ exchanger. The resulting alkalinization, as well as the increased calcium, could lead to increased sensitivity to growth stimulation. Therefore, most of the important pathophysiologic features of the disease are potentially explainable in the context of abnormalities of ion transport.

SECONDARY HYPERTENSION

Approximately 5% of patients with hypertension have secondary hypertension, including renovascular hypertension, hypertension secondary to parenchymal renal disease, Cushing's syndrome, aldosterone-producing tumors, and pheochromocytoma.

RENOVASCULAR HYPERTENSION

CLINICAL CLUES SUGGESTING RENOVASCULAR HYPERTENSION

Systolic/diastolic epigastric, subcostal, or flank bruit

Accelerated or malignant hypertension

Unilateral small kidney discovered by any clinical study

Severe hypertension in child or young adult, or after age 50 y

Sudden development or worsening of hypertension at any age

Hypertension and unexplained impairment of renal function

Sudden worsening of renal function in hypertensive patient

Hypertension refractory to appropriate three-drug regimen

Impairment in renal function in response to angiotensin-converting enzyme inhibitor

Extensive occlusive disease in coronary, cerebral, and peripheral circulation

Figure 7-26. Causes of renal artery stenosis. Lesions of the renal arteries associated with hypertension can be divided into several categories. Atherosclerosis, which tends to occur in older individuals, and fibromuscular hyperplasia, which tends to occur in young women, are the most common causes of significant renal artery stenosis. Other causes are uncommon. Renal artery stenosis occurs in the absence of hypertension and may be present in a hypertensive patient without being the cause of the hypertension. Therefore, the functional significance of the renal artery lesion as a cause of hypertension must be validated by appropriate tests. The clinical characteristics listed here should raise the index of clinical suspicion for renovascular hypertension.

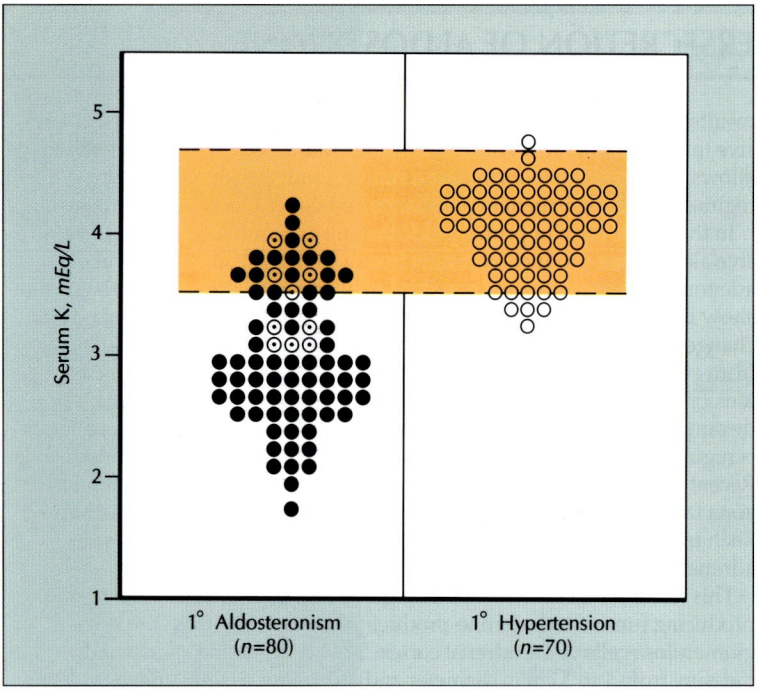

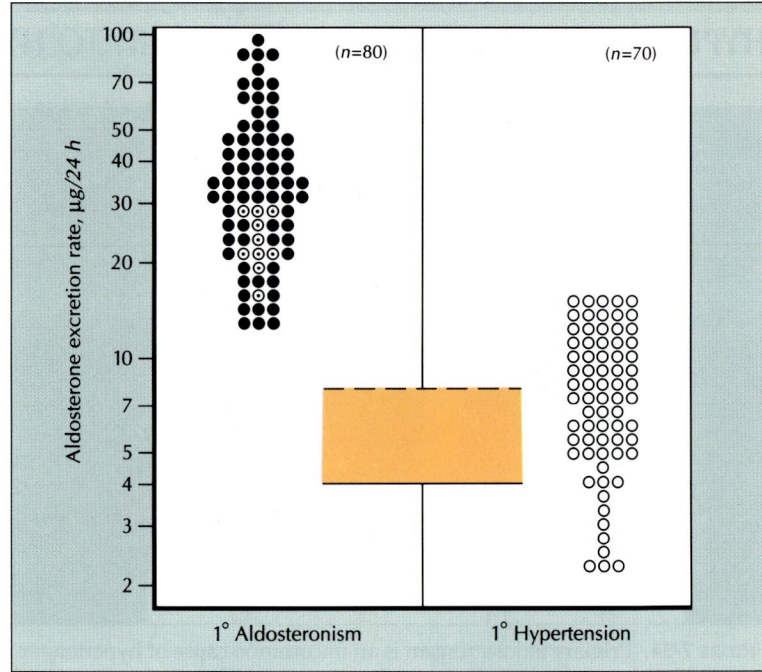

FIGURE 7-36. Serum potassium concentrations in cases of primary aldosteronism and essential hypertension. Patients were age- and sex-matched. No medication had been given for at least 2 weeks, and the patients were on an isocaloric diet containing 110 mEq of sodium and 80 mEq of potassium per day for 5 days. Blood was drawn between 8 AM and 9 AM after an overnight fast and at least 30 minutes of supine rest. Each point represents the mean of at least three determinations. For patients with primary aldosteronism, *solid circles* represent adenomas (*n*=70) and *open circles with dotted centers* represent hyperplasia (*n*=10). The *shaded area* represents 95% confidence intervals (3.5 to 4.6 mEq/L) of values obtained from 60 healthy subjects.

Twenty-two patients (27.5%) with primary aldosteronism (17 with tumors and five with hyperplasia) had fasting serum potassium values of 3.5 mEq/L or greater, while four (5.7%) subjects with essential hypertension had values below 3.5 mEq/L. Serum potassium values below 3.0 mEq/L were usually associated with the presence of a tumor. Ten patients (six of 17 with tumors and four of five with hyperplasia) remained persistently normokalemic, despite intake of high dietary sodium for 3 days. (*Adapted from* Bravo *et al.* [20].)

FIGURE 7-37. Aldosterone excretion rate after 3 days of high dietary sodium intake. Clinical conditions and patient identification are the same as in Fig. 6-16. Urine was collected on the third day of high sodium intake. The level of aldosterone in the urine was measured by a radioimunoassay technique as the pH 1.0 conjugate 18-glucuronide metabolite. The *shaded area* represents the mean (4.0 μg/24 h) and +2 SD (8.0 μg/24 h) of values obtained from 47 healthy subjects. No patient with primary aldosteronism had a value within the 95% normal range. Ten patients (14%) with primary hypertension had values that fell within the range obtained in patients with primary aldosteronism. Using a reference value of greater than 14 μg/24 h after a high sodium intake for 3 days, the sensitivity and specificity of the test were 96% and 93%, respectively. (*Adapted from* Bravo *et al.* [20].)

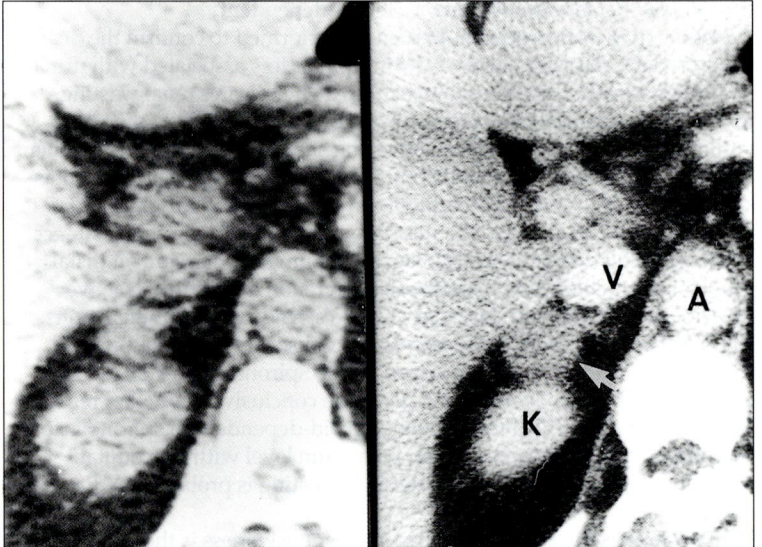

FIGURE 7-38. Computed tomography scan of a right adrenal tumor (*arrow*) before (*left*) and after (*right*) contrast injection. The tumor is located between the vena cava (v) and the upper pole of the kidney (k). A—aorta.

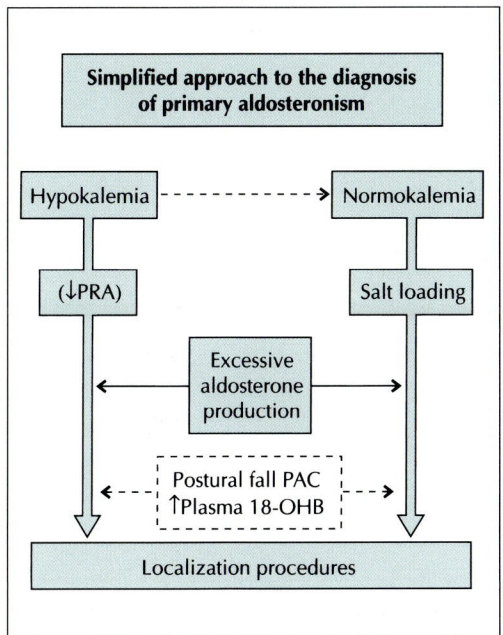

Simplified approach to the diagnosis of primary aldosteronism

- Hypokalemia ----→ Normokalemia
- (↓PRA) | Salt loading
- Excessive aldosterone production
- Postural fall PAC ↑Plasma 18-OHB
- Localization procedures

FIGURE 7-39. A simplified approach to the diagnosis of primary aldosteronism. Priority of evaluation should be given to patients with a history of spontaneous hypokalemia, marked sensitivity to potassium-wasting diuretics, or refractory hypertension in whom other causes of secondary hypertension (*ie*, renal parenchymal disease, renovascular disease, pheochromocytoma) have been eliminated. Patients with significant hypokalemia, suppressed plasma renin activity (PRA) (< 2 ng/mL), or an increased aldosterone excretion rate (> 14 μg/24 h) have unequivocal evidence of primary aldosteronism. Patients with equivocal findings will require salt loading. This evaluation can be accomplished on an outpatient basis by adding 10 to 12 g sodium chloride to the patient's daily diet in addition to determining the values of serum potassium concentration and 24-hour urinary excretion of sodium, potassium, and aldosterone after 7 days of high salt intake. A 24-hour urinary sodium value of at least 250 mEq gives some assurance that the patient has ingested the amount of salt prescribed.

Under these conditions, an aldosterone excretion rate greater than 14 μg/24 h suggests inappropriate aldosterone production. The development of hypokalemia or suppressed PRA are corroborative data, but their absence does not rule out a diagnosis of inappropriate aldoster-one production. Demonstration of a postural decrease in plasma aldosterone concentration (PAC) and overnight recumbent plasma 18-hydroxycorticosterone (OHB) greater than 100 ng/dL indicate the presence of an adenoma. For localization, adrenal computed tomography should be performed first and considered diagnostic if an adrenal mass is clearly identified. When the results of computed tomography are inclusive adrenal venous sampling for aldosterone levels may be performed. (*Adapted from* Bravo [21].)

PHEOCHROMOCYTOMA

IMPORTANT FACTS ABOUT PHEOCHROMOCYTOMAS

About 30% of pheochromocytomas reported in the literature are found either at autopsy or at surgery for an unrelated problem

Thirty-five percent to 76% of pheochromocytomas discovered at autopsy are clinically unsuspected during life

The average age of diagnosis in those whose disease was discovered before death was 48.5 y, while the average in those diagnosed at autopsy was 65.8 y

Death was usually attributed to cardiovascular complications

FIGURE 7-40. *Pheochromocytoma* is a tumor of neuroectodermal origin that produces excessive quantities of catecholamines, thereby causing hypertension with a constellation of signs and symptoms that can mimic several other acute medical and surgical disorders. Early recognition, accurate localization, and appropriate management of benign pheochromocytomas nearly always result in complete cure. If unrecognized, these tumors cause lethal disease that can lead to significant cardiovascular morbidity and mortality and particularly to sudden death during surgical and obstetric procedures.

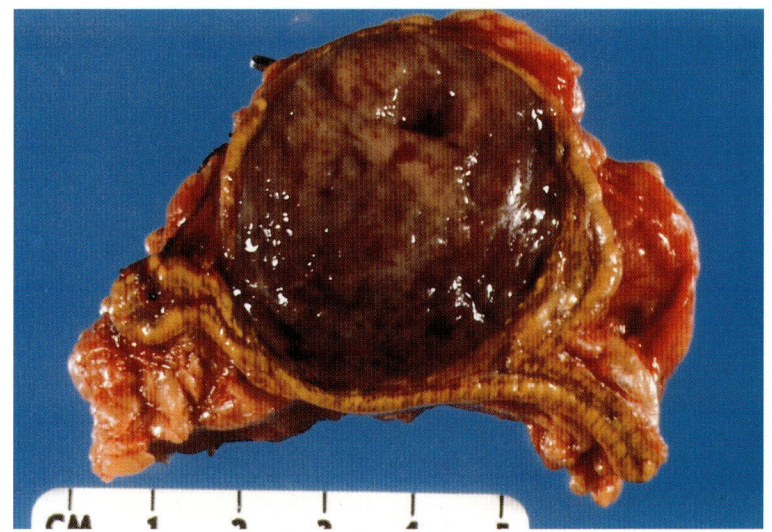

FIGURE 7-41. Typical gross pathologic features of an adrenal pheochromocytoma. The specimen is ovoid and encapsulated, surrounded by a rim of yellow tissue grossly resembling adrenal cortex. The lesion is rubbery to moderately firm and is pale gray to dusky brown. Pheochromocytomas have a strong affinity for chromium salts. Immersion in chromium salt fixative (Zenker's or potassium dichromate solution) changes the tumor from the usual pale-gray appearance to a dark-black color as cytoplasmic catecholamines are oxidized.

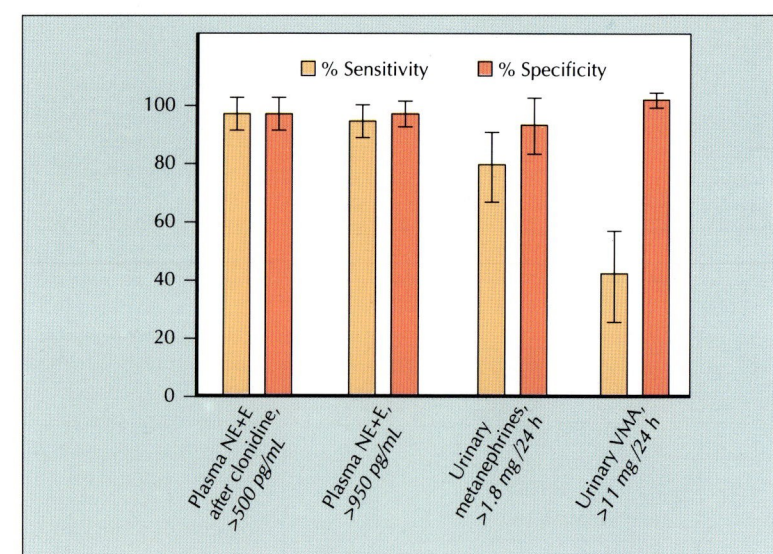

FIGURE 7-42. Priorities for detection of pheochromocytoma. The detection of pheochromocytoma requires a high degree of clinical alertness. Pheochromocytoma usually occurs as a sporadic event. These tumors, have, however, been associated with other clinical syndromes, such as von Recklinghausen's disease, von Hippel-Lindau's disease, Werner's syndrome (MEN type I), Sipple's syndrome (MEN type IIA), mucocutaneous neuroma (MEN type IIB), acromegaly, and Cushing's syndrome. Most patients present with labile hypertension, diaphoresis, headaches, and tachycardia with or without palpitations; however, as many as 30% of all reported cases were unsuspected during life and the tumors were found either at autopsy or during surgery for an unrelated condition.

FIGURE 7-43. Sensitivity and specificity of various tests for pheochromocytoma. Measurement of plasma catecholamines appears to be the most sensitive test, and measurement of urinary vanillylmandelic acid (VMA) seems to be the least sensitive. When levels of catecholamines are elevated, all three tests provide excellent specificity. A combination test of plasma catecholamines and 24-hour urinary metanephrines provides nearly 100% accuracy (sensitivity and selectivity) in the diagnosis of pheochromocytoma. NE+E—norepinephrine plus epinephrine. All values are mean ± 2SE.

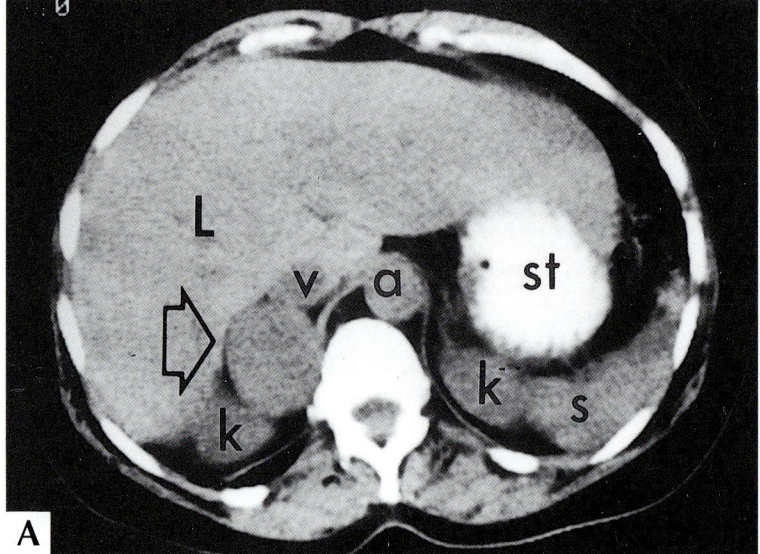

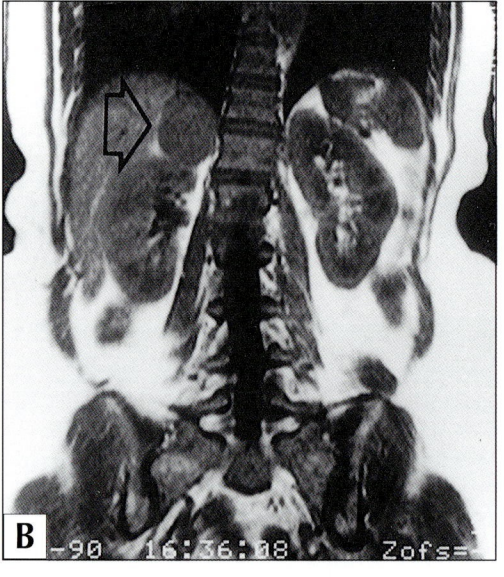

FIGURE 7-44. Three modalities used to localize pheochromocytomas. Computed tomography (CT) can accurately detect tumors larger than 1.0 cm and has a localization precision of approximately 98%, although it is only 70% specific. CT is the most widely applied and accepted modality for the anatomic localization of pheochromocytomas. Magnetic resonance (MR) imaging is equally sensitive to CT and lends itself to *in vivo* tissue characterization, which is not possible with CT. MR imaging is nearly 100% sensitive but is only 67% specific. Scintigraphic localization with radioiodinated ^{131}I-meta-iodobenzylguanidine (MIBG) provides both anatomic and functional characterization. Although this modality is less sensitive than CT and MR imaging, it has a specificity of 100%. Ninety-seven percent of pheochromocytomas are found in the abdominal region, with most found in the adrenal

glands. Less likely sites are the thorax (2% to 3%) and the neck (1%). Multiple tumors may arise in 10% of adults. Familial pheochromocytomas are frequently bilateral or arise from multiple sites. Pheochromocytomas occurring in children are more commonly bilateral and more frequently lie outside the adrenal glands than in adults. Tumor localization not only serves to confirm the diagnosis of pheochromocytoma but also assists the surgeon in planning the surgical strategy. Advances in noninvasive imaging techniques now provide safe and reliable means of localizing pheochromocytomas regardless of their location.

A, CT of the adrenal glands (*arrow*). **B** and **C**, Coronal and sagittal MR imaging sections of the abdomen, respectively. Pheochromocytomas demonstrate high signal intensity on a T_2-weighted image, (*continued*)

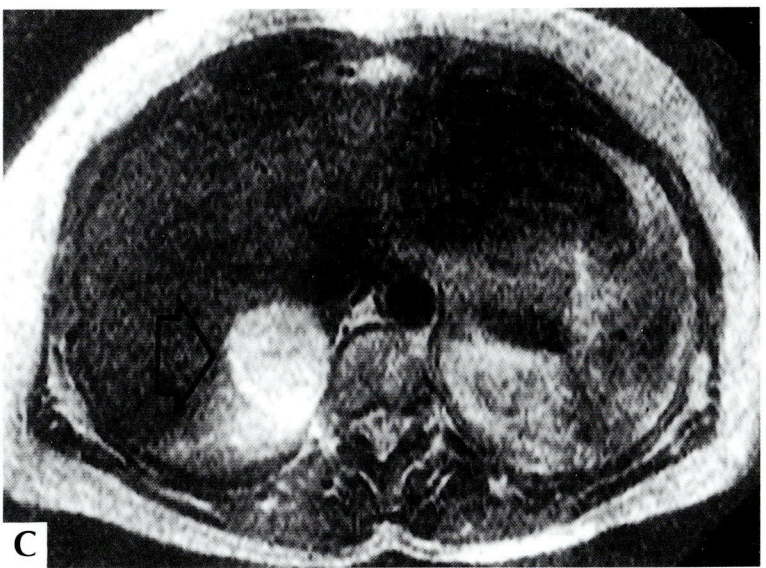
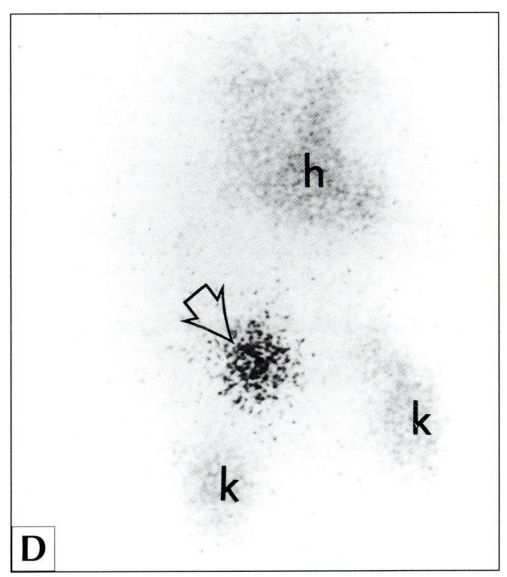

FIGURE 7-44. (*continued*) unlike a benign tumor, which has a low signal intensity. **D**, Scintigraphic localization of a pheochromocytoma (arrow) with radioiodinated 131I-MIBG. This modality provides both anatomic and functional characterization of a tumor. Because 131I-MIBG is actively concentrated in sympathomedullary tissue through the catecholamine

pump, the administration of drugs that block the reuptake mechanism (*eg*, tricyclic antidepressants, guanethidine, labetalol) may result in false-negative results [22]. a—aorta; h—heart; k—kidney; L—liver; s—spleen; st—stomach; v—vena cava. (Part B *from* Bravo [23]; with permission.)

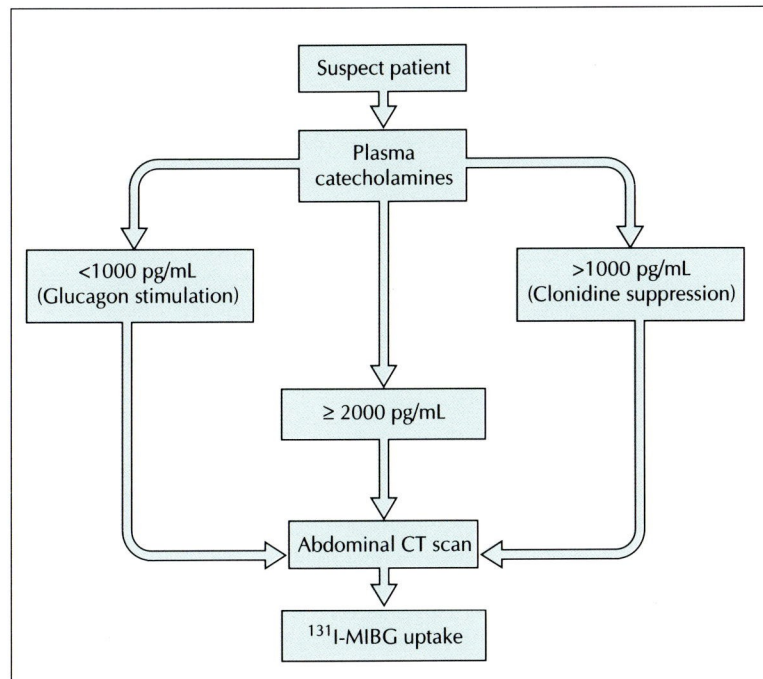

FIGURE 7-45. Diagnostic strategies in pheochromocytoma. Priority of evaluation is given to patients with the signs and symptoms detailed in Fig. 7-42. Concentrations of plasma norepinephrine and epinephrine are measured after the patient has rested in a supine position for at least 30 minutes. Caffeine and nicotine are prohibited for at least 3 hours before testing. Values of 2000 pg/mL or greater are considered pathognomonic for pheochromocytoma. Values between 1000 and 2000 pg/mL require a clonidine suppression test. Abdominal computed tomography (CT) or magnetic resonance imaging is then performed in patients with clinical and biochemical features suggestive of pheochromocytoma. Approximately 5% of patients may have plasma catecholamines of 1000 pg/mL or less. If the clinical presentation strongly suggests pheochromocytoma in these patients, further evaluation should be performed. Such evaluation may include measurement of urinary catecholamine metabolites or a glucagon stimulation test. For patients with arterial pressure greater than 160/100 mg Hg or if coexistent medical problems make sudden increases in blood pressure risky, pretreatment with 10 mg of oral nifedipine, 30 minutes before testing, will attenuate any increases in blood pressure without interfering with catecholamine release. MIBG—meta-iodobenzylguanidine.

NONPHARMACOLOGIC THERAPY

In most patients with hypertension, therapy should begin with or certainly include nonpharmacologic therapy.

TRIAL RESULTS ON EFFICACY OF INTERVENTIONS FOR PRIMARY PREVENTION OF HYPERTENSION

DOCUMENTED EFFICACY	LIMITED OR UNPROVED EFFICACY
Weight loss	Stress management
Reduced sodium intake	Potassium (pill supplementation)
Reduced alcohol consumption	Fish oil (pill supplementation)
	Calcium (pill supplementation)
Exercise	Magnesium (pill supplementation)
	Macronutrient alteration
	Fiber supplementation

FIGURE 7-46. Trial results on the efficacy of interventions for the primary prevention of hypertension. It is ideal to prevent hypertension from becoming clinically evident in genetically susceptible people. We have not yet learned how to select our own genes, but it is possible to manipulate our environment. Not surprisingly, the methods for primary prevention of hypertension are quite similar to those for nonpharmacologic treatment of established hypertension [24].

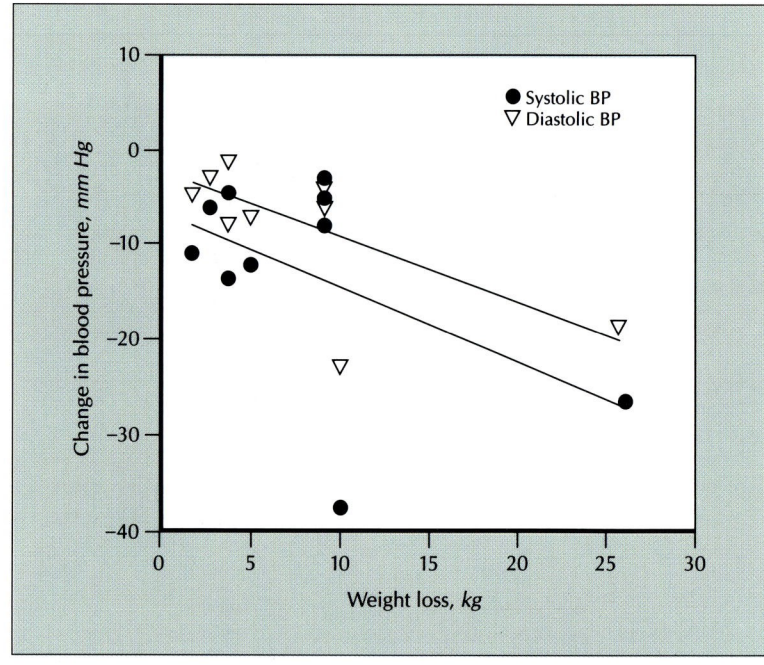

FIGURE 7-47. Regression of blood pressure (BP) following weight loss. Excellent studies have demonstrated that weight reduction, even without sodium restriction, is generally associated with substantial reductions in BP. Either the BP normalizes or the amount of drug required for normalization is reduced. The regression of change in systolic and diastolic BP on weight loss from 10 studies was reviewed by Johnston [25]. Although there is a great deal of scatter, greater weight loss does seem to correlate with greater reduction in BP ($r=0.50$ and $r=0.66$ for systolic and diastolic BP, respectively). The regression lines for systolic (lower) and diastolic (upper) pressures are nearly parallel.

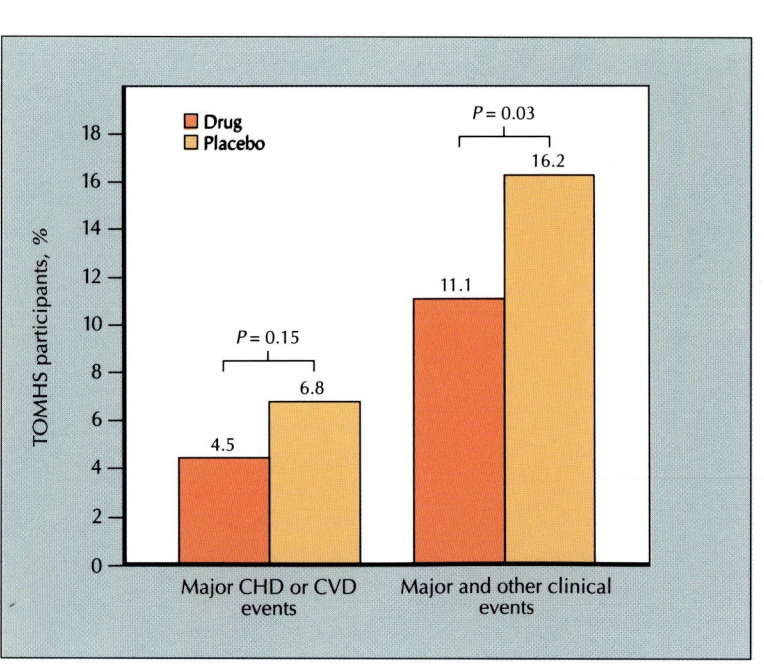

FIGURE 7-48. Despite the substantial reduction in blood pressure (-9.1/-8.6 mm Hg) achieved in the Treatment of Mild Hypertension Study patients with nutritional-hygienic intervention alone, the greater reduction achieved by the addition of drug therapy to nutritional-hygienic intervention (-15.9/-12.3 mm Hg) was sufficient to reduce major coronary heart disease (CHD) and cerebrovascular disease (CVD) events more than that achieved by nutritional-hygienic intervention alone [26]. This difference did not achieve statistical significance, but when major and all other clinical events were combined, drug treatment was significantly more effective than nonpharmacologic therapy alone. Other clinical events included hospitalization for cerebral transient ischemic attacks, definite angina or intermittent claudication, and peripheral arterial occlusive disease.

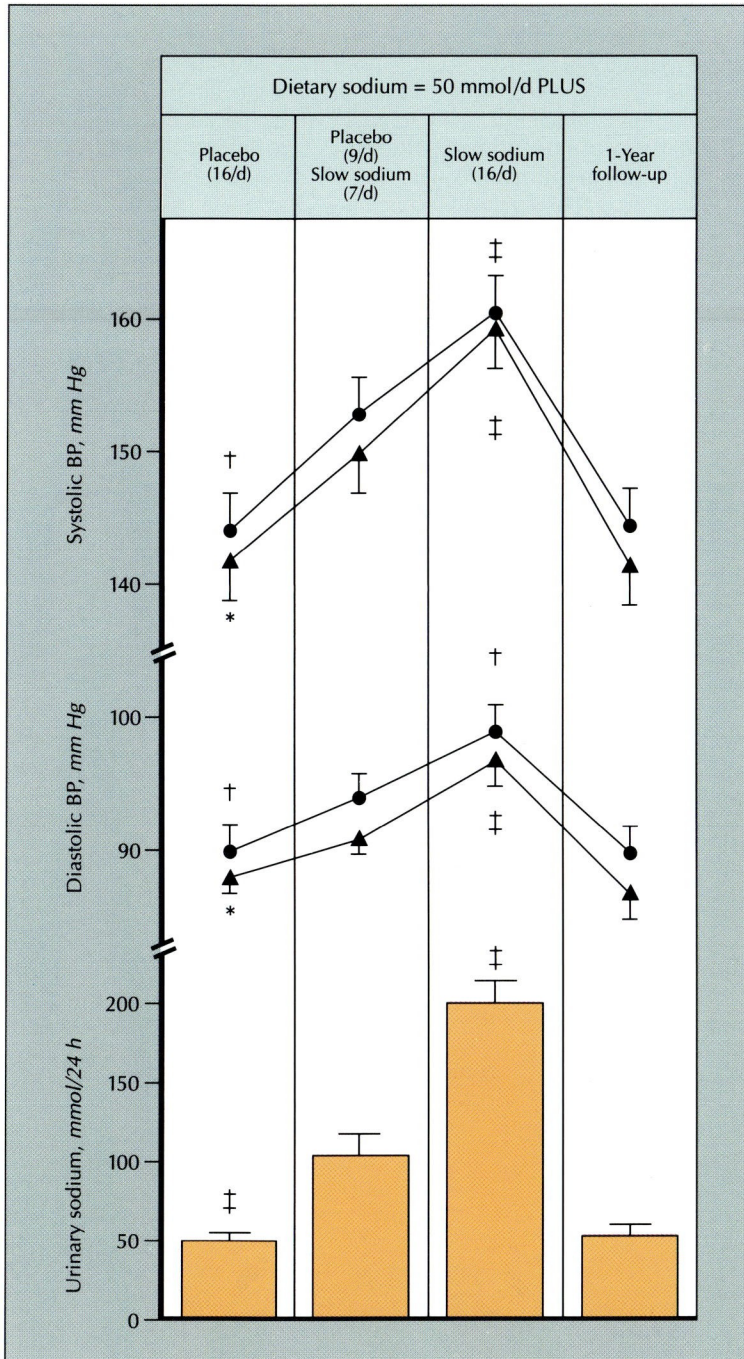

FIGURE 7-49. Data from one of many studies demonstrating the pressor effect of additional dietary sodium. These patients were placed on a sodium-restricted diet (about 50 mmol/d) to which either placebo or slow-release sodium tablets were added. Both systolic and diastolic blood pressures increased with the addition of sodium and returned to baseline when the supplement was discontinued. Patient samples included 19 patients (*closed circles*), three of whom required the addition of antihypertensive medications, and 16 patients (*closed triangles*) who were not taking medications. *Asterisks* indicate *P*<0.05; *daggers* indicate *P*<0.01; and *double daggers* indicate *P*<0.001 compared with the phase of seven slow-release tablets per day. *T-bars* indicate standard error. (*Adapted from* MacGregor et al. [27].)

NONPHARMACOLOGIC (NUTRITIONAL-HYGIENIC) THERAPY

ADVANTAGES

May reduce blood pressure substantially without drugs

Enhances efficacy of drug therapy

May prevent or mitigate adverse drug effects (*eg*, hypokalemia, hyperlipidemia)

May regress left ventricular hypertrophy

DISADVANTAGES

Labor-intensive, expensive

Requires high patient and provider motivation

Requires continuous monitoring and reinforcement

May not protect against coronary artery disease and cardiovascular disease, including stroke, as well as does the addition of drugs

FIGURE 7-50. Nonpharmacologic (nutritional-hygienic) therapy is of great potential value. However, there are disadvantages to its use as well.

PRINCIPLES OF PHARMACOLOGIC THERAPY

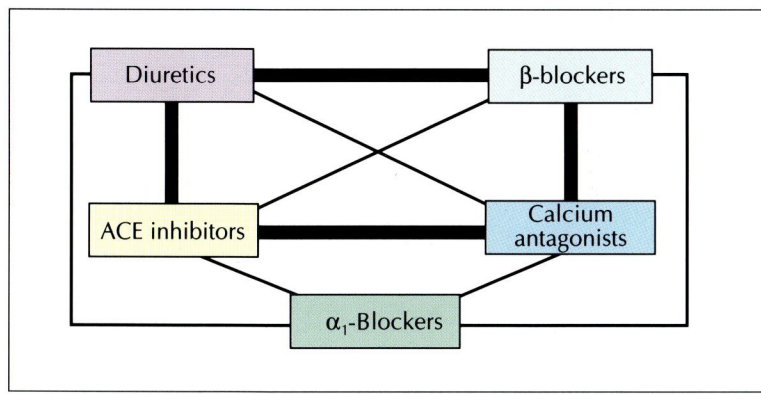

FIGURE 7-51. First-line antihypertensive drugs. Different classes of antihypertensive agents are proposed as first-line treatment for hypertension, *ie*, diuretics, β- (and α-) adrenergic blockers, angiotensin-converting enzyme (ACE) inhibitors, and calcium antagonists [28,29]. These agents reduce blood pressure by various mechanisms. They are therefore more or less effective, depending on the prevailing pathogenic factors in a given hypertensive patient. The angiotensin receptor blockers (ARBs) have been listed next to the ACE inhibitors. At the moment, they appear to be equivalent in efficacy with a lower frequency of adverse events and dropout associated with the ARBs. There is no reliable way to predict a positive response (*ie*, normalized blood pressure) to a specific therapeutic approach. A patient may respond favorably to one class of drugs exclusively or to several types of antihypertensive agents. Some patients may remain hypertensive regardless of the drug used as monotherapy. When necessary, different types of antihypertensive agents can be combined. Some drug associations are particularly effective (*thick lines*) [30].

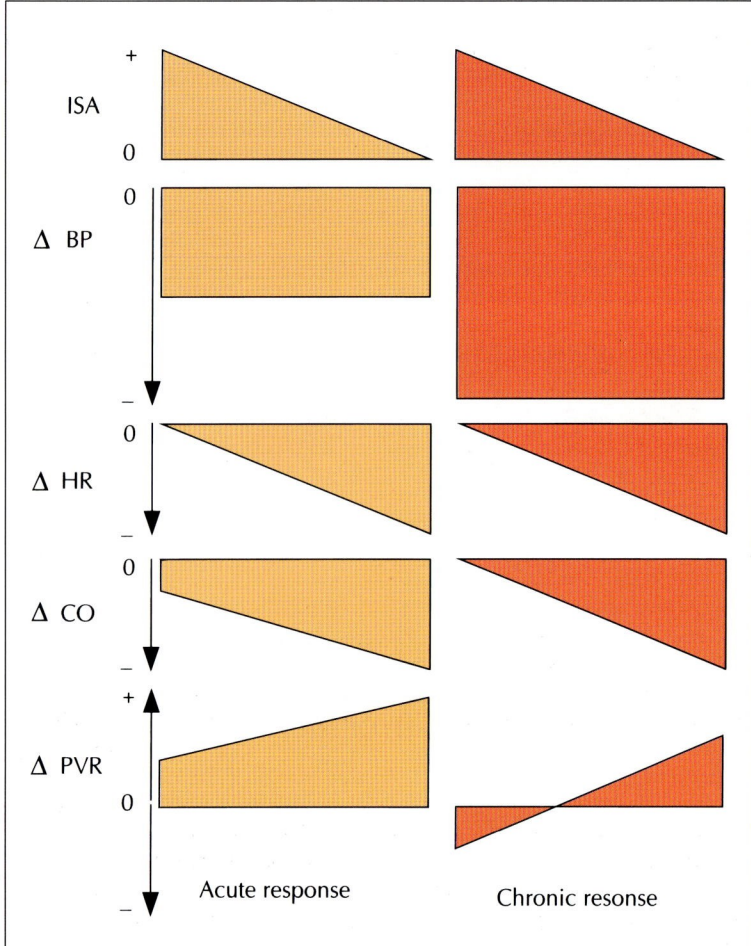

FIGURE 7-52. Hemodynamic response to β-adrenoceptor blockade. Blood pressure (BP) is determined by cardiac output (CO) multiplied by peripheral vascular resistance (PVR). Responses to β-adrenoceptor blockade, both acute and chronic, have been organized according to the amount of intrinsic sympathomimetic activity (ISA) shown by the individual agents. At initiation of treatment, heart rate (HR) and CO are reduced. This effect is most prominent in compounds with the least pronounced ISA [31]. These changes are accompanied by an increase in PVR that is inversely proportional to the degree of sympathomimetic activity. Although the blood pressure fall shortly after first administration (acute response) is modest, with continued treatment the blood pressure fall becomes substantially larger in many patients (chronic response). The magnitude of the fall in heart rate and cardiac output and the reactive rise in PVR vary with the degree of ISA, as is shown in this figure, but these responses do not account for the long-term fall in blood pressure.

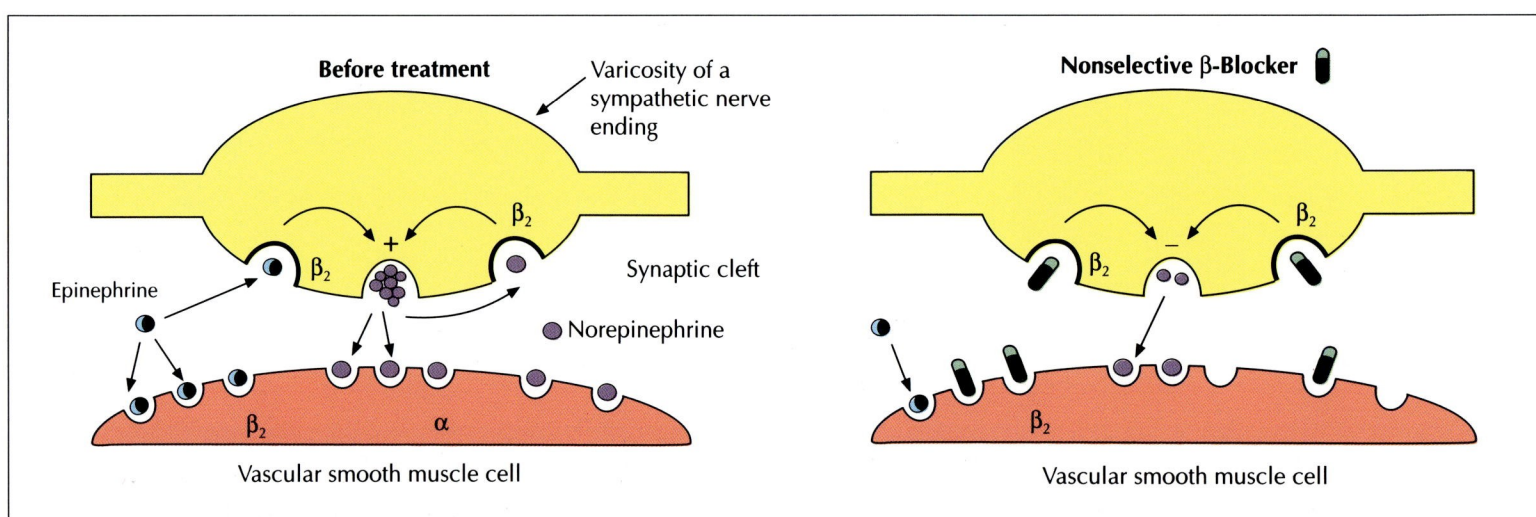

FIGURE 7-53. Reduced release of norepinephrine during blockade of presynaptic β-adrenoceptors. β₂-adrenoceptors are located on varicosities of sympathetic nerve endings. Activation of these receptors enhances the neurally induced release of norepinephrine. Blockade of presynaptic β₂ receptors causes a decrease in norepinephrine discharge (*right panel*). This effect may be an important contributor to the antihypertensive action of β-blockers.

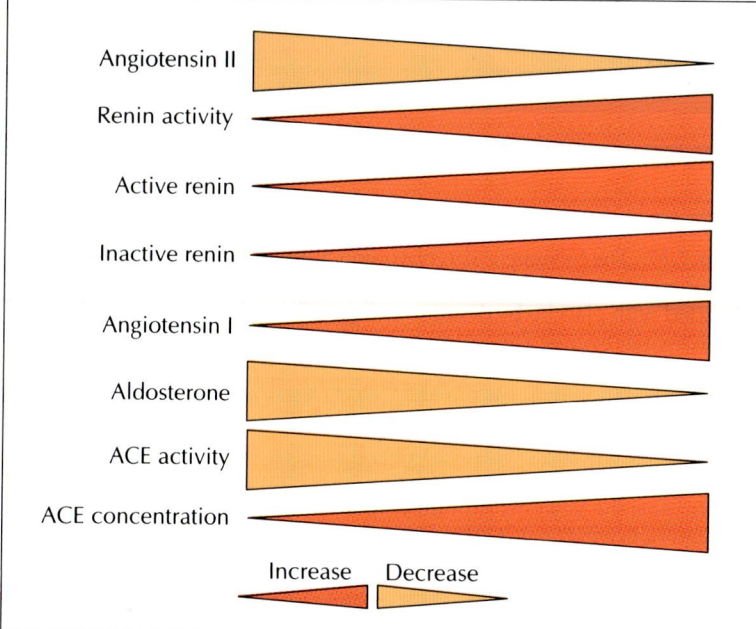

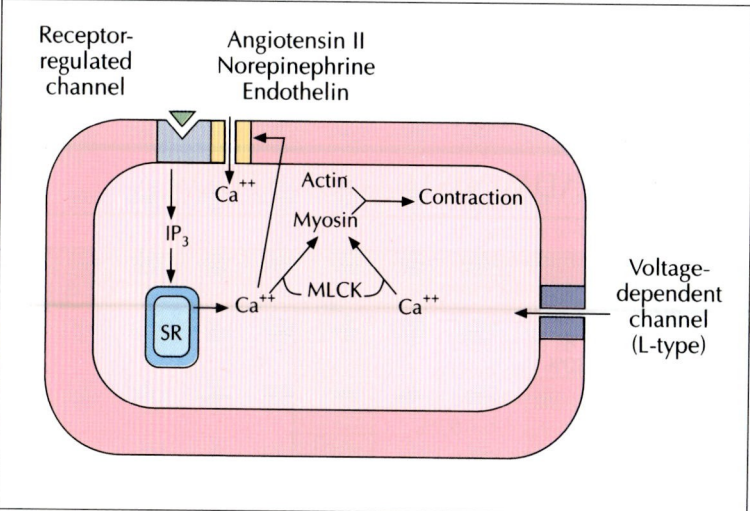

FIGURE 7-54. Effects of chronic angiotensin-converting enzyme (ACE) inhibition on the components of the renin-angiotensin system. Angiotensin II nearly disappears from the circulation during peak ACE inhibition [32]. Angiotensin II normally exerts a negative inhibitory feedback on renin secretion. During blockade of angiotensin II generation, plasma renin activity as well as active and inactive renin concentrations increase. The hyperreninemia is accompanied by a rise in plasma angiotensin I levels. Angiotensin II is a physiologic stimulus of aldosterone secretion. The plasma levels of this salt-retaining hormone are reduced during ACE inhibition. There is an induction of ACE synthesis during long-term treatment with ACE inhibitors.

FIGURE 7-55. Mechanism of action of calcium antagonists. Increased free calcium in the cytoplasm of vascular smooth muscle cells leads to vasoconstriction [33,34]. The calcium ion, after binding to calcium-binding proteins, activates a myosin light-chain kinase (MLCK), causing phosphorylation of myosin filaments followed by an interaction of these filaments with actin filaments and finally cell contraction. The calcium ion can enter the vascular smooth muscle cell by two main channels. The receptor-regulated channels cause, upon activation with an agonist (*eg*, angiotensin II, norepinephrine, endothelin), the formation of inositol trisphosphate (IP_3). This intracellular messenger triggers the release of calcium from the sarcoplasmic reticulum (SR). The rapid calcium mobilization by this pathway stimulates then sustains entry of calcium through the channel. Calcium antagonists block voltage-dependent channels. These channels allow the entry of calcium in response to cell depolarization.

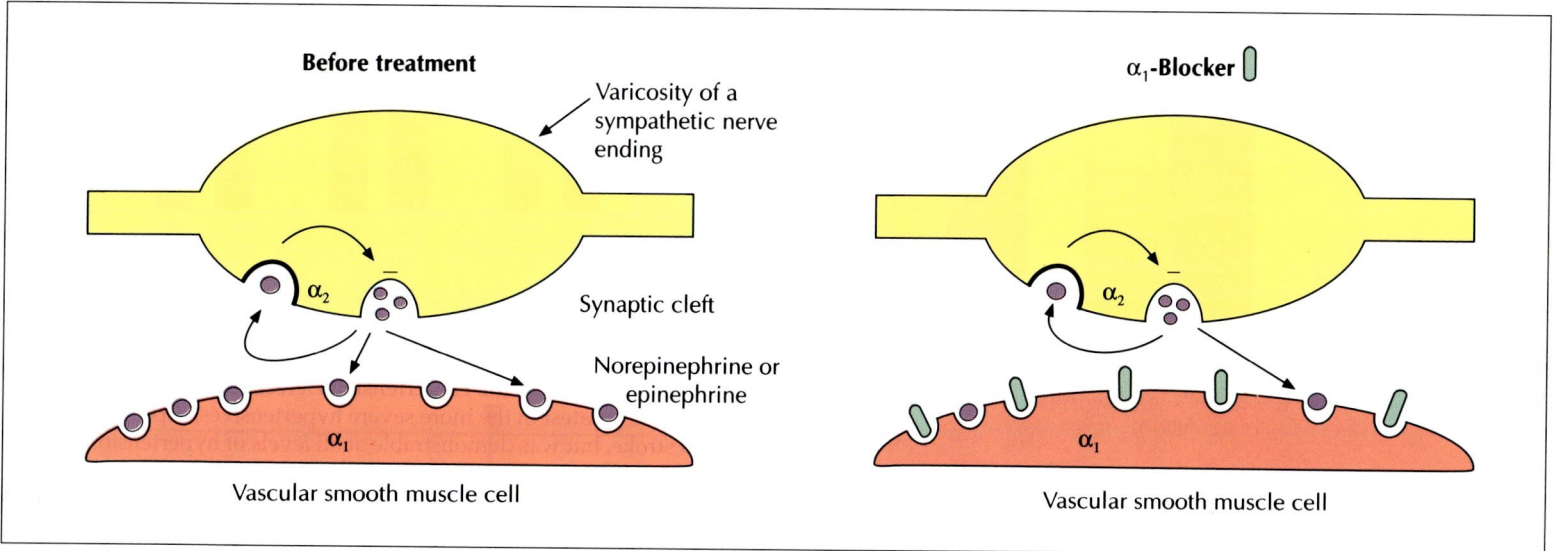

FIGURE 7-56. α_1-Adrenoceptor blocking agents. α_1-Blockers (doxazosin, prazosin, terazosin) lower blood pressure by preventing catecholamine-induced vasoconstriction [35]. In this illustration, norepinephrine released from the sympathetic nerve ending is depicted as *circles*, and the α_1-adrenergic blocking agent as an *oval*. The competitive action is confined to the vascular smooth muscle cell. These agents selectively block postsynaptic α_1-adrenoceptors. Catecholamines can still activate presynaptic α_2-receptors and thus exert an inhibitory action on norepinephrine release by the sympathetic nerve terminal. This probably accounts for the lack of reflex heart rate acceleration during α_1-adrenoceptor blockade. α_1-Blockers induce dilation of both arteries and veins. The effect on the capacitive system accounts for the prominent fall in postural blood pressure that occurs in some patients; this effect often limits the utility of these agents. α_1-Blockers are effective in reducing the symptoms of benign prostatic hypertrophy, which makes them an attractive choice in hypertensive elderly men with that disorder.

SITUATIONS IN WHICH AUTOMATED NONINVASIVE AMBULATORY BLOOD PRESSURE MONITORING DEVICES MAY BE USEFUL

"Office" or "white-coat" hypertension: blood pressure repeatedly elevated in office setting but repeatedly normal out of office

Evaluation of drug resistance

Evaluation of nocturnal blood pressure changes

Episodic hypertension

Hypotensive symptoms associated with antihypertensive medications or autonomic dysfunction

Carotid sinus syncope and pacemaker syndromes

FIGURE 7-72. Situations in which automated noninvasive ambulatory blood pressure monitoring devices may be useful. For carotid sinus syncope and pacemaker syndromes, electrocardiographic monitoring should also be employed.

CAUSES OF LACK OF RESPONSIVENESS TO THERAPY

A

Nonadherence to therapy

Cost of medication

Instructions not clear and/or not given to patient in writing

Inadequate or no patient education

Lack of involvement of patient in treatment plan

Side effects of medication

Organic brain syndrome (*eg,* memory deficit)

Inconvenient dosing

FIGURE 7-73. Causes of lack of responsiveness to antihypertensive therapy, including nonadherence (**A**), drug-related causes (**B**), and associated conditions (**C**).

B

Drug related causes

Doses too low

Inappropriate combinations (*eg,* two centrally acting adrenergic inhibitors)

Rapid inactivation (*eg,* hydralazine)

Drug interactions

Nonsteroidal anti-inflammatory drugs

Oral contraceptives

Sympathomimetics

Antidepressants

Adrenal steroids

Nasal decongestants

Licorice-containing substances (*eg,* chewing tobacco)

Cocaine

Cyclosporine

Erythropoietin

C

Associated conditions

Increasing obesity

Alcohol intake more than 1 oz/d of ethanol

Secondary hypertension

Renal insufficiency

Renovascular hypertension

Pheochromocytoma

Primary aldosteronism

Volume overload

Inadequate diuretic therapy

Excess sodium intake

Fluid retention from reduction of blood pressure

Progressive renal damage

Pseudohypertension

HYPERTENSION IN PREGNANCY

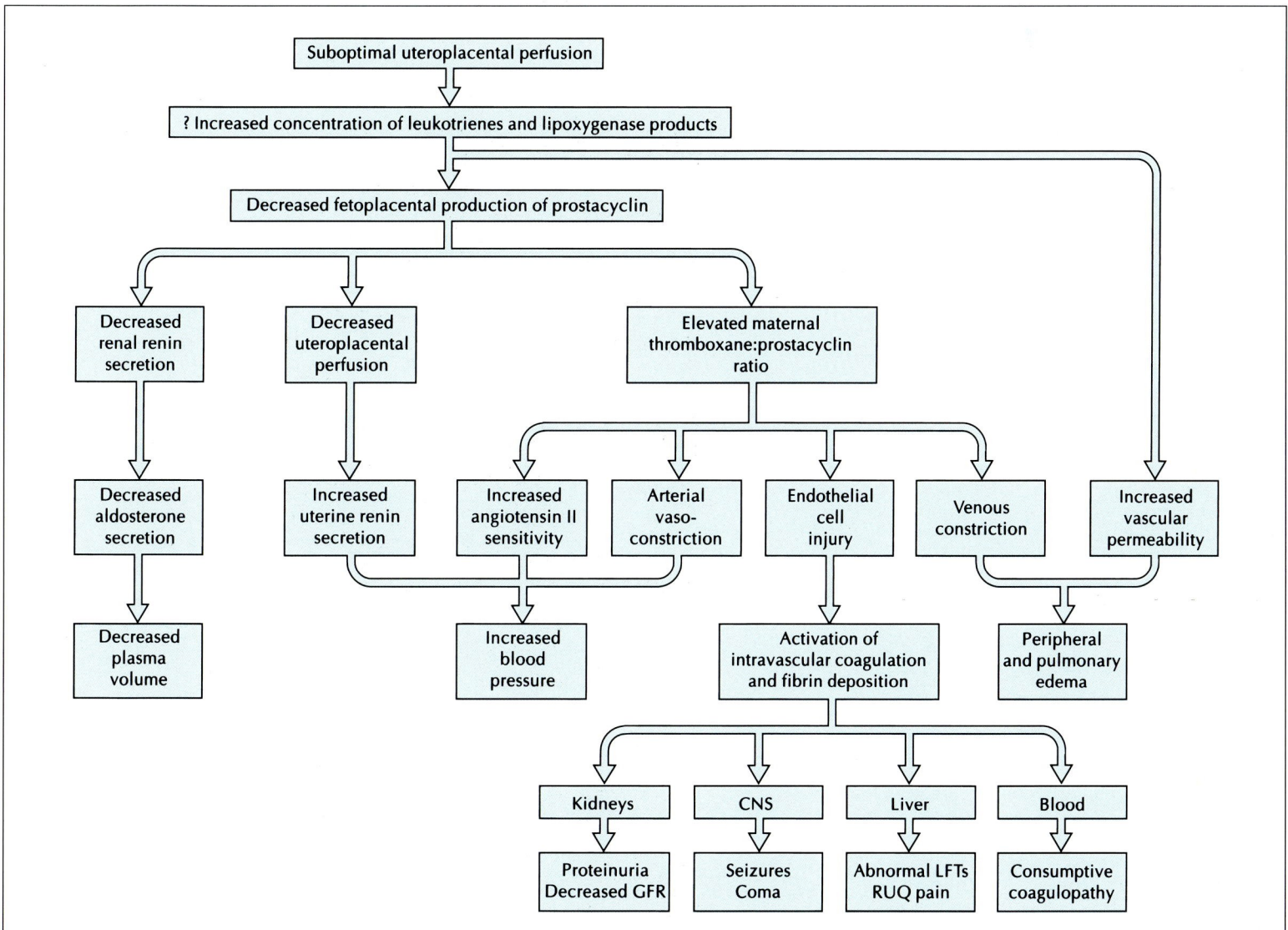

FIGURE 7-74. Scheme proposed to explain some of pathophysiologic factors thought to be operative in preeclampsia and their consequences [52]. Note that hypertension is but one feature of this complex illness. CNS—central nervous system; GFR—glomerular filtration rate; LFTs—liver function tests; RUQ—right upper quadrant.

CLASSIFICATION SCHEME FOR HYPERTENSION IN PREGNANCY

- Gestational hypertension or proteinuria

  Gestational hypertension: DBP > 110 once or 90 mm Hg twice, at least 4 h apart

  Gestational proteinuria: > 300 mg/24 h or two clean voided urines showing 2+ (1 g/L) dipstick proteinuria

  Gestational proteinuric hypertension (ie, preeclampsia)

- Chronic hypertension or chronic renal disease (*previously diagnosed*)

- Unclassified hypertension or proteinuria (usually from insufficient antenatal information)

- Eclampsia (convulsions during pregnancy or within 7 d of delivery not caused by convulsive disorders)

FIGURE 7-75. Classification of hypertensive disorders of pregnancy [53]. Knowledge of blood pressure before the 20th week of pregnancy is necessary to identify chronic hypertension. DBP—diastolic blood pressure.

DRUG THERAPY OF HYPERTENSION IN PREGNANCY

Recommended	Methyldopa—initial drug of choice against which all other antihypertensive agents must be tested; used for the longest time in the treatment of hypertension of pregnancy, so it has the best long-term follow-up data supporting its lack of toxicity; also lowers the number of midtrimester abortions in hypertensive women compared with placebo
	Hydralazine—used extensively, usually with methyldopa, and considered safe for mother and fetus by most obstetricians
	β-blockers (typically atenolol and labetalol)—used with caution and concern about growth retardation, fetal bradycardia, and the ability of the fetus to withstand hypoxic stress
	Nifedipine—used in Europe but teratogenic in rats (at 30 × the recommended dose in humans); used mostly in preterm labor
Not recommended	Diuretics—cause volume depletion, which has been associated with poor fetal outcomes
Contraindicated	ACE inhibitors—associated with lethal acute renal failure in neonates of women treated in the third trimester

FIGURE 7-76. Drug therapy for hypertension in pregnancy, according to the Working Group on High Blood Pressure in Pregnancy [54]. Angiotensin-converting enzyme (ACE) inhibitors are contraindicated, and both dietary sodium restriction and the use of diuretics are controversial and not recommended unless such agents were necessary in the pregravid state.

HYPERTENSION IN CHILDREN AND THE ELDERLY

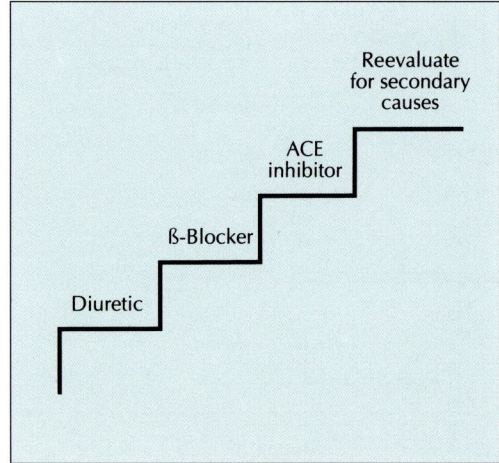

FIGURE 7-77. Treatment algorithm for hypertension in children, based on the 1987 Working Group Report [55]. This scheme closely follows earlier recommendations for using "stepped-care" therapy in adults. Since 1987, many pediatricians have also been considering the use of angiotensin-converting enzyme (ACE) inhibitors or calcium antagonists for the initial treatment of elevated blood pressures in children, particularly because many children develop impaired exercise tolerance with β-blockers and some physicians are concerned about the long-term metabolic effects of thiazide diuretics [56].

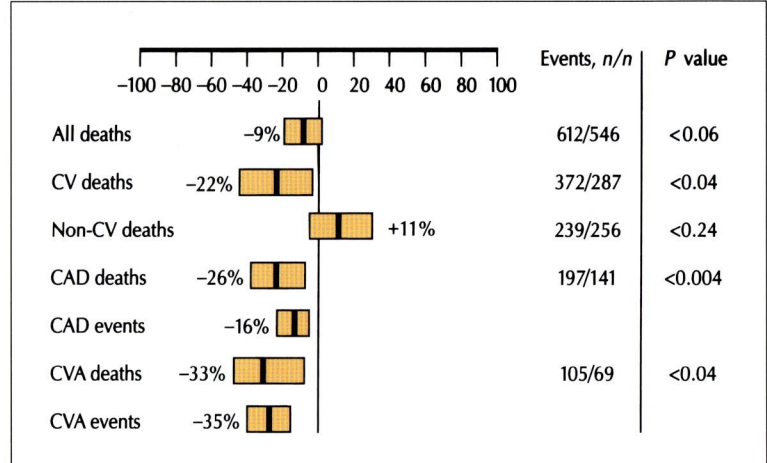

FIGURE 7-78. Results of a meta-analysis of six hypertension trials in the elderly, according to types of clinical event [57]. Unlike the situation in younger patients, the treatment groups (using diuretics and β-blocking agents) received nearly all of the expected beneficial reductions in fatal and nonfatal [58] cerebrovascular (CVA) and coronary artery diseases (CAD). Noncardiovascular (CV) deaths were not increased by effective antihypertensive therapy.

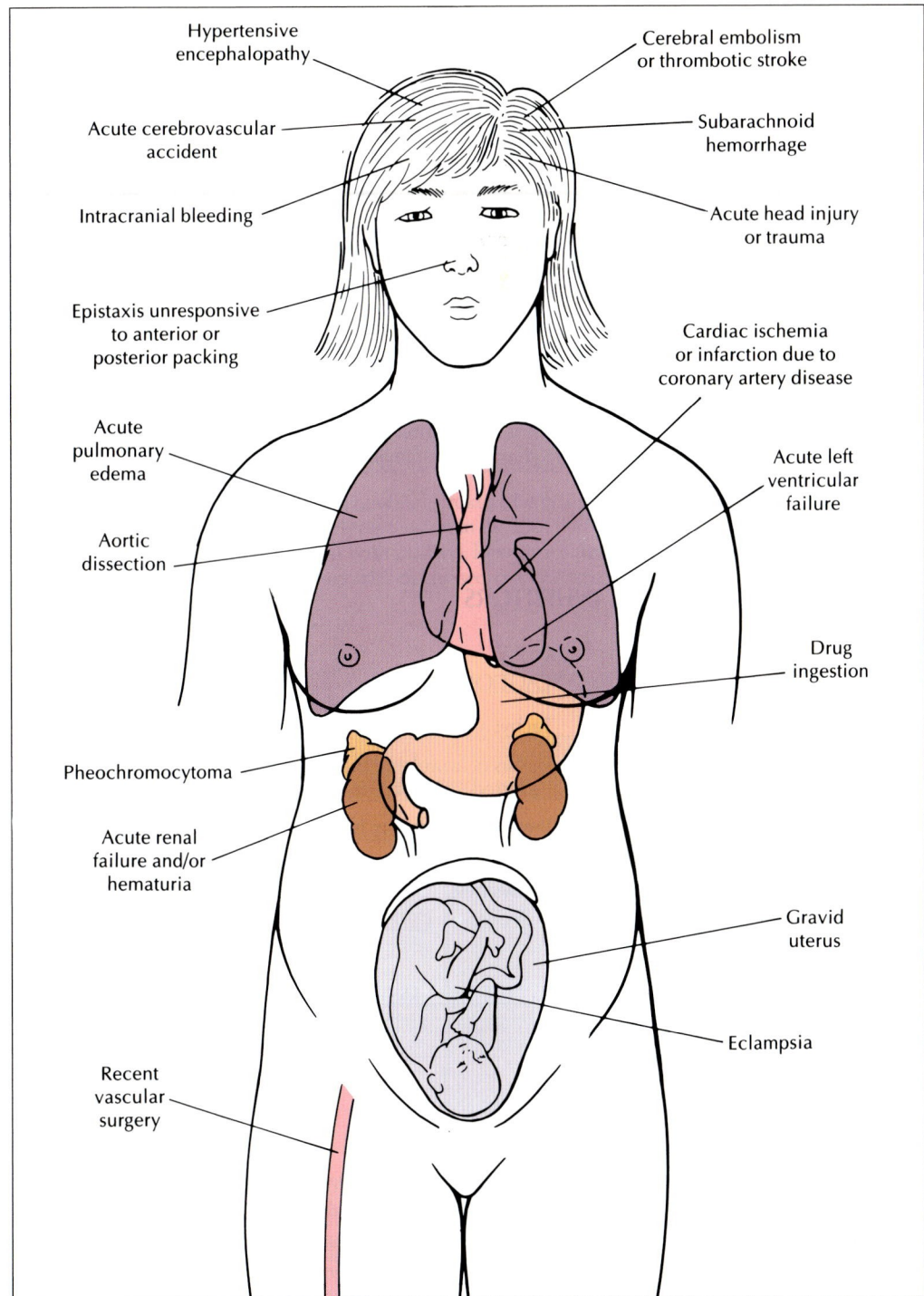

FIGURE 7-79. Common clinical conditions that are often considered hypertensive emergencies. Severe *acute* target organ damage is the major distinguishing factor between emergencies and urgencies.

Hypertensive encephalopathy

Cerebral embolism or thrombotic stroke

Acute cerebrovascular accident

Subarachnoid hemorrhage

Intracranial bleeding

Acute head injury or trauma

Epistaxis unresponsive to anterior or posterior packing

Cardiac ischemia or infarction due to coronary artery disease

Acute pulmonary edema

Acute left ventricular failure

Aortic dissection

Drug ingestion

Pheochromocytoma

Acute renal failure and/or hematuria

Gravid uterus

Eclampsia

Recent vascular surgery

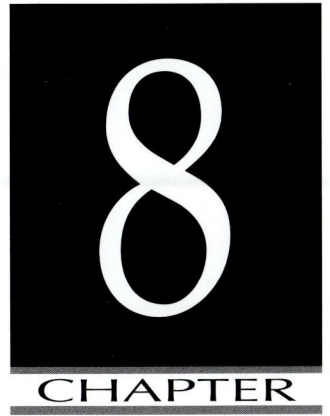

8 CHAPTER

VALVULAR HEART DISEASE

Edited by Shahbudin H. Rahimtoola

Manuel J. Antunes, Allen P. Burke, Blase A. Carabello,
Melvin D. Cheitlin, Andrew Farb, Gary L. Grunkemeier,
David T. Kawanishi, John S. MacGregor, Peter C. Nishan,
Rick A. Nishimura, Robert A. O'Rourke, Sumanth D. Prabhu,
Albert Starr, Renu Virmani

MITRAL STENOSIS

PATHOPHYSIOLOGY

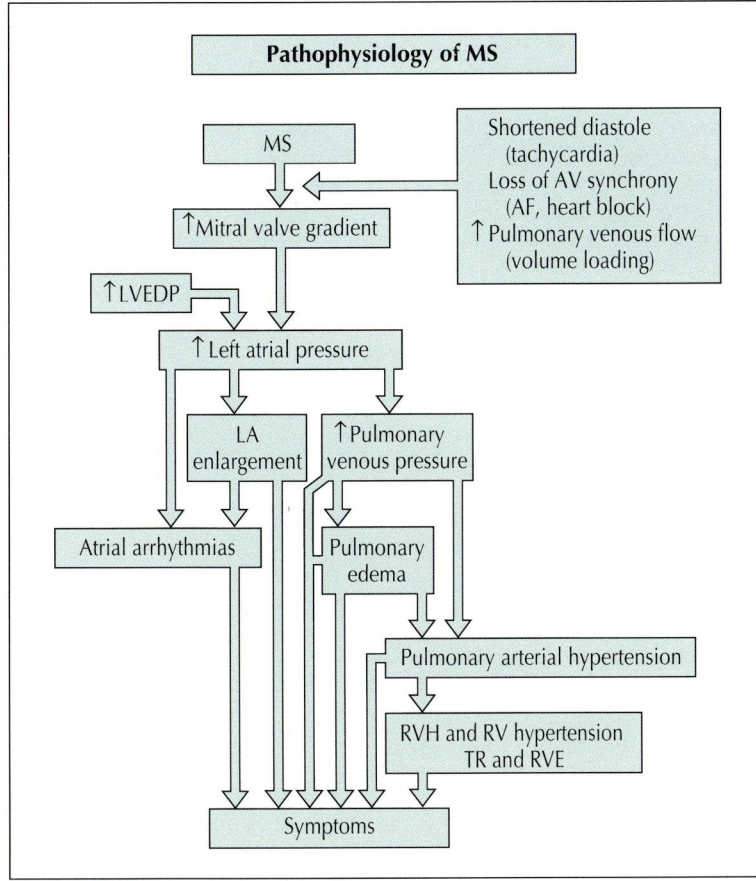

FIGURE 8-1. Pathophysiology of mitral stenosis (MS). MS results in a diastolic pressure gradient between the left atrium (LA) and the left ventricle (LV). The actual gradient depends on the mitral valve area (MVA) and the mitral valve *flow per diastolic second*. As a result, there is an elevation of LA pressure and, therefore, also of pulmonary venous pressure. Physiologic and pathologic changes—such as tachycardia and atrial fibrillation (AF) (which shorten diastole and may also result in loss of effective atrial contraction) or pregnancy, volume loading, and left-to-right shunts (at ventricular and aortopulmonary levels), which increase pulmonary venous flow—increase the mitral valve gradient and LA and pulmonary venous pressures. An increased LV end-diastolic pressure (LVEDP) also results in further increase of LA pressure.

An elevated LA pressure has several important effects, including enlargement of the LA, atrial arrhythmias, and an increase of pulmonary venous pressure. Pulmonary venous hypertension may result in pulmonary edema and pulmonary arterial hypertension. Pulmonary arterial hypertension and right ventricular (RV) hypertension result in RV hypertrophy (RVH) and may result in tricuspid regurgitation (TR) and RV enlargement (RVE). All of these changes contribute to producing symptoms. In addition, a fixed or even reduced cardiac output also contributes to the symptomatic state of the patient. AV—atrioventricular. (© Copyright SH Rahimtoola, MB, FRCP, MACP, MACC.)

PATHOLOGY

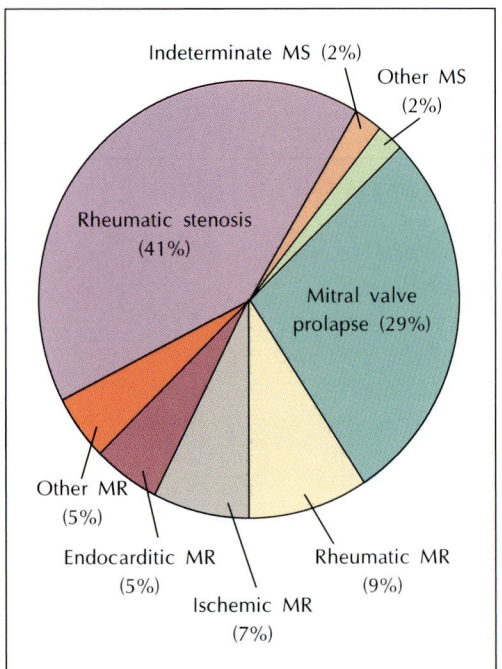

Figure 8-2. Causes of congenital and acquired mitral valve (MV) disease. Pathologic findings noted in MV excisions. MR—mitral regurgitation; MS—mitral stenosis. (*Adapted from* Dare *et al.* [1].)

PHYSICAL SIGNS

PHYSICAL SIGNS IN MS

EXAMINATION	SIGN
General	Low cardiac output: pink-purple facies, peripheral cyanosis, cool extremities
Arterial	Small-volume pulse
	Absent or reduced pulse in any vascular territory
Venous	Jugular venous distension
	Hepatojugular reflux
	Prominent *a* wave
	Prominent *v* wave
Cardiac palpation	Inconspicuous apical impulse
	Palpable mitral valve closure (S_1)
	Palpable diastolic thrill at apex
	Palpable pulmonic valve closure (P_2)
	RV lift
Cardiac Auscultation	Accentuated S_1
	Opening snap
	Diastolic rumbling murmur
	Presystolic murmur
	Accentuated P_2
	Pulmonic ejection click
	Pulmonic regurgitation (Graham-Steell) murmur
	RV S_4/S_3
Pulmonary	Egophony at tip of left scapula
	Rales

Figure 8-3. Physical signs of mitral stenosis (MS). In severe MS with a low cardiac output at rest, hypoperfusion may be suggested on general inspection of the patient; a characteristic pink-purple complexion was described by Wood [2]. The extremities may be cool and cyanotic. In such severe cases, the small stroke volume results in a perceptibly diminished pulse volume. An elevated right atrial (RA) pressure is apparent from distention of the jugular veins, or such distention may be elicited by compression of the abdomen. The elevated RA pressure is a result of fluid retention associated with heart failure, right ventricular (RV) hypertension, or tricuspid regurgitation. The *a* wave is prominent in the presence of RV hypertension and the *v* wave is prominent with tricuspid regurgitation.

Palpation of the precordium may reveal an inconspicuous apical impulse, and mitral valve closure may be felt (a palpable S_1). A loud diastolic rumbling murmur may be felt as a thrill at the apex; this can be better appreciated if the apex is brought more into proximity of the chest wall by placing the patient in the left lateral decubitus position. With pulmonary arterial hypertension or RV dilatation, a parasternal RV lift may be present. When the RV is markedly dilated, the left ventricular (LV) apical impulse may be displaced posteriorly and the RV impulse may be mistaken for the LV apex. Also in the presence of severe pulmonary arterial hypertension, pulmonic valve closure (P_2) may be palpable in the second left parasternal intercostal space.

On auscultation, a loud S_1, an opening snap, and a mid-diastolic rumbling murmur with presystolic accentuation are considered the cardinal signs of MS [3,4] (*see* Fig. 8-4). With pulmonary arterial hypertension, the intensity of P_2 is increased; in severe pulmonary arterial hypertension, a pulmonary ejection click and a diastolic murmur of pulmonary valve regurgitation may be present (Graham Steell murmur). Auscultation of the posterior chest rarely reveals an area of egophony at the lower tip of the left scapula, a result of marked left atrial enlargement [5]. Rales may be present when there is pulmonary congestion or pulmonary edema.

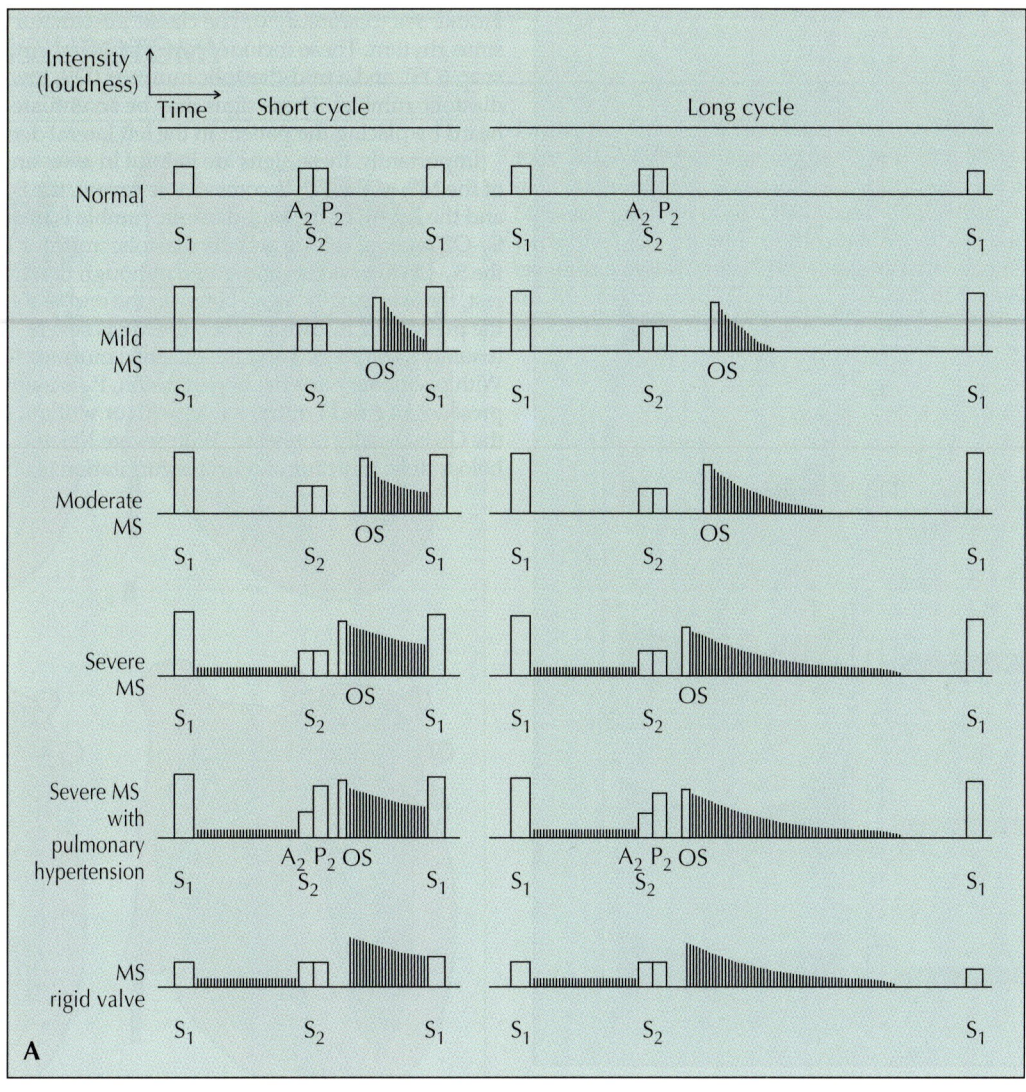

FIGURE 8-4. A, The classic auscultatory signs of mitral stenosis (MS) in atrial fibrillation (AF). The auscultatory findings are much more variable on a beat-to-beat basis in AF. The presystolic murmur is usually absent. The loud S_1 and the OS are still heard. In the short cycles, the duration of diastole is short and the mid-diastolic rumble occupies the whole of diastole (*left panel*). In the long cycles (*right panel*) the duration of the mid-diastolic murmur is related to the severity of MS (*panel A*). As the MS becomes more severe, the length of this murmur is increased. In AF, with a slow ventricular response and very long R-R intervals, the diastolic rumble may not occupy the whole diastolic period and the presystolic murmur is absent. Thus, one may get the impression that the MS is moderate rather than severe. Increasing the heart rate, *eg*, with brief physical exertion, may produce more characteristic auscultatory findings. Alternatively, when the ventricular rate in AF is rapid or in short cycles, the auscultatory findings may suggest a more severe degree of MS than is really the case (*left panel*). (*continued*)

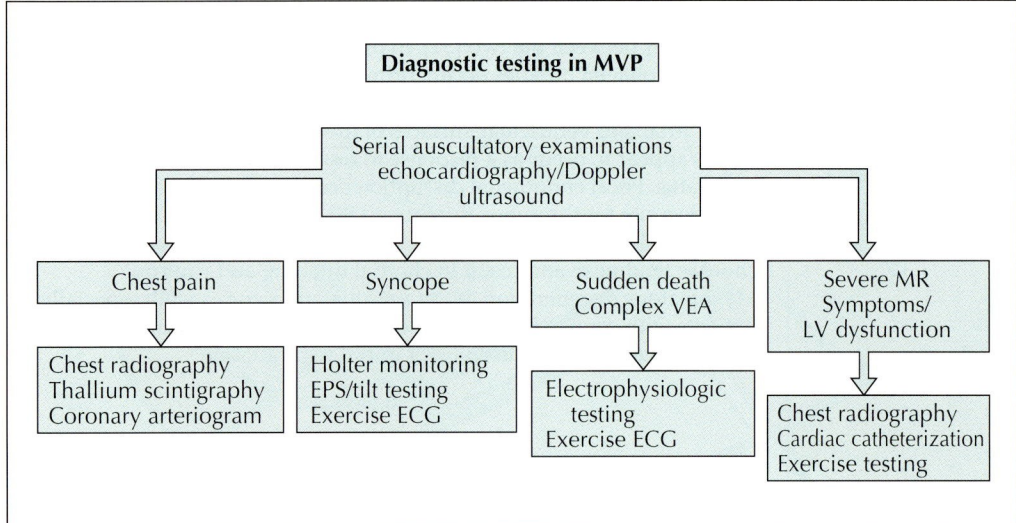

Diagnostic testing in MVP

Serial auscultatory examinations
echocardiography/Doppler
ultrasound

Chest pain → Chest radiography / Thallium scintigraphy / Coronary arteriogram

Syncope → Holter monitoring / EPS/tilt testing / Exercise ECG

Sudden death / Complex VEA → Electrophysiologic testing / Exercise ECG

Severe MR Symptoms/ LV dysfunction → Chest radiography / Cardiac catheterization / Exercise testing

FIGURE 8-24. Diagnostic testing in mitral valve prolapse (MVP). The diagnosis of MVP is based on the presence of typical auscultatory findings detected during carefully performed serial examinations. Echocardiography (M-mode, two-dimensional, and Doppler) is the single most useful test in the definition of MVP. It is used to assess natural history and prognosis, the presence of associated conditions (*eg*, atrial septal defect, hypertrophic cardiomyopathy), the need for antibiotic prophylaxis, and the degree of mitral regurgitation (MR). Echocardiography should *not* supplant the physical examination in the diagnosis of MVP; up to 10% of patients diagnosed with MVP by typical auscultatory findings will have a non-diagnostic two-dimensional echocardiogram [35]. Electrocardiography (ECG) is routinely performed to assess for ventricular preexcitation and resting ST- and T-wave abnormalities. The tests listed in the lowest level of the flow diagram are not required for the diagnosis of MVP, but they are useful in assessing certain symptoms and complications that can occur in this disorder. EPS—electrophysiology; LV—left ventricular; MR—mitral regurgitation; VEA—ventricular ectopic arrhythmia.

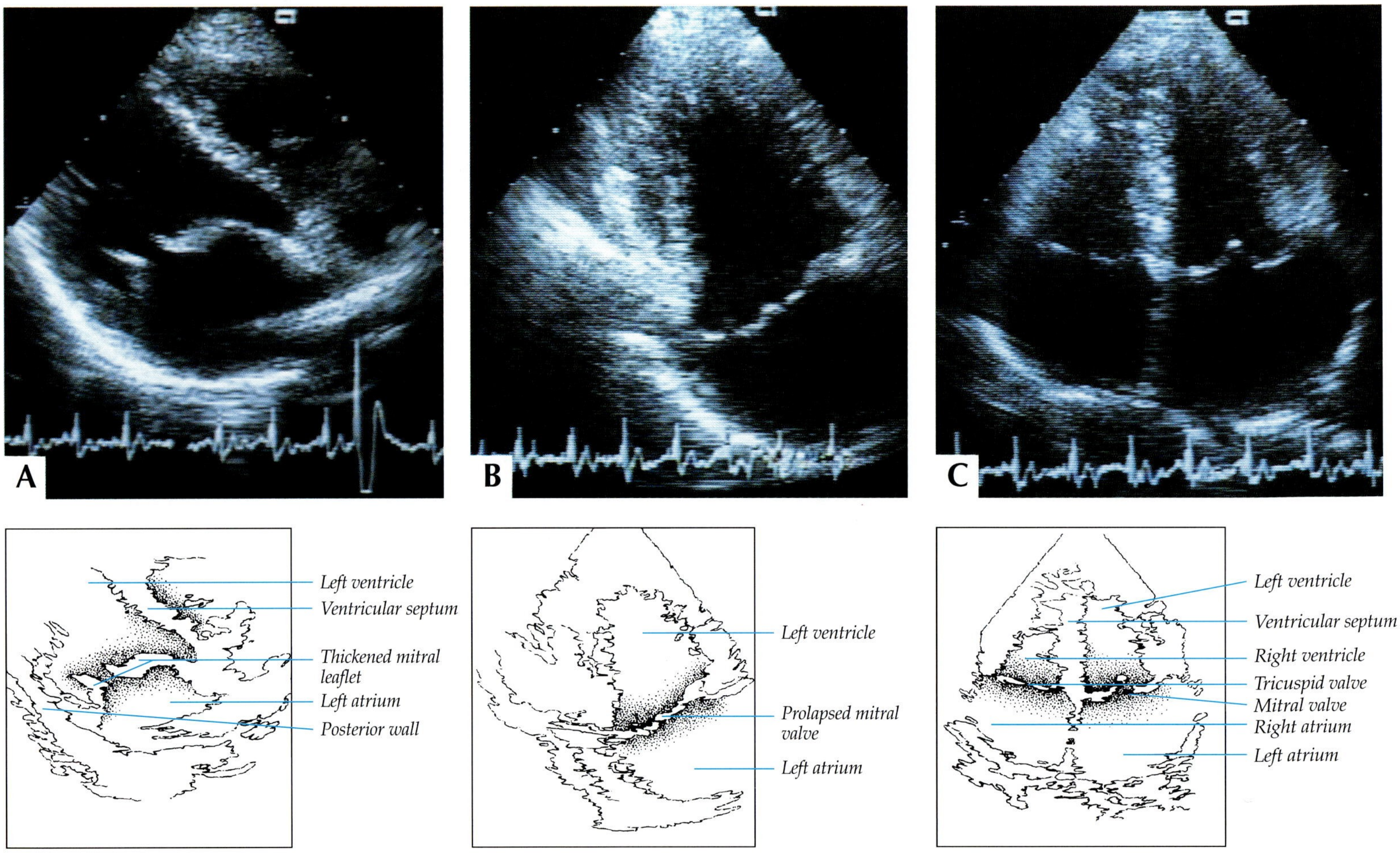

A

Left ventricle
Ventricular septum
Thickened mitral leaflet
Left atrium
Posterior wall

B

Left ventricle
Prolapsed mitral valve
Left atrium

C

Left ventricle
Ventricular septum
Right ventricle
Tricuspid valve
Mitral valve
Right atrium
Left atrium

FIGURE 8-25. Two-dimensional echocardiographic and Doppler ultrasound images from a 55-year-old man with classic mitral valve prolapse and associated tricuspid valve prolapse. The parasternal long axis view shows significant leaflet thickening of both mitral leaflets (**A**). The apical long axis view shows prolapse of both leaflets and the coaptation point beyond the annular plane (**B**).The apical four-chamber view displays a systolic prolapse of both the mitral and tricuspid valves (**C**). (*continued*)

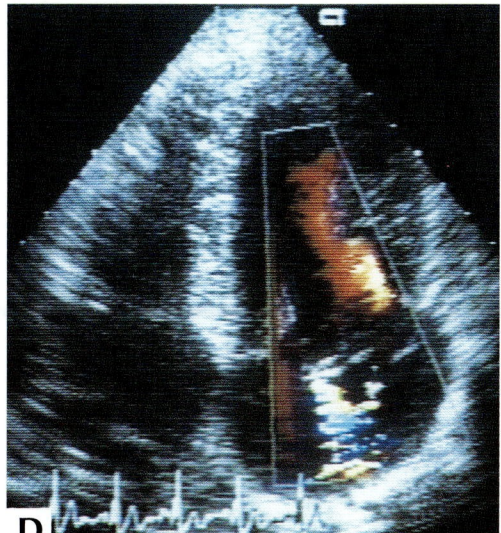
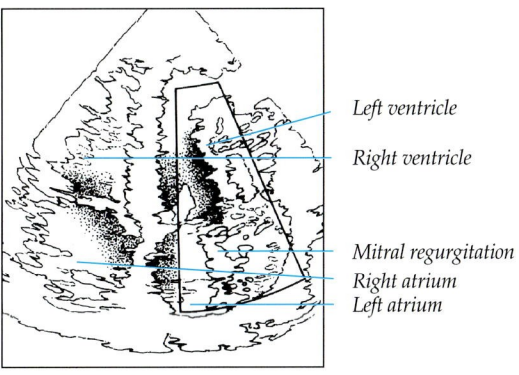

FIGURE 8-25. (*continued*) Color flow Doppler mapping in the left atrium demonstrates central mitral regurgitation (**D**). Tricuspid regurgitation was noted as well (not shown).

Left ventricle

Right ventricle

Mitral regurgitation
Right atrium
Left atrium

D

MANAGEMENT

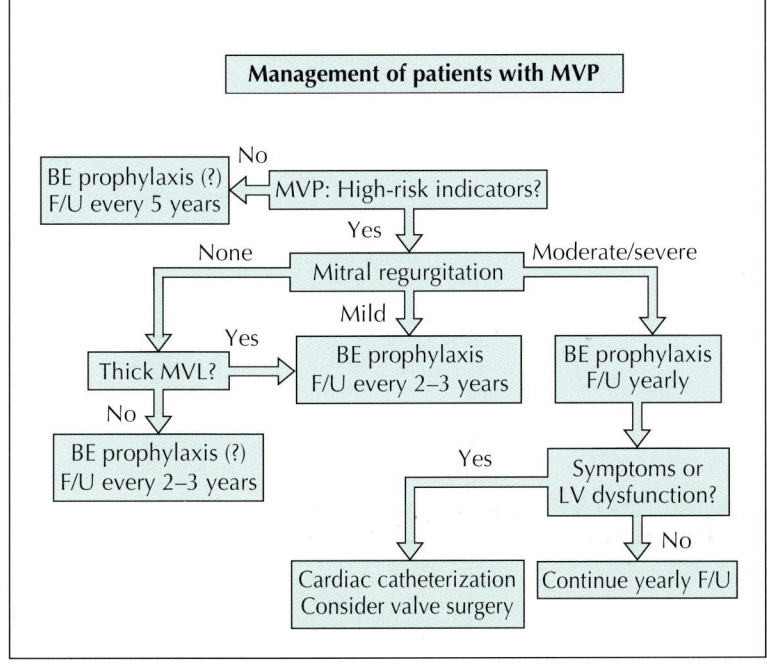

Management of patients with MVP

MVP: High-risk indicators? — No → BE prophylaxis (?) F/U every 5 years

Yes ↓

Mitral regurgitation — Moderate/severe → BE prophylaxis F/U yearly

None / Mild

Thick MVL? — Yes → BE prophylaxis F/U every 2–3 years

No ↓ BE prophylaxis (?) F/U every 2–3 years

Symptoms or LV dysfunction? — Yes → Cardiac catheterization Consider valve surgery

No → Continue yearly F/U

FIGURE 8-26. Management of patients with mitral valve prolapse (MVP). High-risk characteristics in MVP patients are additive, that is, the more indicators present, the greater the total risk. The majority of patients with MVP are asymptomatic and have no or minimal high-risk indicators. They are treated with reassurance and can lead a normal life [36,37]. Clinical and echocardiographic assessment every 5 years is reasonable to determine passage into a higher-risk group. If any high-risk indicators are present, patients can be further stratified based on the presence of mitral regurgitation (MR). Some authorities advocate prophylaxis for bacterial endocarditis (BE) only if MVP is associated with MR or thickened mitral valve leaflets (MVL). However, given the variability of physical findings and the dynamic nature of MR in MVP, prophylaxis may be reasonable in all patients with MVP. Patients with MVP and severe MR should be managed in the same manner as patients with severe MR due to other causes. The decision to proceed with valve surgery is based on the presence of symptoms or impairment of left ventricular (LV) systolic function. Mitral valve reconstructive surgery can often be used in lieu of valve replacement to correct regurgitant floppy valves [38–40]. Compared to valve replacement, valve repair is associated with a lower operative and late mortality, lower long-term thromboembolic risk, and lower BE risk [38,40]. F/U—follow-up.

PATHOLOGY

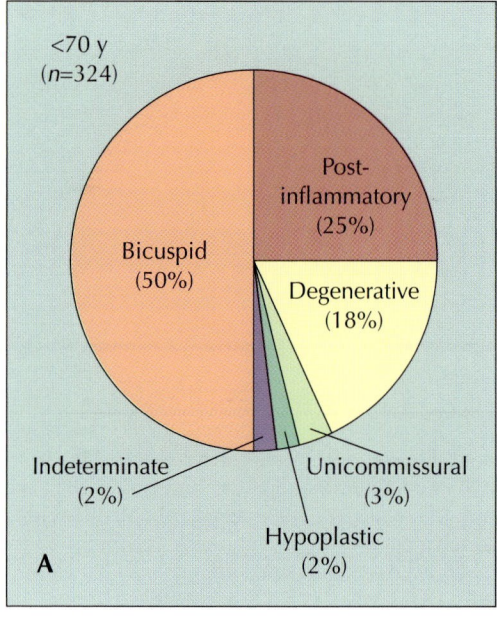 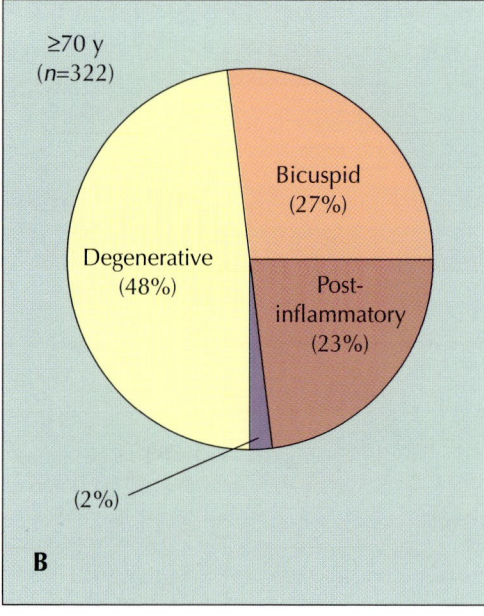

FIGURE 8-27. Causes of aortic stenosis (AS). **A,** Among patients 70 years of age or younger, calcification of congenitally bicuspid valves accounted for half of the surgical cases of AS. **B,** Conversely, degenerative calcification accounted for almost half the cases of AS in patients 70 years of age or older [10]. (*Adapted from* Passik *et al.* [41].)

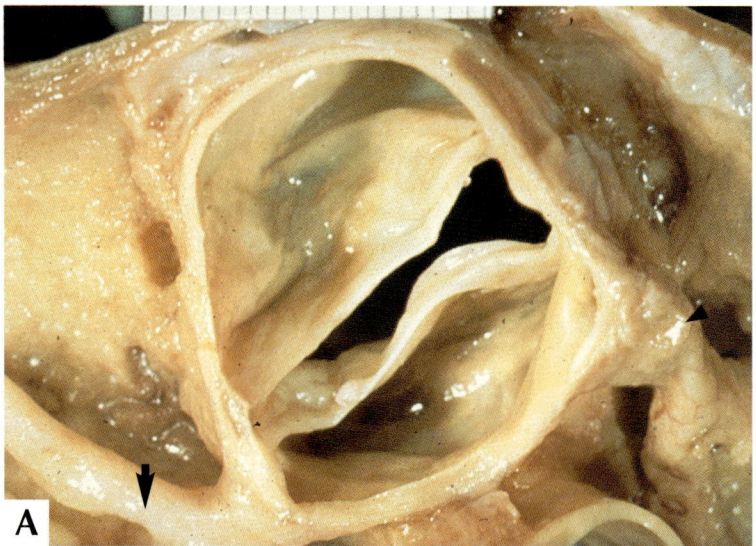 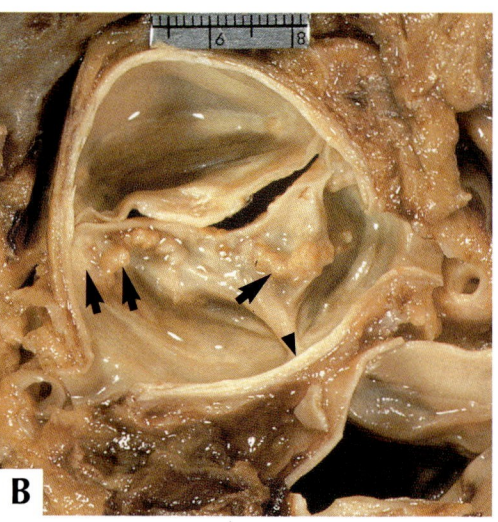

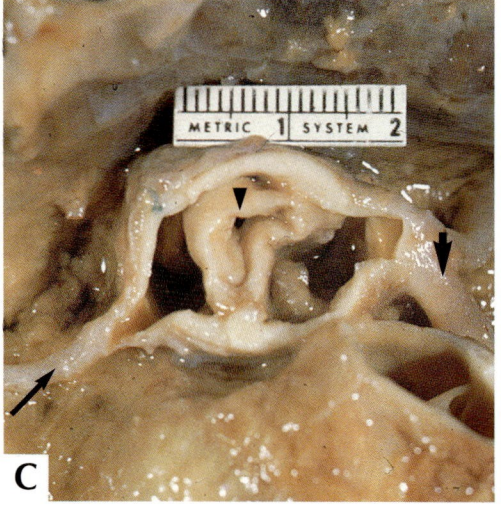

FIGURE 8-28. Congenital aortic valve (AV) disease. **A,** A normally functioning bicuspid AV with two commissures and the two leaflets, which are almost equal in size in a 58-year-old man who died of metastatic lung carcinoma. The commissures are located right and left and both coronary ostia arise from the anterior aortic sinus. Note the absence of raphe in either leaflet. The right coronary artery is denoted by an *arrow*; the left coronary artery is denoted by an *arrowhead*.

B, A mildly calcified congenitally bicuspid AV in a 69-year-old man. Note a nonstenotic functionally normal bicuspid valve with mild calcification (*arrows*) and a raphe (*arrowhead*) in the anterior leaflet.

C, A bicuspid dysplastic and fibrotic AV (*arrowhead*) from a 24-year-old woman who had a commissurotomy 5 years before death. She was found dead in the hospital while awaiting repeat surgery. The commissures are located anterior and posterior and the leaflets are right and left with the right coronary artery (*long arrow*) and the left coronary artery (*short arrow*) arising from the right and left coronary sinuses. Patients with dysplastic bicuspid valves usually become symptomatic early in life, whereas those with calcified and fibrotic bicuspid valves usually present in the fifth to seventh decade.

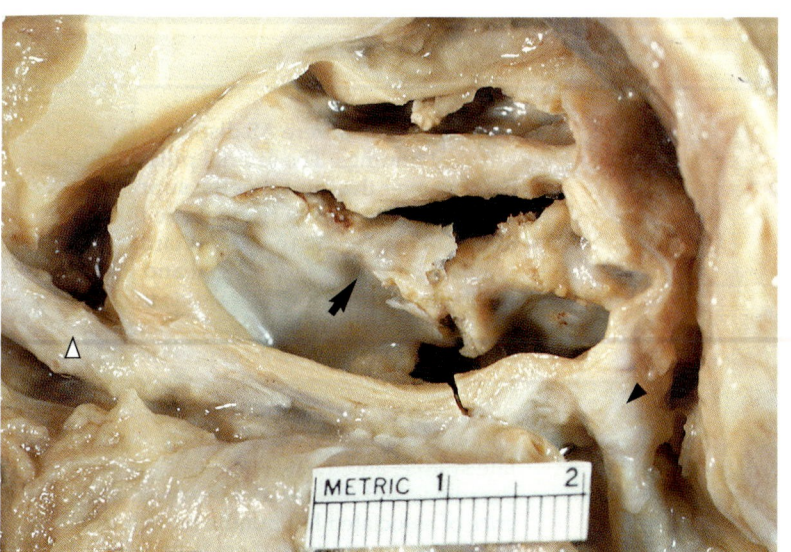

FIGURE 8-29. Bicuspid aortic valve (AV): congenital versus acquired. Congenital bicuspid stenotic AV with calcified and fibrotic raphe (*arrow*). The patient was in his fifth decade. Note that leaflets are anterior and posterior, and there is a rudimentary commissure in the anterior leaflet that does not reach the level of the true commissures. *Asterisk* shows calcified nodules; *black arrowhead* shows right commissure; *white arrowhead* shows left commissure.

Shown here is a calcified fibrotic congenital bicuspid aortic stenosis (AS) (*arrow*). No raphe is identified. Note the marked thickening of the valve leaflets, which are similar in size. The patient was a woman in her forties with symptomatic AS. *White arrowhead* shows right coronary artery; *black arrowhead* shows left coronary artery.

PATHOPHYSIOLOGY

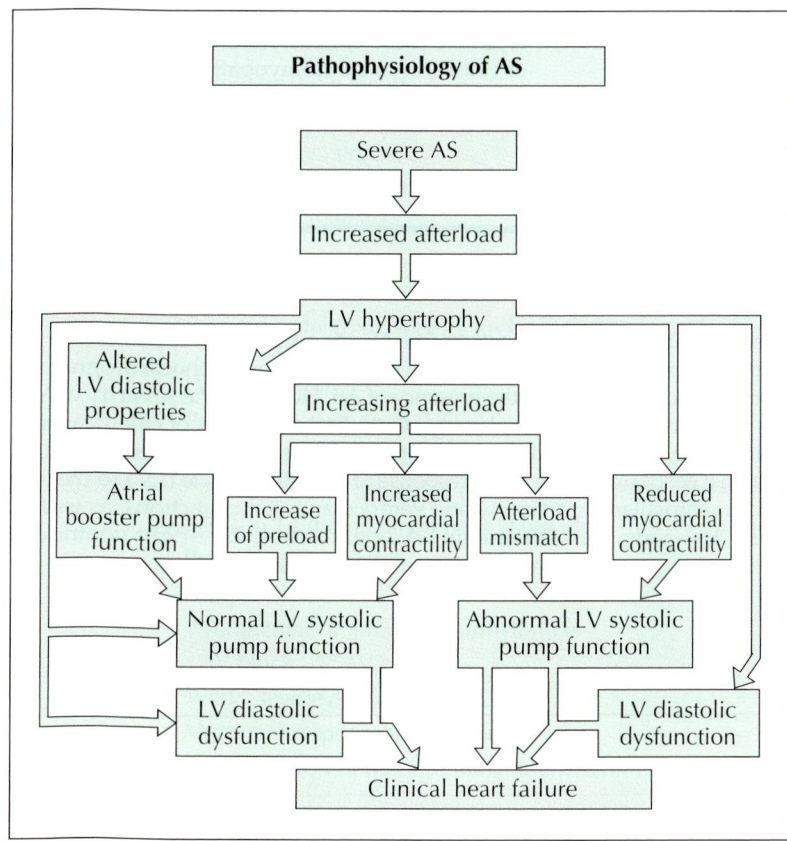

FIGURE 8-30. Pathophysiology of aortic stenosis (AS). With reduction in the aortic valve area (AVA), energy is dissipated during the transport of blood from the left ventricle (LV) to the aorta. The AVA has to be reduced by 50% of normal before a measurable gradient can be demonstrated. When a pressure gradient develops between the LV and the ascending aorta, LV pressure rises and LV wall stress (afterload) increases. This could result in an impairment of LV function. The heart responds by becoming hypertrophied and myocardial stress remains normal. LV mass in patients with severe AS undergoing valve replacement averages 229 g/m² (normal mass, 105 g/m²) [42]; at autopsy, LVs weighing as much as 1000 g have been reported. LV volume remains within the normal range; therefore, there is considerable thickening of the LV wall. As a result of the LV hypertrophy, LV systolic pump function remains normal. LV hypertrophy may alter the LV diastolic properties and there is increased resistance to LV filling. As a result, LV end-diastolic pressure is elevated; but this cannot be used as a measure of LV failure. Powerful atrial contraction produces the required LV filling [43,44] and fiber length (atrial booster pump function). Because atrial systole occupies only a small part of the cardiac cycle, there is only a transient increase in left atrial pressure; therefore, mean left atrial pressure remains in the normal range [43] or is only minimally increased.

As LV afterload continues to increase, the LV uses two additional compensatory mechanisms, namely, increase of preload and increase of myocardial contractility. Both of these help maintain normal LV systolic pump function.

When the limit of the preload reserve has been reached (afterload mismatch) [45] or myocardial contractility is reduced, LV systolic pump function becomes abnormal.

Clinical heart failure is usually a result of abnormal LV systolic pump function; diastolic dysfunction may also be present in some patients. Clinical heart failure in those with normal systolic pump function is a result of LV diastolic dysfunction. (© Copyright SH Rahimtoola, MB, FRCP, MACP, MACC.)

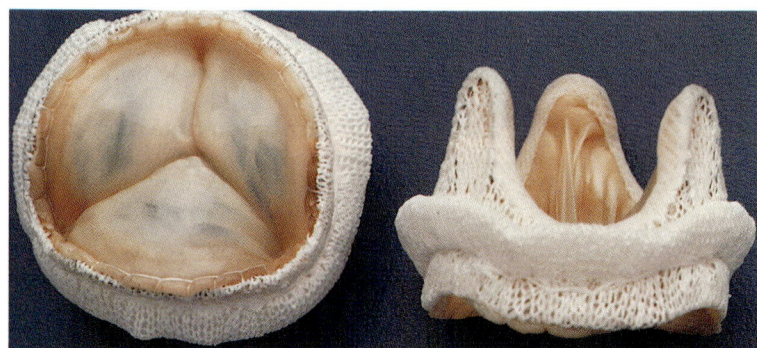

FIGURE 8-57. Carpentier-Edwards stented porcine valves: Standard, SAV, and Duraflex. The Carpentier-Edwards (Standard) (Baxter Healthcare Corporation, Irvine, CA) porcine bioprosthesis was released for general marketing shortly after the Hancock valve. The frame of the valve is a flexible wire stent made of Elgiloy, intended to reduce stresses on the leaflets and orifice. A flexible Mylar cylinder surrounds and supports the Elgiloy frame. The annulus is asymmetrically shaped, to obliterate the septal ridge of the porcine right coronary cusp.

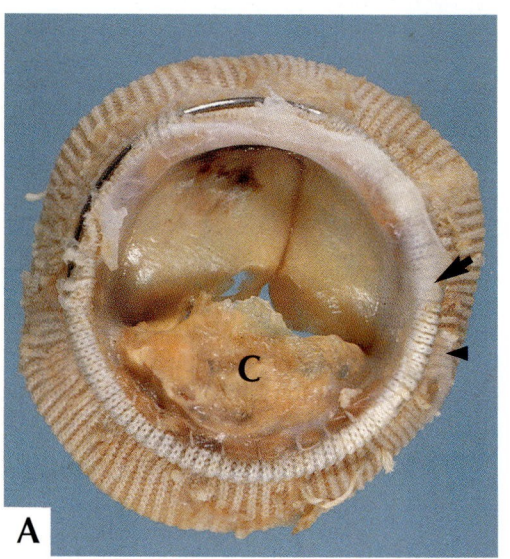

FIGURE 8-58. Bioprosthetic valves, degenerative changes. **A,** Mineralization occurs in virtually all bioprosthetic valves, especially in children and young adults. In this case calcification (C) was limited primarily to one cusp. The porcine AV is asymmetric, the right coronary cusp being larger, with a muscle shelf that results in less complete opening and accelerated calcification after xenotransplantation. The stent and sewing ring are denoted by the *arrow* and *arrowhead*, respectively. **B,** Perforation, bioprosthetic valve. This Hancock valve had been in the mitral position for 5 years. The patient died soon after hospitalization for sudden-onset congestive heart failure. There is a linear type II perforation (*arrows*) at the base of the cusp that does not involve the free edge.

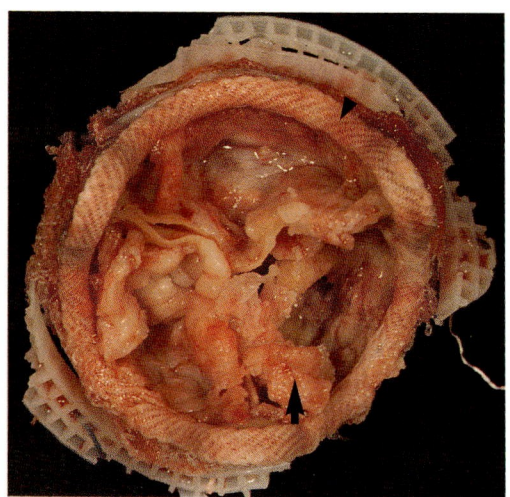

FIGURE 8-59. Bioprosthetic valve, endocarditis. Porcine valve viewed from aortic aspect is shown in this figure. Note destruction of valve leaflets by infectious vegetation (*arrow*). The infectious agent was *Staphylococcus epidermidis*; the valve was moved 1 month after insertion. Endocarditis occurs at a rate of about 5% at 5 years, and up to five times this rate in patients originally operated for endocarditis. Early infections are usually secondary to perioperative contaminants, whereas infections after 60 days result from bacteremic seeding. *Arrowhead* denotes cloth-covered stent.

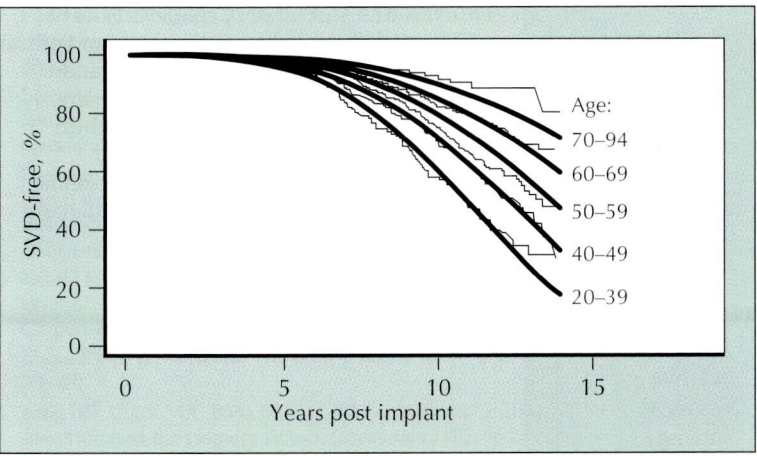

FIGURE 8-60. Actual versus actuarial freedom from structural valve deterioration (SVD). Time-related curves are required for the comparisons of biologic valves to incorporate the nonconstant risk of structural failure.

It is important to understand that the usual actuarial curve gives the percentage free of an event at a given time, provided that the patients do not die (*ie*, that the risk of death has been eliminated). But many patients will die before their valve would have failed, so that the percent of patients who *actually* experience tissue failure will be lower than the usual *actuarial* estimates [71].

Shown here are the usual *actuarial* failure-free curves for 4910 operative survivors of isolated aortic or mitral replacement with Hancock or Carpentier-Edwards porcine valves from two centers (Stanford and Vancouver), followed up to 15 years, for a total of almost 30,000 valve-years [72]. The curves are stratified by age group, and a Weibull regression model based on patient age and valve position (*smooth lines*) was used to fit the actuarial Kaplan-Meier curves (*jagged lines*). Older patients have a much lower risk than younger patients.

An additional 164 patients with double valves from these same institutions were not used in the modeling above, but their risk of valve failure was as predicted based on the model for isolated valves only. Thus, the risk for a valve to fail does not seem to be influenced by the existence of a comparison valve in the same patient. (*Adapted from* Grunkemeier *et al.* [72].)

VALVE SELECTION FOR INDIVIDUAL PATIENTS

RECOMMENDATIONS FOR VALVE REPLACEMENT WITH A MECHANICAL PROSTHESIS

INDICATION	CLASS
Patients with expected long life spans	I
Patients with a mechanical prosthetic valve already in place in a different position than the valve to be replaced	I
Patients in renal failure, on hemodialysis, or with hypercalcemia	II
Patients requiring warfarin therapy because of risk factors* for thromboembolism	IIa
Patients age ≤65 years for AVR and age ≤70 years for MVR[†]	IIa
Valve re-replacement for thrombosed biologic valve	IIb
Patients who cannot or will not take warfarin	III

RECOMMENDATIONS FOR VALVE REPLACEMENT WITH A BIOPROSTHESIS

INDICATION	CLASS
Patients who cannot or will not take warfarin	I
Patients ages ≥65 years* needing AVR who do not have risk factors for thromboembolism[†]	I
Patients considered to have possible compliance problems with warfarin therapy	IIa
Patients ages >70 years[‡] needing MVR who do not have risk factors for thromboembolism	IIa
Valve re-replacement for thrombosed mechanical valve	IIb
Patients ages <65 years[‡]	IIb
Patients in renal failure, on hemodialysis, or with hypercalcemia	III
Adolescent patients who are still growing	III

*Risk factors: AF, severe LV dysfunction, previous thromboembolism, and hypercoagulable conditions.

[†]The age at which patients may be considered for biosprosthetic valves is based on the major reduction in the rate of structural valve deterioration after age 65 years and the increased risk of bleeding in this age group.

[‡]The age at which patients should be considered for bioprosthetic valves is based on the major reduction in the rate of structural valve deterioration after age 65 years and the increased risk of bleeding in this age group.

FIGURE 8-61. Selection of prosthesis for individual patients (**A**). The general principles in valve selection derive from the fundamental difference between the mechanical and biologic valves. Mechanical valves are extremely durable yet require lifetime anticoagulation to mitigate thromboembolic complications. Biologic valves have not eliminated thromboembolism, but they achieve rates comparable to those of mechanical valves without anticoagulation; however, they have limited lifetimes. Beyond this fundamental difference between types of valves, patient-specific factors influence the results as much as valve-specific factors.

Valve repair (not covered in this review) should be considered preferable to replacement for the mitral position [73,74]. Repair can also be considered for the aortic position [75]. Homografts or the Ross procedure may also be considered, especially for very young patients. However, the vast majority of patients requiring replacement will be served by one of the commercially available prostheses.

When prosthetic replacement is necessary, some general recommendations can be made with regard to valve selection, based on the above fundamental difference between valve types. A biologic valve would be preferred for a patient who cannot, or does not want to take, anticoagulants, who desires pregnancy, or who has a short life expectancy. A mechanical valve would be preferred for a patient who will be receiving anticoagulants for another reason (*eg*, previous stroke or infarction, atrial fibrillation, mechanical valve in another position), who is in renal failure or on dialysis, or who has a long life expectancy. AF—atrial fibrillation; AVR—aortic valve replacement; LV—left ventricle; MVR—mitral valve replacement. (*Adapted from* Bonow *et al.* [76].)

9 CHAPTER

CONGENITAL HEART DISEASE

Edited by Robert M. Freedom

Leland N. Benson, Christine Boutin, Scott D. Flamm,
Michael D. Freed, Charles B. Higgins, Paul R. Julsrud,
Luc C. Jutras, Ira A. Parness, P. Syamasundar Rao,
Stephen P. Sanders, Jeong-Wook Seo, Norman H. Silverman,
Gil Wernovsky, Shi-Joon Yoo

Congenital heart disease occurs in approximately one percent of live births. In this chapter, the pathophysiology, diagnosis, and treatment of many important congenital malformations of the heart are illustrated.

ATRIAL SEPTAL DEFECT

Atrial septal defect is a very common anomaly that occurs more frequently in females than males. There are three principal forms of atrial septal defect. Defects of the sinus venosus type occur in the superior portion of the atrial septum. They are usually associated with anomalous connection of the pulmonary veins of the right lung to the right atrium near the entry of the superior vena cava. Ostium secundum defects occur in the region of the foramen ovale, whereas ostium primum defects occur in the lower portion of the septum.

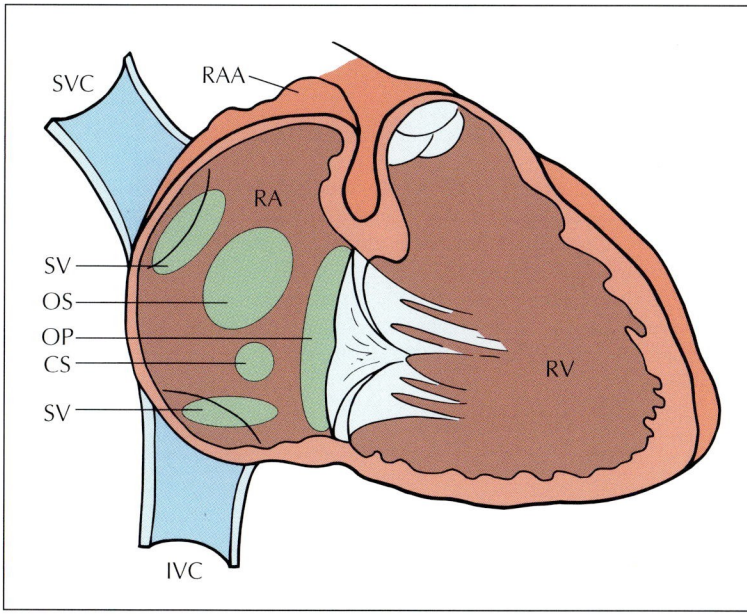

FIGURE 9-1. Diagrammatic representation of the sites of communication between the atria, shown from the perspective of the right atrium (RA). The RA, right ventricle (RV), superior vena cava (SVC), and inferior vena cava (IVC) are shown. The tricuspid valve apparatus lies between the RA and RV. The classic site of an ostium secundum (OS) atrial septal defect is shown in the confines of the fossa ovalis, the commonest site for interatrial communications. The defects result from a deficiency of septum primum. The ostium primum (OP) defect lies adjacent to the atrioventricular valve. The upper sinus venosus (SV) defect occurs adjacent to SVC, while the lower SV defect occurs adjacent to the IVC. Interatrial communications also occur through the coronary sinus (CS), related to a deficiency of the CS septum and entering through the mouth of the CS. In most patients with this defect, ultrasound is the primary mode of diagnosis. This can be confirmed by a variety of techniques, including magnetic resonance imaging [1]. RAA—right atrial appendage.

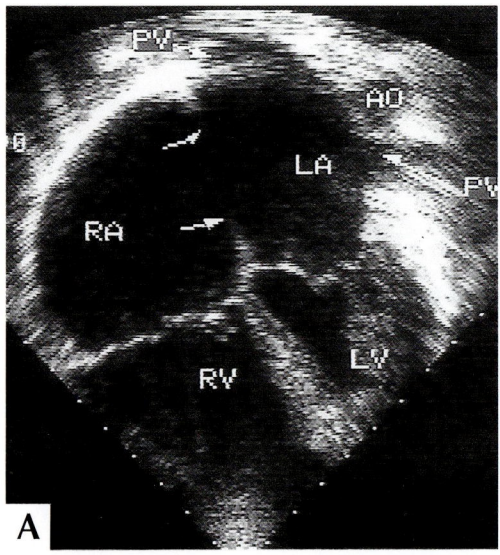

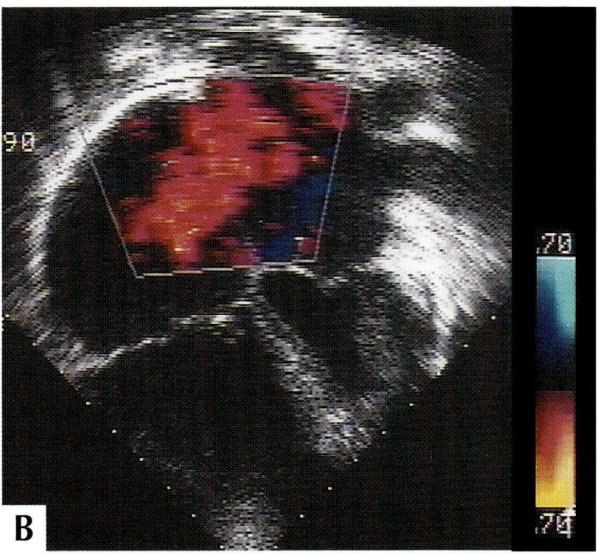

FIGURE 9-2. A, Apical four-chamber view of the left and right heart structures in a patient with a large ostium secundum atrial septal defect is shown (*arrows*). The pulmonary vein (PV) can be seen to enter the corners of the left atrium (LA), while the descending aorta (AO) is straddled by these two venous entry sites. **B,** During the Doppler color flow study the diastolic frame shows transatrial flow across this large defect. The color scale on the lower left-hand part of the frame demonstrates the color assignment toward the transducer in yellow-orange, and flow away from the transducer in blue hues. The Nyquist limit, the velocity range defined by the map, is indicated at 0.70 m/s. LV—left ventricle; RA—right atrium; RV—right ventricle.

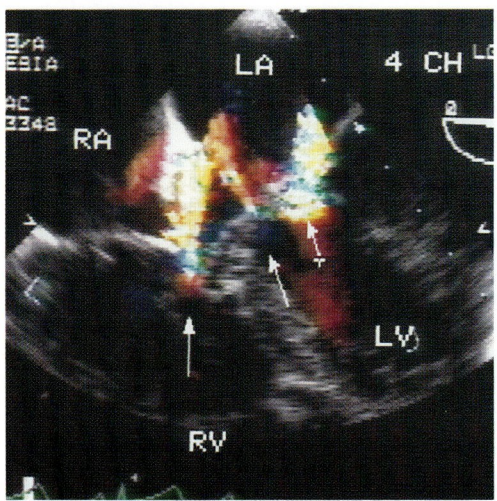

FIGURE 9-3. In this transesophageal frame of the four chambers of the heart in a patient with an ostium primum atrial septal defect taken in late systole, three regurgitation jets can be identified arising through the AV valve (*arrows*). There is lateral regurgitation between the left ventricle (LV) and left atrium (LA), probably arising from the junction between the mural leaflets and the opposed anlagen of the anterosuperior and posteroinferior bridging leaflets. There is a central jet adjacent to the atrial septum probably arising through the "cleft" between the bridging leaflets, and a separate jet between the right ventricle (RV) and right atrium (RA). Color flow Doppler study has revolutionized the definition of the shunting patterns in this group of lesions by allowing one to observe the pattern of shunt flow through the AV valve, the atrial and ventricular communication. The detection of shunting patterns is important surgically as well as prognostically [2–4]. Atrial and ventricular shunting patterns can be observed and the magnitude of the shunt size at the atrial or ventricular level estimated.

It is remarkable that there is so vast a degree of variability in the regurgitant patterns in valves that appear morphologically similar but have such a wide degree of functional impairment. Color flow is now the primary mode for Doppler ultrasound study in this condition. The AV valve regurgitation through the left side of the commissure most frequently is directed centrally and is part of the so-called LV-to-RA shunt. Less frequently the jet is directed more leftward and then becomes an LV-to-LA shunt. Ebels *et al.* [5] have suggested that this is related to the relative hypoplasia of the mural leaflet of the left component of the AV valve [2,4,5]. The regurgitation from the RA to the RV may be substantial as well.

VENTRICULAR SEPTAL DEFECT

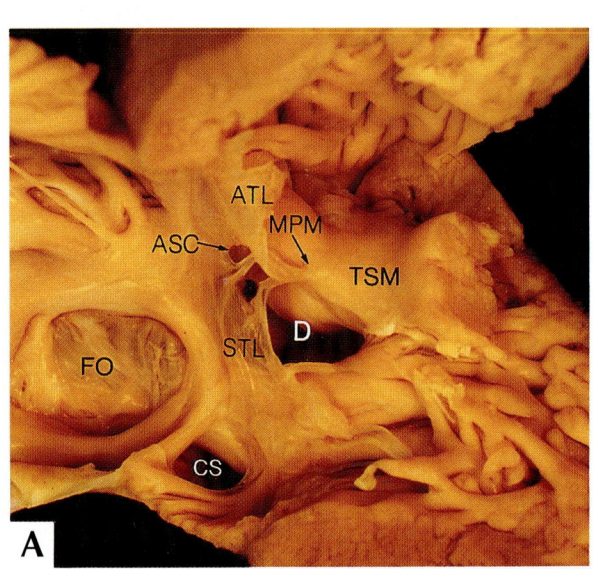

FIGURE 9-4. Perimembranous ventricular septal defects extending toward the inlet of the right ventricle (RV). Ventricular septal defect may occur as an isolated defect or as one component of a more complex congenital anomaly. Single defects usually occur in the membranous septum (perimembranous ventricular septal defect). Small defects at birth commonly close in early childhood. Large isolated defects may produce left ventricular failure in infancy and severe pulmonary hypertension in childhood leading to Eisenmenger's syndrome. **A,** RV aspect of a specimen. The defect (D) involves the inlet ventricular septum (IS) along the septal leaflet of the tricuspid valve (STL). It abuts on the anteroseptal commissure (ASC) superiorly. The medial papillary muscle (MPM) is seen at the anterosuperior aspect of the defect. (*continued*)

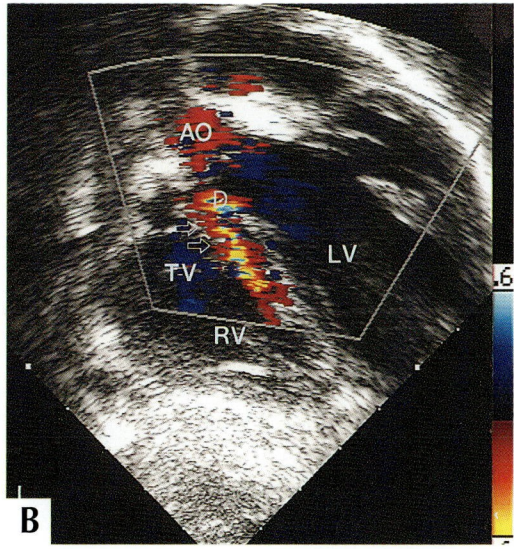
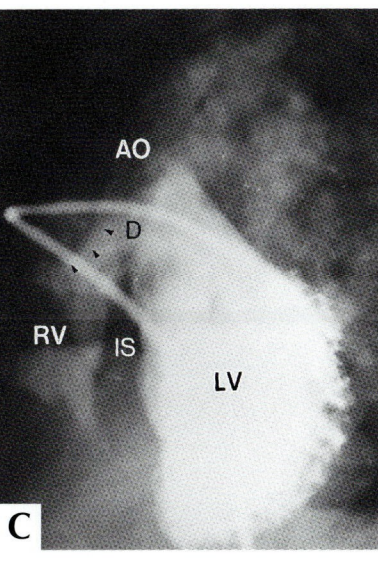

FIGURE 9-4. (*continued*) **B,** Color Doppler echocardiogram in the subxyphoid long-axis plane from a different patient. The defect is located immediately below the aortic valve. The color-coded shunt flow (*arrows*) can be seen between the septal leaflet of the tricuspid valve (TV) and the IS. **C,** Left ventriculogram in long-axial oblique projection from another patient. The defect is seen immediately below the aortic valve. The initial shunt flow opacifies the inlet part of the RV between the septal leaflet (*arrowheads*) of the TV and the IS. AO—aorta; ATL—anterior leaflet of the TV; CS—coronary sinus; FO—fossa ovalis; LV—left ventricle; TSM—trabecula septomarginalis. (Part C *from* Yoo and Choi [6]; with permission.)

ATRIOVENTRICULAR SEPTAL DEFECT

Atrioventricular septal defects (AVSDs) are malformations characterized by varying degrees of incomplete development of the inferior portion of the atrial septum, the superior portion of the ventricular septum, and the mitral or tricuspid valve. The lesions include atrial septal defect of the ostium primum type, high ventricular septal defects, mitral regurgitation, and tricuspid regurgitation. These may occur singly or in any combination.

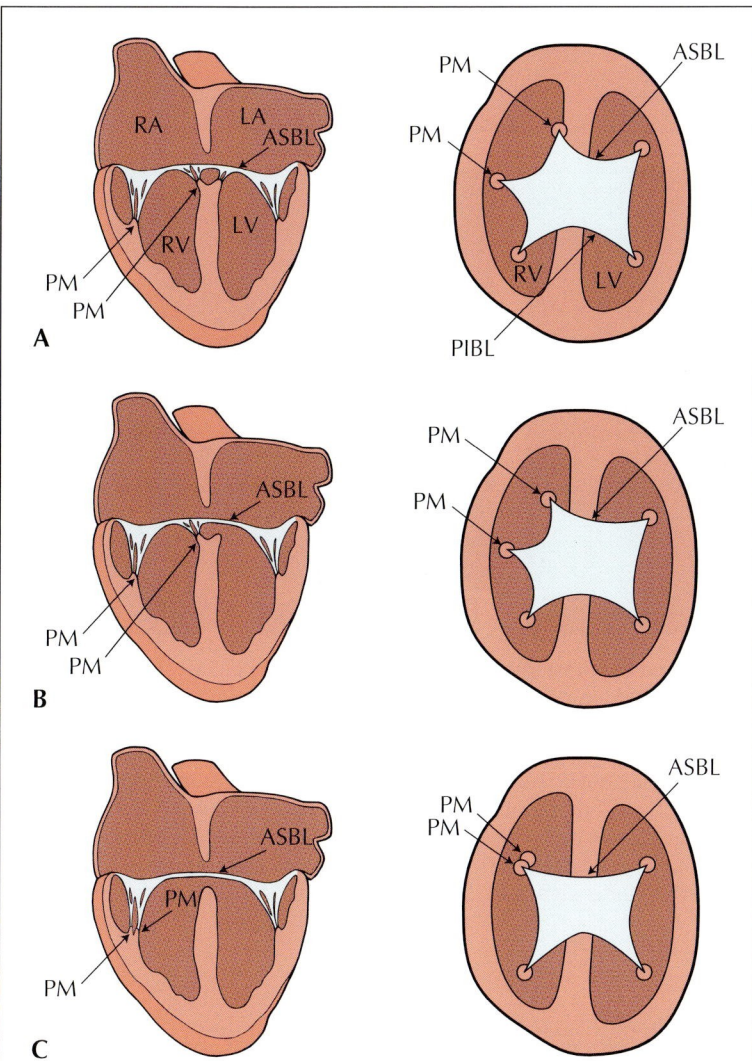

FIGURE 9-5. The classification of complete AVSDs, popularized by Rastelli *et al.* [7], is based on the morphology of the anterosuperior bridging leaflet (ASBL), which can be displayed exquisitely echocardiographically. This diagram of a complete AVSD depicts the types of AV valve attachments of the ASBL that are identifiable echocardiographically and fit the surgical description of Rastelli. The *left-hand panels* are four-chamber views, while the *right-hand panels* are equivalent to subcostal short-axis or parasternal short-axis views.

A, Rastelli type A defect. Here the ASBL can be seen to be attached to the papillary muscle (PM) lying on the crest of the septum between the left (LV) and right (RV) ventricles. In the subcostal view, the posteroinferior bridging leaflet (PIBL) is depicted to be attached to the crest of the septum. **B,** Rastelli type B defect. The ASBL is not attached to the septum, but to PM arising from the RV. **C,** Rastelli type C defect. The ASBL is attached to PM, which also supports the other leaflet of the tricuspid valve yielding a free-floating nonattached leaflet. The *arrows* in the *right-hand panels* indicate how the PM attachment is from a septally attached (type A) to RV-originating PM (type B), and PM fused with the anterior PM within the RV (type C).

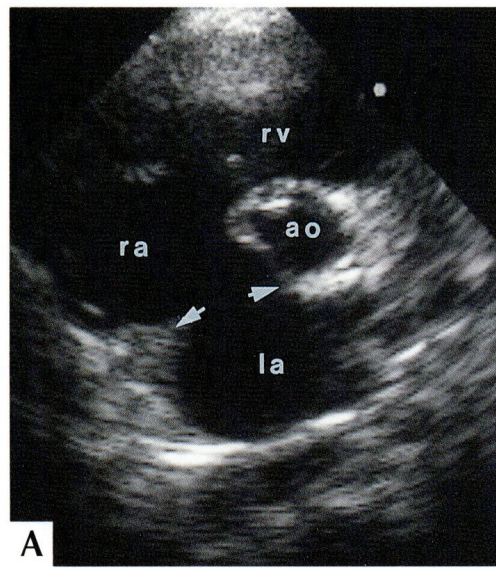 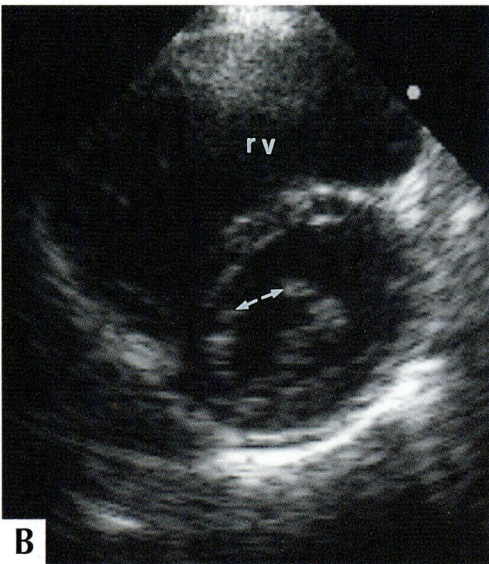 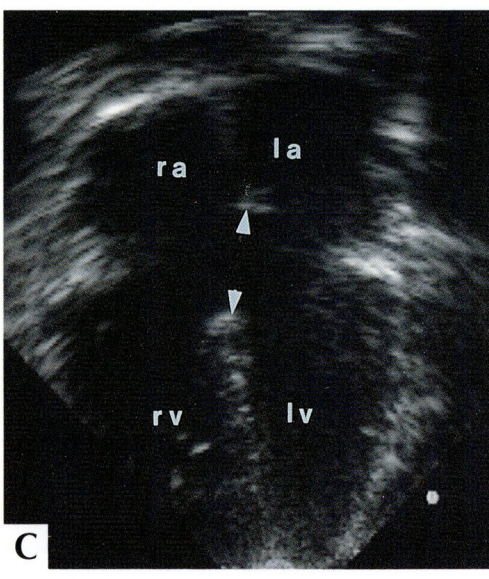

Figure 9-6. Transthoracic echocardiography can provide an accurate preoperative hemodynamic and morphologic evaluation of the wide spectrum of atrioventricular septal defects (AVSDs) [5,8–10]. Subcostal, parasternal short- and long-axis, and apical four-chamber views are complementary in assessing the extent of the atrial and ventricular communications, as well as the morphology, competency, and chordal attachments of the atrioventricular valves. The degree of septal malalignment, ventricular size, and outflow tract obstruction are also well defined by echocardiography. All of these different aspects of AVSDs, in addition to associated anomalies, must be addressed before surgical repair. **A,** Parasternal short-axis view illustrating the large primum defect component (*arrows*). In this patient, no

ventricular septal defect was present. **B,** Parasternal short-axis view at the level of the papillary muscles (PMs). This view is ideal to evaluate the number of PMs, the distance separating them, and the cleft in the anterior bridging leaflet. In AVSDs the PMs, particularly the posteromedial muscle, are rotated counterclockwise from their normal position. This patient has two distinct PMs and the cleft is typically oriented toward the right ventricular (rv) outflow tract (*arrows*). **C,** Apical four-chamber view of a patient with a complete AVSD with the common atrioventricular valve open in diastole. Large atrial and ventricular communications are present (*arrowheads*), and there is no atrioventricular septal malalignment. Both ventricles are well developed. ao—aorta; la—left atrium; lv—left ventricular; ra—right atrium.

SUBAORTIC STENOSIS

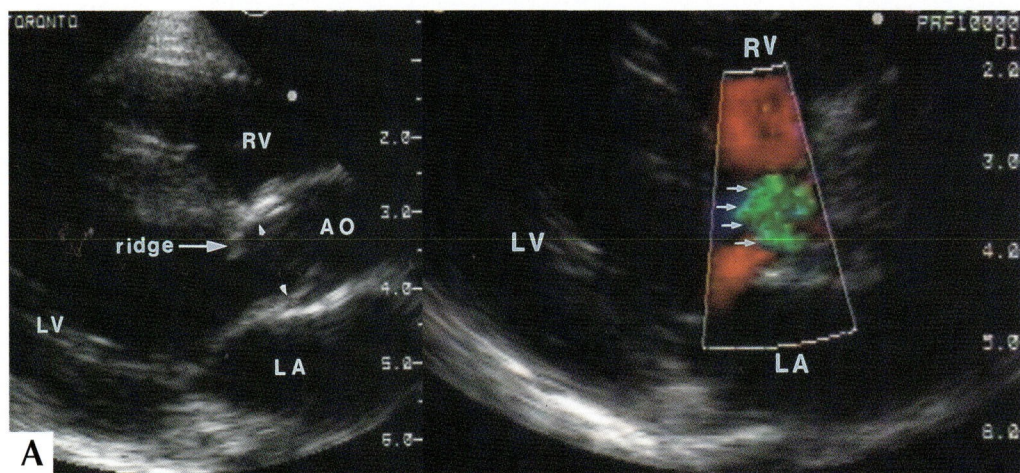 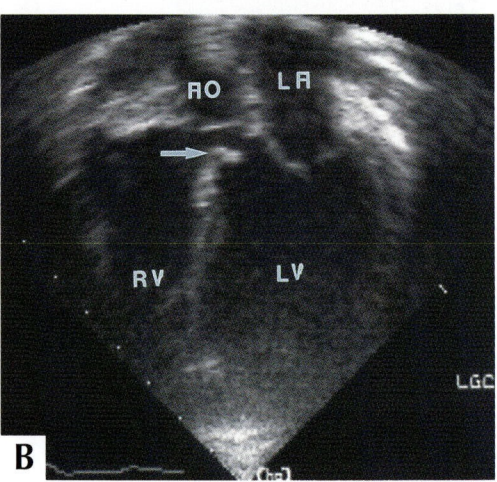

FIGURE 9-7. Although obstruction at the level of the aortic valve (congenital valvular aortic stenosis) is the most common form of congenital obstruction to left ventricular outflow, congenital subaortic stenosis due to a subaortic membrane or ridge is important to recognize since it can be readily corrected surgically. Subvalvular aortic stenosis can be the result of a discrete fibrous membrane, a thicker fibromuscular circumferential ridge, or a long tubular subaortic stenosis. This type of left ventricular (LV) outflow tract obstruction is frequently associated with ventricular septal defect, coarctation of the aorta (AO), and tubular hypoplasia of the aortic transverse arch. Optimal visualization of the subvalvular aortic stenosis can

be achieved in parasternal long-axis and apical five-chamber views. **A,** Parasternal long-axis view of a patient with subaortic stenosis caused by a fibrous ridge in close proximity to the aortic valve (*arrowheads*). Because of the parallel orientation of the membrane with the ultrasound beam part of the ridge may not be fully imaged in this view (*left*). Color Doppler mapping is useful in confirming the LV outflow tract obstruction created by this ridge (*arrows* on *right*). **B,** The apical five-chamber view allows good delineation of the circumferential nature of the fibrous membrane beneath the aortic valve inserting at the mitral aortic junction (*arrow*). (*continued*)

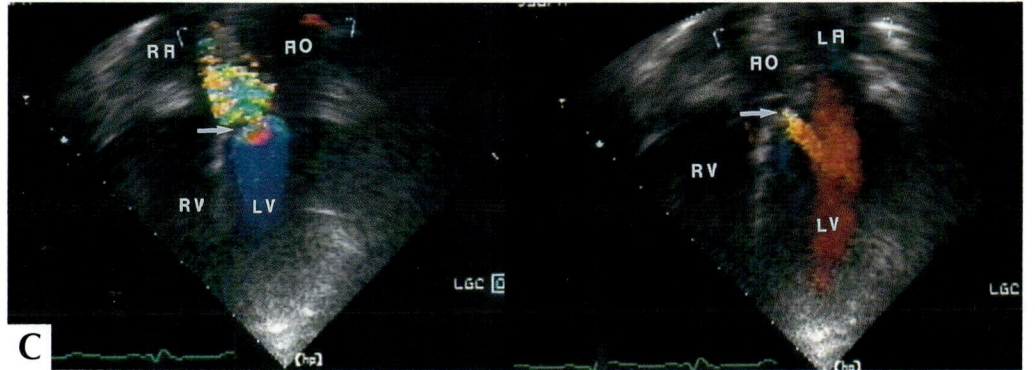

FIGURE 9-7. (*continued*) **C,** The presence of this subaortic ridge, its close proximity to the aortic valve, and the jet through the stenosis are responsible for progressive damage to the aortic valve. Color Doppler interrogation in apical five-chamber view in the same patient illustrates the systolic flow turbulence created by the stenotic subaortic membrane (*left*), and the red diastolic aortic valve regurgitation jet directed toward the LV apex as a result of jet lesion of the aortic valve (*right*) [11,12]. *Arrows* indicate the level of the subaortic membrane. LA—left atrium; RA—right atrium; RV—right ventricle.

COARCTATION OF THE AORTA

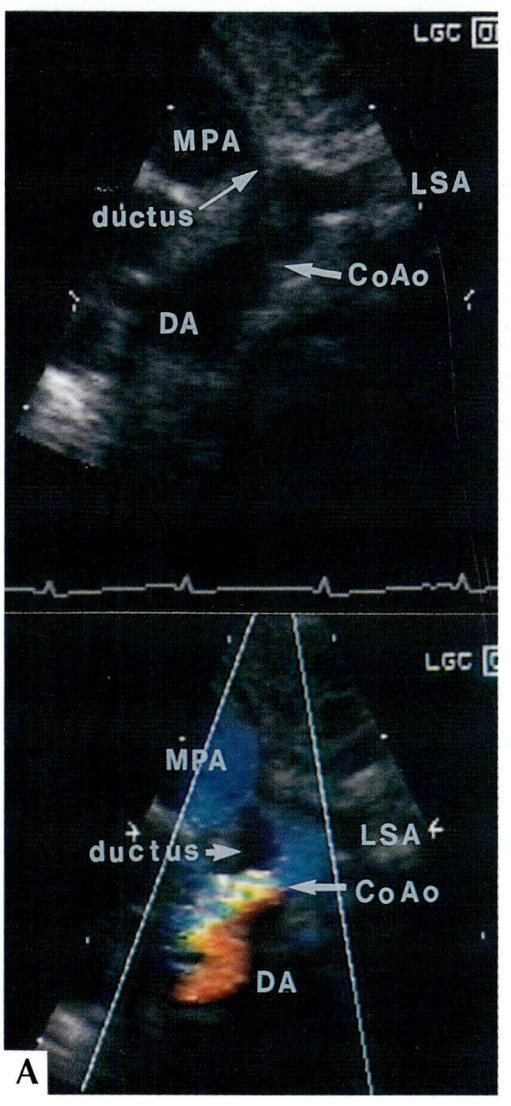

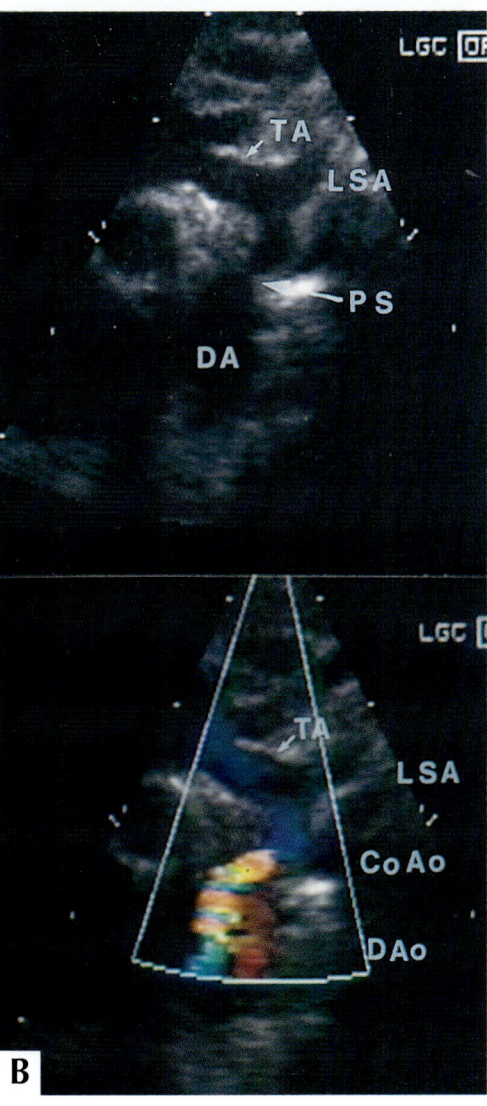

FIGURE 9-8. Coarctation of the aorta (CoAo). In this anomaly, which occurs twice as commonly in males as in females, there is constriction of the aorta, most commonly distal to the origin of the left subclavian artery. It is an important form of secondary hypertension. **A,** The ductal cut view with the transducer in the left subclavicular region is the best to show the relation between the site of coarctation created by the posterior shelf and the ductus arteriosus and the origin of the left subclavian artery (LSA) (*top*). Color Doppler reveals turbulent flow beginning at the level of coarctation. In this patient, the ductus arteriosus was closed as demonstrated by the absence of color signal in it (*bottom*). **B,** Coarctation of the aorta is also very well imaged from the suprasternal long-axis view. In this view the relation of the coarctation with ductus arteriosus is not well defined but the diameter of the transverse arch, which is often hypoplastic, can be well evaluated (*top*). As mentioned previously, color Doppler revealed the exact site of obstruction (*bottom*). (*continued*)

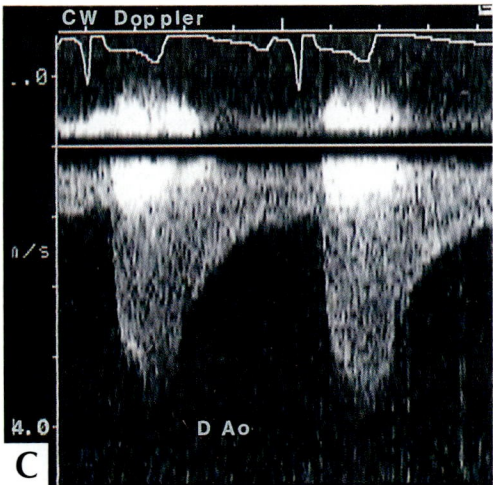

C

FIGURE 9-8. (*continued*) **C,** Continuous-wave Doppler examination of the descending aorta (DA/DAo) from the suprasternal notch of a patient with severe coarctation of the aorta. This negative signal represents flow away from the transducer. This is a typical flow signal observed in patients with coarctation of the aorta, with high-velocity systolic flow (3.7 m/s) continuing in diastole, representing the persistent gradient across the site of obstruction [13]. MPA—main pulmonary artery; PS—posterior shelf; TA—transverse arch.

EBSTEIN'S ANOMALY

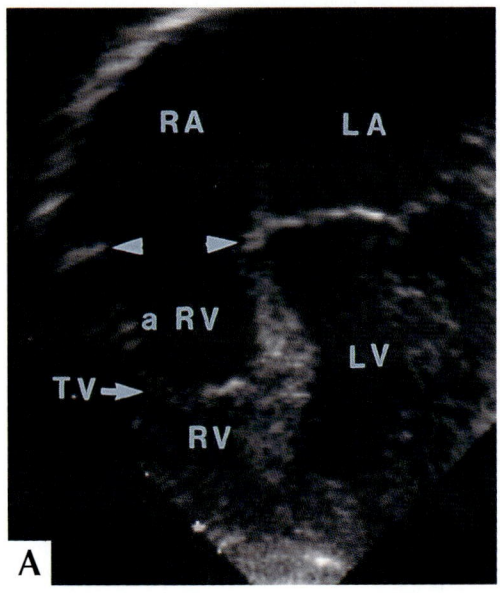

A

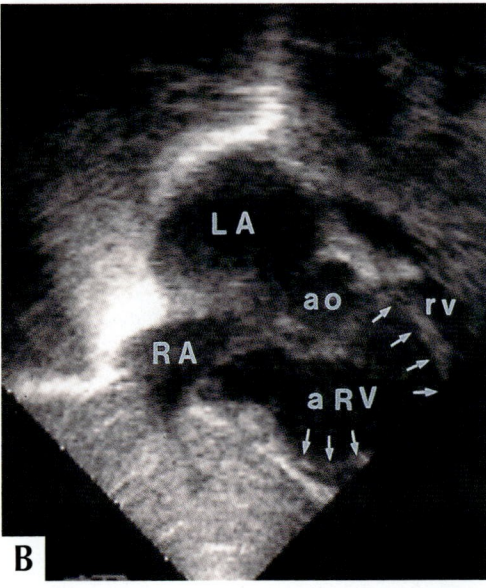

B

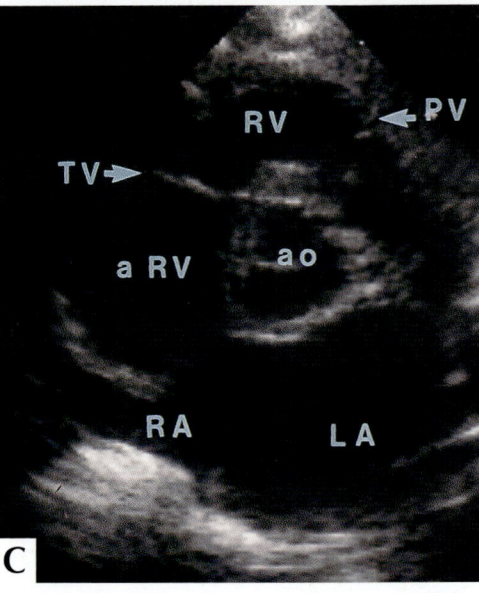

C

FIGURE 9-9. Patients with Ebstein's anomaly often are cyanotic due to right-to-left atrial shunting, and they frequently develop symptoms secondary to tricuspid regurgitation and right ventricular dysfunction due to hypoplasia of this chamber; paroxysmal atrial tachycardia is common as well. Surgical treatment includes prosthetic replacement of the tricuspid valve or creation of a competent unicuspid tricuspid valve by insertion of an anterior leaflet into the tricuspid annulus. Ebstein's anomaly of the tricuspid valve (TV) is characterized by dysplasia of the leaflets with downward displacement of the septal and posterior leaflets from the annulus. This results in atrialization of a portion of the right ventricle (aRV). Although the superoanterior leaflet is not displaced, its distal attachments are abnormal and may promote significant hemodynamic abnormalities. **A,** Apical four-chamber view of a patient with Ebstein's anomaly with severe inferior displacement of the TV septal leaflet. This view is the best to diagnose Ebstein's malformation. The anterosuperior and septal leaflets can be seen, and the degree of aRV can be evaluated as well as the severity of TV stenosis and/or regurgitation. *Arrowheads* indicate the right atrioventricular groove. **B,** Subcostal sagittal view, where inferior leaflets and the saillike anterior leaflet with its abnormal attachments can be visualized. Size and patency of the RV outflow tract can also be assessed in this plane. *Arrows* indicate the extent of the "atrialized" portion of the RV. **C,** Parasternal short-axis view showing the septal leaflet plastered down to the septal surface resulting in a displacement of the TV and partial aRV. The anterior leaflet is also visualized in this view [14,15]. ao—aorta; LA—left atrium; LV—left ventricle; PV—pulmonary valve; RA—right atrium.

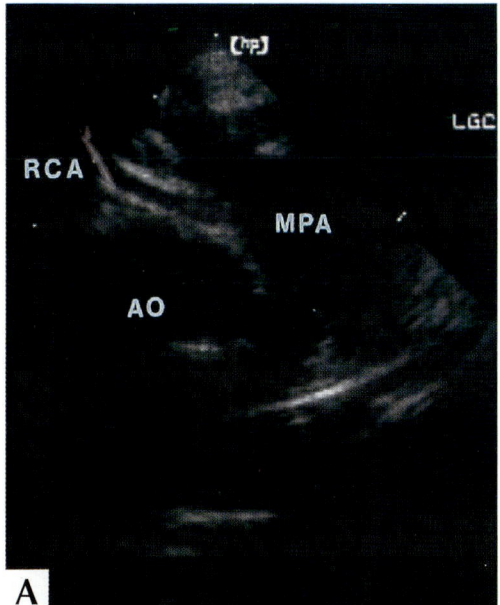

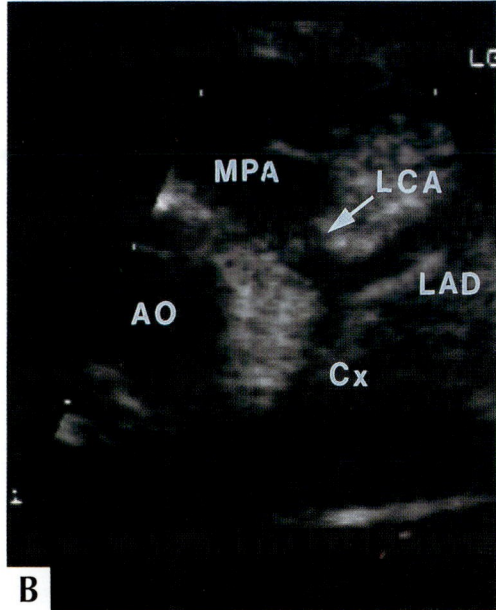

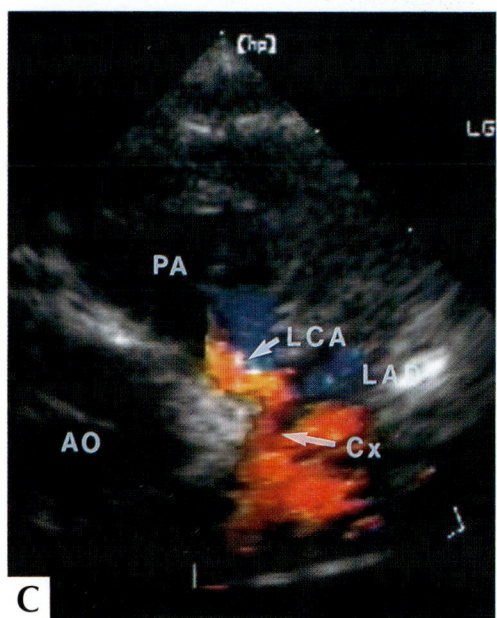

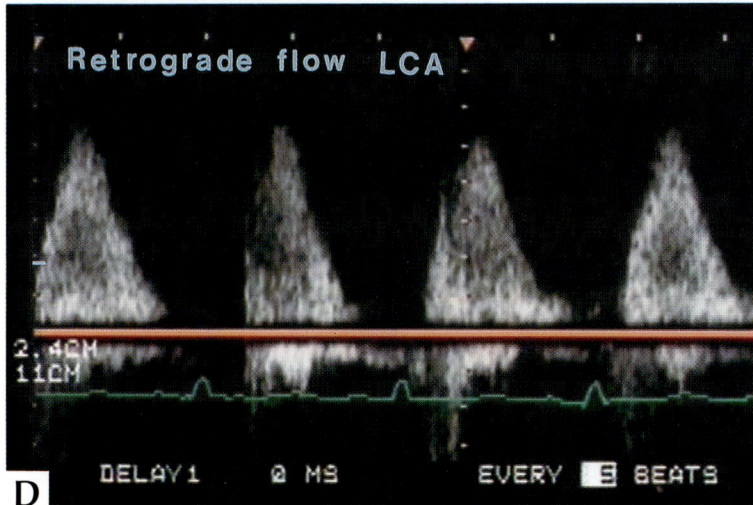

FIGURE 9-10. Infants with anomalous origin of the left coronary artery present with myocardial infarction and congestive heart failure as well as angina-like symptoms that may be misinterpreted as colic. The electrocardiogram shows deep Q waves and ST- and T-wave alterations in leads 1,

aVL, V5, and V6. The chest roentgenogram usually demonstrates enlargement of the left atrium and left ventricle. Medical treatment consists of the management of heart failure, and surgical treatment involves reimplanting the left coronary artery into the aortic root. Echocardiography is critical to the diagnosis. The anomalous origin of the left main coronary artery (LCA) from the main pulmonary artery (MPA) results in progressive steal of the myocardial blood supply by retrograde flow from the coronary arteries into the pulmonary trunk as the pulmonary vascular bed resistance decreases. It is mandatory to eliminate a diagnosis of anomalous origin of the LCA when echocardiographic signs such as poorly contractile and dilated left ventricle with evidence of endocardial fibroelastosis and mitral valve regurgitation are present. **A,** One of the most pathognomonic echocardiographic signs is the diffuse dilation of the right coronary artery (RCA). **B,** Parasternal short-axis view with clockwise rotation of the transducer illustrating the LCA originating from the MPA trunk usually from the posterior surface. In some cases, the coronary ostium is difficult to visualize properly, and Doppler interrogation has proven to be very helpful in defining the origin and direction of the coronary blood supply. **C,** In the parasternal short-axis view, color Doppler examination reveals retrograde flow in the left anterior descending (LAD; *blue*) and the circumflex (Cx; *red*) coronary arteries going toward the MPA. **D,** In the same position, pulsed Doppler interrogation confirmed the retrograde diastolic flow in the LCA [16]. AO—aorta; PA—pulmonary artery.

TETRALOGY OF FALLOT

PATHOPHYSIOLOGY

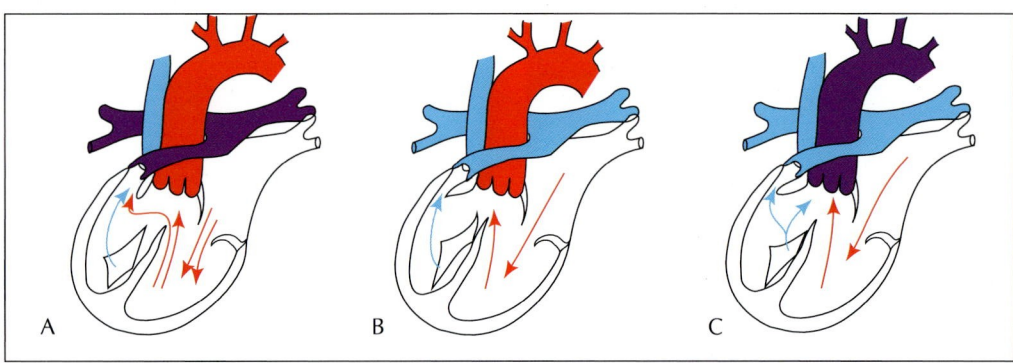

the degree of PS determines the amount of pulmonary blood flow. Perhaps surprisingly in ToF, PS may be mild enough to allow a net left-to-right shunt (A), even to the extent of causing symptoms and signs of pulmonary overcirculation [17]. If the degree of PS is moderate (B), the circulation may be balanced with minimal shunting in either direction. As PS becomes more severe (C), right-to-left shunting at the level of the VSD increases, causing increasing cyanosis. With critical stenosis or atresia, pulmonary blood flow becomes dependent on alternate sources of supply. Patients may present with moderate, severe, or critical PS in infancy; others may present "pink" and then undergo "transformation" into the cyanotic form of ToF as the degree of stenosis progresses [18].

FIGURE 9-11. Pathophysiology of Tetralogy of Fallot (ToF). The physiology of ToF serves as the paradigm of VSD in association with pulmonary stenosis (PS). Because the VSD is usually nonrestrictive,

IMAGING

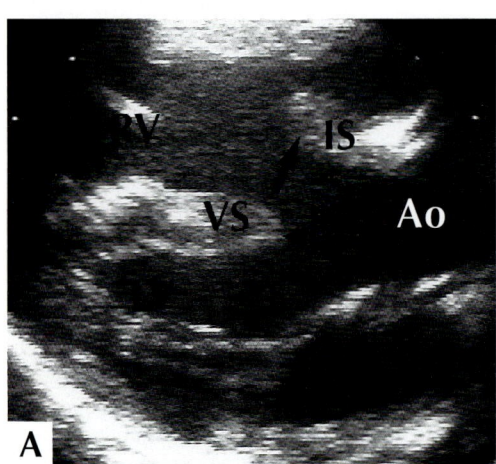

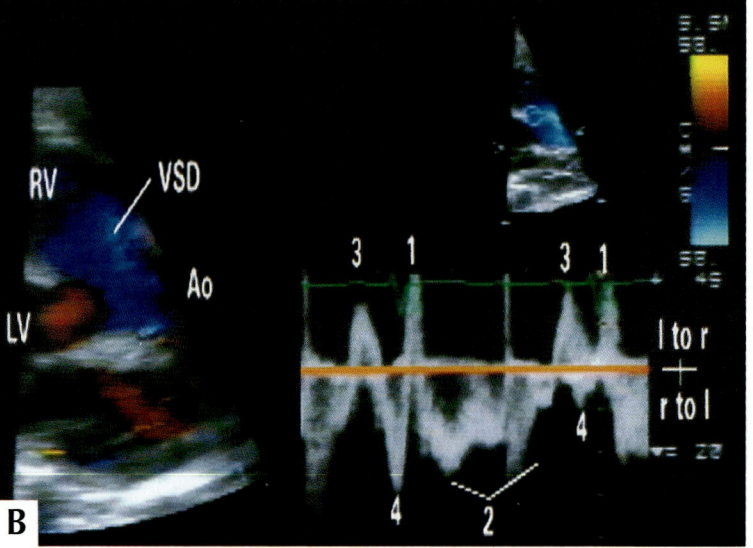

FIGURE 9-12. Parasternal long-axis views of the VSD in Tetralogy of Fallot (ToF). **A,** In ToF, the aorta (Ao) overrides the large defect left between the crest of the ventricular septum (VS) (*arrowhead*) and the anteriorly deviated infundibular septum (IS) (*arrow*). The latter "squeezes" the pulmonary infundibulum causing subpulmonary stenosis. **B,** Although color flow

mapping of the VSD in ToF demonstrates predominantly RV to LV shunting, this pulsed wave spectral display reveals complex phasic bidirectional shunting (phases 1 and 3, left to right; phases 2 and 4, right to left). Additional muscular VSDs occasionally may complicate ToF or TAC. LA—left atrium; LV—left ventricle; RV—right ventricle.

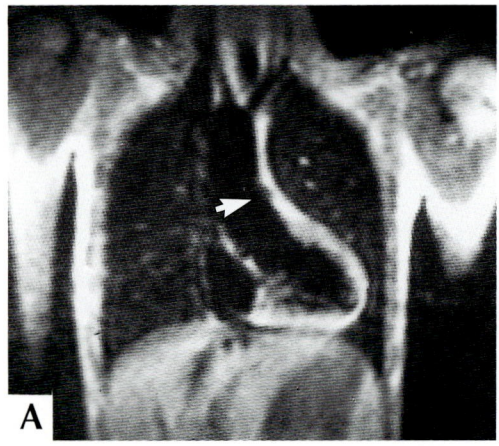

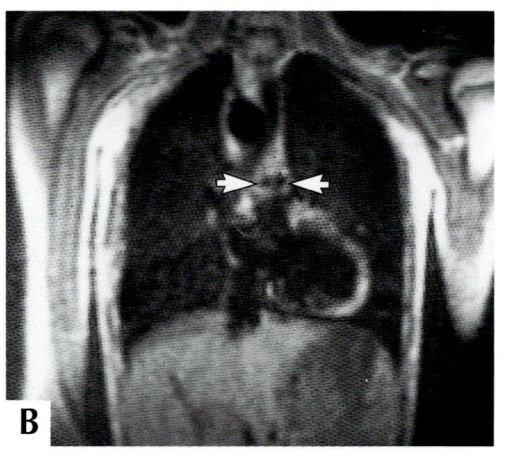

FIGURE 9-13. Tetralogy of Fallot (ToF) with pulmonary valve atresia. Shown are coronal MR images beginning anteriorly at the level of the ascending aorta (*arrow*) (**A**) and progressing posteriorly. The hypoplastic right and left pulmonary arteries (4 mm in diameter) are demonstrated (*arrows* in **B**) and the presence of a pulmonary artery confluence (*arrow*) can be ascertained (**C**). (*continued*)

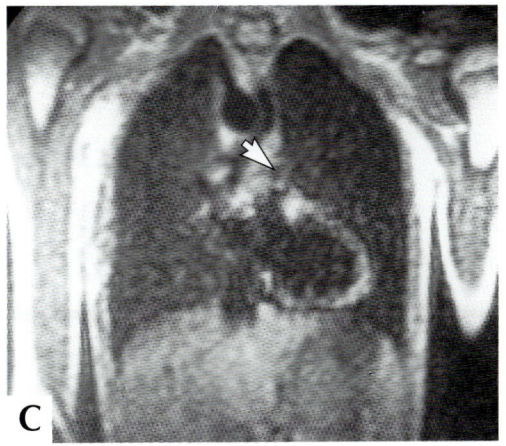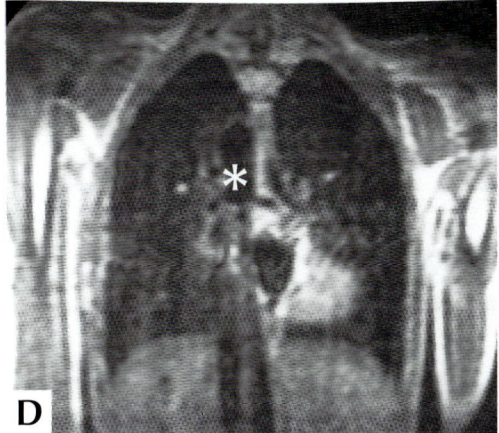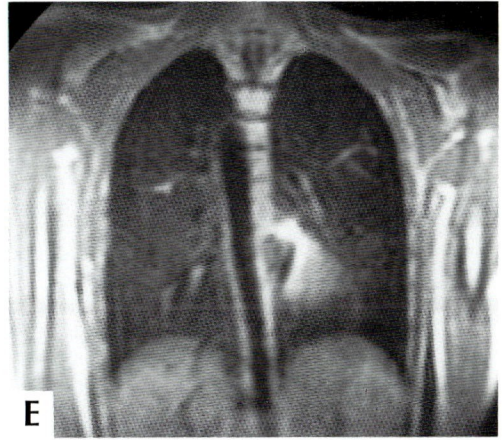

FIGURE 9-13. (*continued*) Although systemic to pulmonary collateral arteries are shown to arise from the upper descending thoracic aorta (*asterisk* in **D**), the extent of the pulmonary arterial tree supplied and the degree of possible arborization abnormality present await definition by standard radiographic angiographic investigation. The most posterior image (**E**) demonstrates the right-sided descending aorta.

CLINICAL PRESENTATION

CLINICAL PRESENTATION OF TOF

DIAGNOSIS	AGE AT PRESENTATION	CLINICAL FINDINGS	CHEST RADIOGRAPHY	ECG	HYPEROXIA TEST (PASS: $PO_2 \geq 150$ TORR WHEN $FIO_2 = 1.0$)
ToF with moderate sub-PS	Day 1 of life	Loud SEM; cyanosis proportional to degree of PS	"Boot-shaped" cardiac silhouette with scooped-out MPA segment; normal or decreased PBF	RV hypertrophy (upright T waves in V_1 after 3–5 d of age)	Pass or fail depending on degree of PS
ToF pulmonary atresia	1st day to months depending on source(s) and amount of PBF	Cyanosis, if too little PBF, classically with closing ductus arteriosus; CHF and continuous murmurs if too much PBF from collaterals	"Boot-shaped" cardiac silhouette with absent MPA segment; usually decreased PBF; may have abnormal PBF pattern if aortopulmonary collaterals are present	Same as ToF; may also develop LV hypertrophy if there are excessive aortopulmonary collaterals and PBF	Fail
ToF with AV canal defect	Day 1 of life	Often, trisomy 21; loud SEM; cyanosis proportional to the degree of PS	Similar to ToF; ± RA enlargement if AV valve incompetence	RV hypertrophy + superior frontal plane axis with counterclockwise looping	Pass or fail depending on degree of PS
ToF with absent pulmonary valve syndrome	Day 1 of life	Air trapping + CO_2 retention improved in prone position; classic loud to-and-fro murmur of PS and PR	Cardiac enlargement, bilateral hyperinflation, aneurysmal hilar PAs	Same as ToF	Fail, but picture confused by associated hypoventilation

FIGURE 9-14. Clinical presentation of Tetralogy of Fallot (ToF). This table presents the salient clinical features, common signs, symptoms, and initial laboratory evaluation of ToF, TAC, and their major variations. The "hyperoxia" test [19] involves evaluating the arterial partial pressure of oxygen (PO_2) of the patient 20 minutes after administration of 100% fraction of inspired oxygen (FiO_2), and requires normal ventilation for meaningful interpretation. AV—atrioventricular; CHF—congestive heart failure; LV—left ventricular; MPA—main pulmonary artery; PA—pulmonary artery; PBF—pulmonary blood flow; PR—pulmonary regurgitation; PS—pulmonary stenosis; RA—right atrium; RV—right ventricular; SEM—systolic ejection murmur.

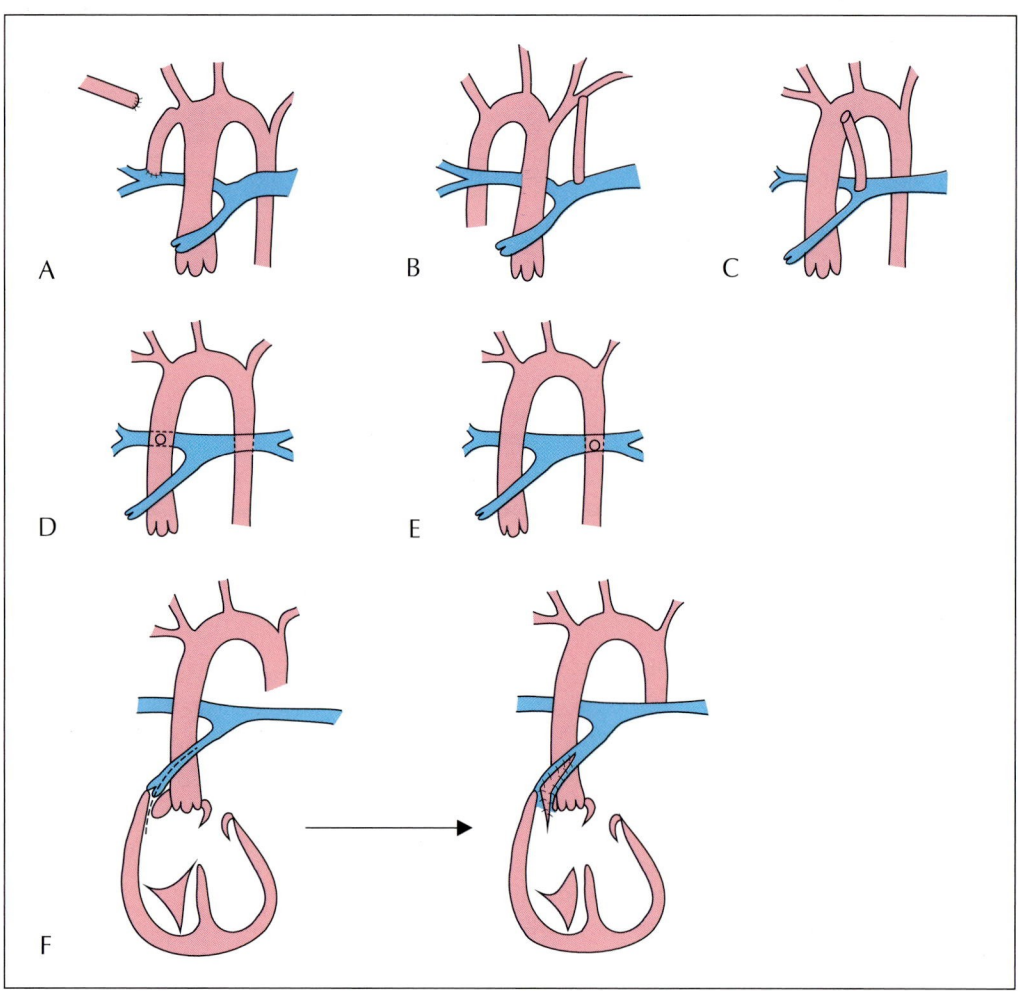

FIGURE 9-15. Palliative surgery for Tetralogy of Fallot (ToF). In most cases, complete surgical correction is the treatment of choice for ToF. However, a number of palliative procedures are also possible. **A–E,** Various palliative shunt procedures that do not require cardiopulmonary bypass. These shunts are designed to increase pulmonary blood flow and allow growth of the branch pulmonary arteries (PAs), but must be small enough to restrict transmission of aortic pressure to the PAs. The classic Blalock-Taussig (B-T) shunt (**A**) devised by dividing the subclavian artery and anastomosing it to the ipsilateral branch PA, usually on the side opposite the arch. The modified (*left*) B-T shunt (**B**) involves interposition of a prosthetic tube graft between the ipsilateral subclavian artery and branch PAs. The "central shunt" (**C**) has many variations and is usually created by placing a prosthetic tube graft between the ascending aorta and the area of the PA bifurcation. The Waterston (**D**) and Potts (**E**) shunts involve creation of direct "window" anastomoses between the right PA and the overlying ascending aorta or the left PA and the underlying descending aorta, respectively. The Waterston and Potts shunts have largely been abandoned because they were associated with a high incidence of complications such as pulmonary vascular disease and/or severe branch PA distortion. **F,** In patients with severe branch PA hypoplasia, which is associated more frequently with ToF and pulmonary atresia, a transannular outflow patch can be performed without closure of the VSD, improving pulmonary blood flow, and allowing access for subsequent transcatheter balloon angioplasty of branch PA stenoses.

TRUNCUS ARTERIOSUS COMMUNIS

In truncus arteriosus communis, a single vessel forms the outlet for both ventricles and gives rise to both the systemic and pulmonary arteries.

CLASSIFICATION OF TRUNCUS ARTERIOSUS

	Collett-Edwards	VanPraagh
	Type 1	Type A1
	Type 2	Type A2
	Type 3	Type A2
	Type 4	Tetralogy of Fallot with pulmonary atresia
	Subtype of type 3	Type A3
	Subtype of types 1 or 2	Type A4
	Type "5" (incomplete form of TAC)	Type B2
	Not encountered	Type B3

FIGURE 9-16. The classification schemes of persistent truncus arteriosus communis (TAC) as devised by Collett and Edwards [20] and VanPraagh and VanPraagh [21]. The existence of two different popular classification schemes that employ similar numerical labeling is a recipe for confusion. This figure contrasts the classification schemes of the variants of TAC encountered by these two groups of investigators. A basic disagreement over the embryologic origin of the two defects partly underlies the differing approaches to nomenclature and categorization [22–24].

Collett and Edwards [20] call the defect "persistent truncus arteriosus" and classify the anomaly according to the origin of the branch pulmonary arteries (PAs). In type 1 TAC, the branches arise from a main pulmonary artery (MPA) component; in type 2, the branches arise adjacent to one another without a distinct MPA component; and in type 3, the branches arise remotely from one another. Collett and Edwards claim that each stage, in ascending numerical order, represents persistence of an even earlier embryonic phase of development. Type 4, in which true mediastinal branch PAs are absent and "collateral" arteries from the descending aorta supply the lungs, probably does not fulfill the criteria for TAC. VanPraagh and others [25] have argued that Collett-Edwards type 4 TAC is really tetralogy of Fallot with pulmonary atresia, a view with which Edwards [24] later agreed.

VanPraagh and VanPraagh [21] omit "persistent" from the name TAC, believing that the defect is not the consequence of *persistence* of the embryonic truncus, but rather is a variant of pulmonary infundibular and (often) valvar atresia associated with solitary aortic trunk, and completely absent aorticopulmonary septum. They first divide TAC according to whether a VSD is present (type A) or absent (type B). Type B TAC in their scheme has separate semilunar valves and an intact ventricular septum, a defect that other authorities classify as the complete form of aorticopulmonary septal defect [26]. Types A1 and A2 are identical to types 1 and 2 of Collett-Edwards. The VanPraagh scheme assigns a separate category, type A3, to highlight the rare but important group of TAC with absence or discontinuity of either branch PA. In this situation, the involved lung derives its supply from a ductus or an aortopulmonary collateral vessel. Type A4 of VanPraagh comprises the uncommon but serious group in which there is associated aortic arch interruption or coarctation. Other rare but important variants not covered in either classification include TAC with atrioventricular canal defect [27], TAC with restrictive aorticopulmonary or VSD components [28], or a common truncal valve with intact ventricular septum [29], among others [30].

PATHOPHYSIOLOGY

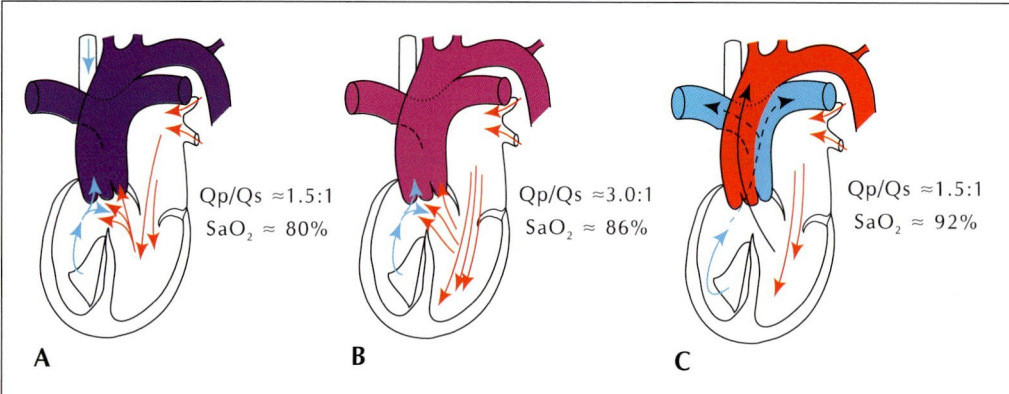

$Qp/Qs \approx 1.5:1$
$SaO_2 \approx 80\%$

$Qp/Qs \approx 3.0:1$
$SaO_2 \approx 86\%$

$Qp/Qs \approx 1.5:1$
$SaO_2 \approx 92\%$

A   **B**   **C**

FIGURE 9-17. Pathophysiology of TAC. The physiology of TAC depends in part on the presence or absence of *streaming*, separating oxygenated from deoxygenated blood despite the absence of anatomic aortopulmonary septation. Such streaming, when it occurs, is presumably related to favorable spatial orientation of the branch pulmonary arteries relative to the VSD and results in unexpectedly high arterial oxygen saturation (SaO_2). More typically, however, physiology in TAC is analogous to single ventricle in which there is common mixing of oxygenated and deoxygenated blood (at the level of the VSD in TAC). The SaO_2 is wholly dependent on the ratio of pulmonary-to-systemic blood flow (Qp/Qs), which in turn is inversely proportional to the pulmonary:systemic resistance ratio (Rp/Rs). As the elevated pulmonary vascular resistance (PVR) of the newborn falls, pulmonary blood flow increases associated with parallel increases in SaO_2 and symptoms of congestive heart failure.

A, Mixing of oxygenated with deoxygenated blood at the level of the VSD. With only mildly reduced PVR, symptoms of congestive heart failure are absent or mild. **B,** As pulmonary flow increases, consequent to a falling Rp/Rs ratio in the first weeks of life, more oxygenated blood mixes with the deoxygenated blood, resulting in a more highly oxygen-saturated systemic mixture. Unfortunately, this improved SaO_2 is at the expense of pulmonary overcirculation and consequent heart failure. **C,** The less common situation in which the oxygenated and deoxygenated blood streams cross each other with little mixing, allowing excellent systemic oxygen saturation irrespective of the amount of pulmonary blood flow. This situation may allow the patient to pass a "hyperoxia" test and to have a high SaO_2 without the expected signs and symptoms of pulmonary overcirculation.

IMAGING

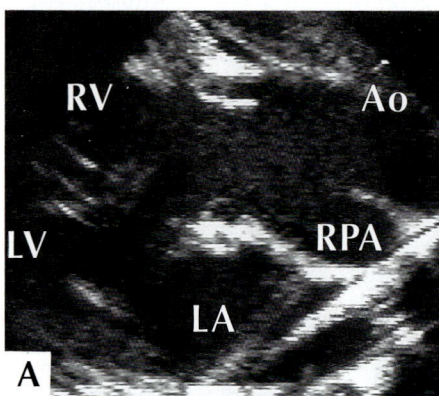

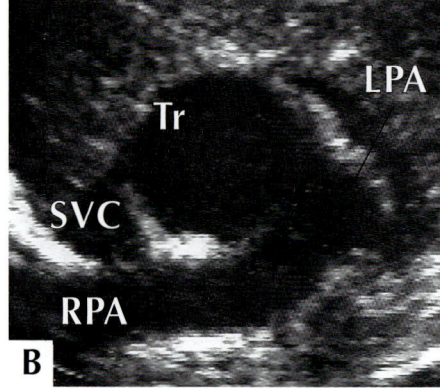

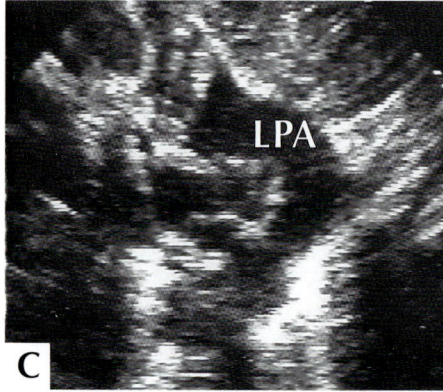

FIGURE 9-18. Imaging of TAC with separate origins of branch pulmonary arteries from the truncus (type A2 of the VanPraagh classification). **A,** A parasternal long-axis view shows excellent systolic excursion of the thin truncal valve overriding the crest of the ventricular septum. **B,** The course of the right pulmonary artery (RPA) posterior to the truncus (Tr) is best displayed in a high parasternal transverse plane. The right pulmonary artery (RPA) arises from the posterior aspect of the truncus, immediately to the right of the left pulmonary artery (LPA) takeoff. **C,** Angling just superior to the RPA orifice and rotating counterclockwise displays the course of the LPA. Not infrequently, it is difficult by any imaging modality to distinguish between adjacent separate branch pulmonary artery origins from the truncus versus a very short MPA component, a situation somewhat facetiously referred to as type A "1 and 1/2." Ao—aorta; LA—left atrium; LV—left ventricle; RV—right ventricle.

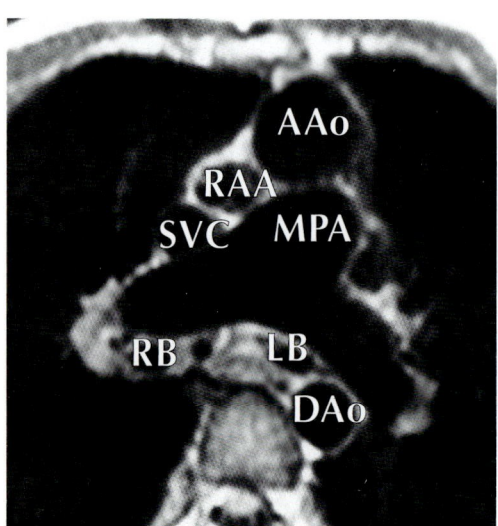

FIGURE 9-19. Axial spin-echo image showing a patient with d-transposed great arteries. The ascending aorta (AAo) is clearly seen anterior to the main pulmonary artery (MPA). Caudal images allow us to follow the AAo to the right ventricle and the MPA to the left ventricle. Although the coronary arteries are often seen in thin axial images, in many cases, their small size compared with the image thickness makes it difficult to define their precise anatomy and course. DAo—descending aorta; LB—left mainstem bronchus; RAA—right atrial appendage; RB—right mainstream bronchus; SVC—superior vena cava.

Complete Transposition of the Great Arteries

In complete transposition of the great arteries, the aorta arises from the right ventricle, and the pulmonary artery arises from the left ventricle to the left and posterior to the aorta. In most cases there is an interatrial septal defect and a patent ductus arteriosus. Patients are characterized by severe cyanosis, congestive heart failure, and in the absence of aortic stenosis, the development of pulmonary vascular changes.

SURGICAL TREATMENT

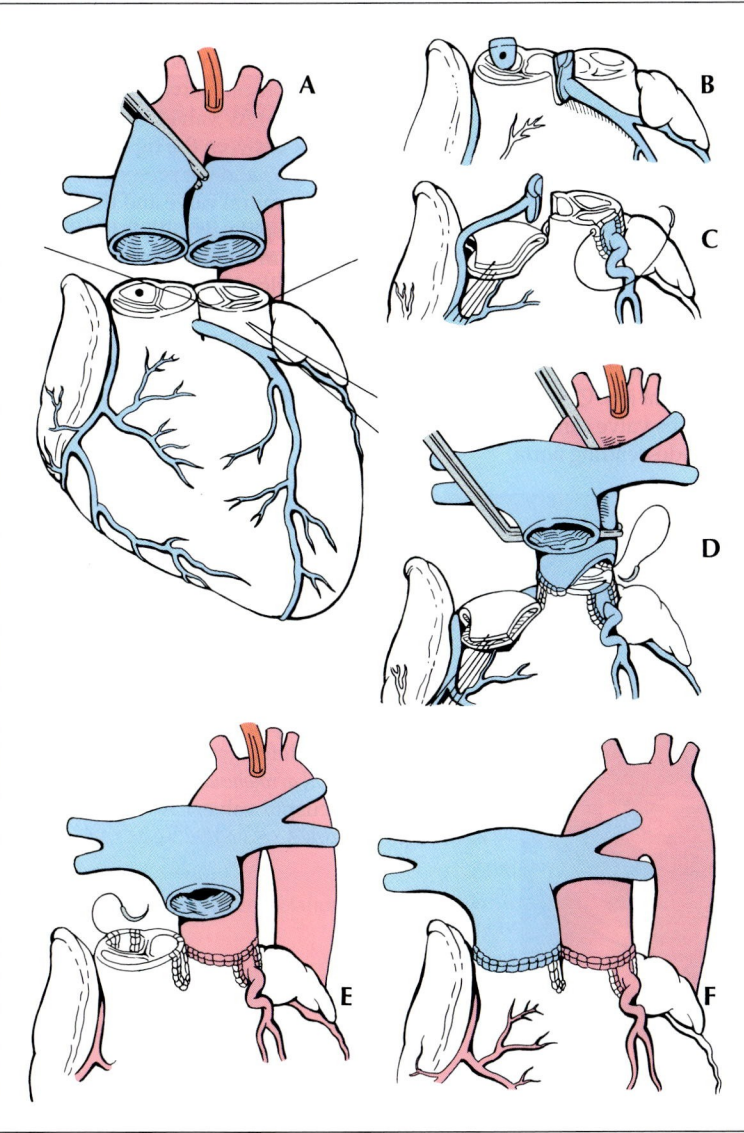

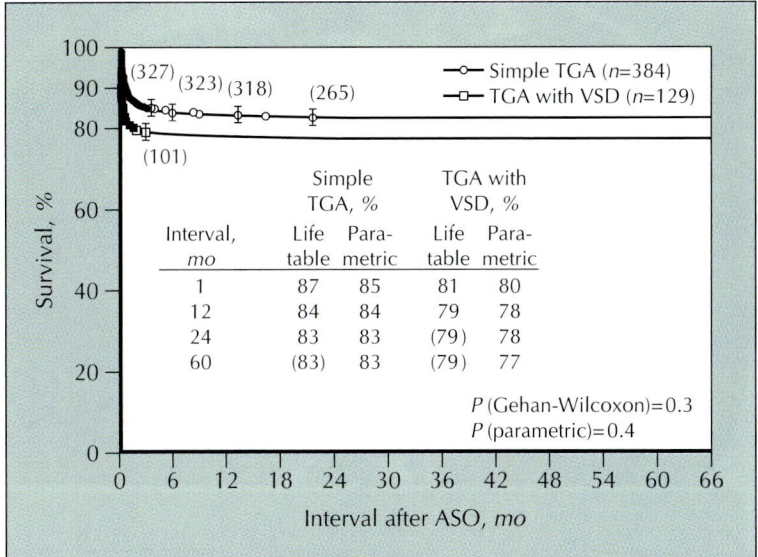

FIGURE 9-21. Operative mortality and risk factors for death. This graph shows survival after the ASO in patients with transposition of the great arteries (TGA) with intact ventricular septum (simple TGA) or TGA with ventricular septal defect (VSD). The *circles* and *squares* and the *t-bars* represent actuarial estimates based on reported experience from a multi-institutional study of outcomes after surgery for TGA conducted by the Congenital Heart Surgeons Society [37]. "Life table" refers to the actual Kaplan-Meier depiction; "parametric" refers to the average risk-adjusted survival obtained in the 513 patients repaired at 22 separate institutions from January 1, 1985 through March 1, 1989. Recent surgical results have improved significantly [38,39]. (*Adapted from* Kirklin *et al.* [37].)

FIGURE 9-20. Technique of the arterial switch operation (ASO). The anatomic challenges of arterial switching have been met by the application of novel surgical techniques [31–35] with many individual modifications. **A,** The great arteries are transected in a manner that allows eventual reanastomosis of the distal aortic segment to the proximal pulmonary artery (PA) (neoaortic root). **B,** Transfer of the coronary arteries to this pulmonary segment is facilitated by their excision from the aortic sinus with a cuff of adjacent aortic wall. **C,** Posterior translocation of the coronary "buttons" with incorporation into the neoaortic root. **D,** The proximal neoaortic root is connected to the distal aorta by an end-to-end anastomosis; Lecompte's innovative maneuver [32] passes the previously anterior aorta behind the bifurcation of the PA. **E,** The coronary artery "donor sites" are patched with glutaraldehyde-treated pericardium. **F,** The distal PA is directly anastomosed to the neopulmonary root. Alternatively, the right ventricular–PA connections can be established by using an interposed prosthetic tubular conduit [33]. (*Adapted from* Castañeda *et al.* [36].)

BALLOON ATRIAL SEPTOSTOMY

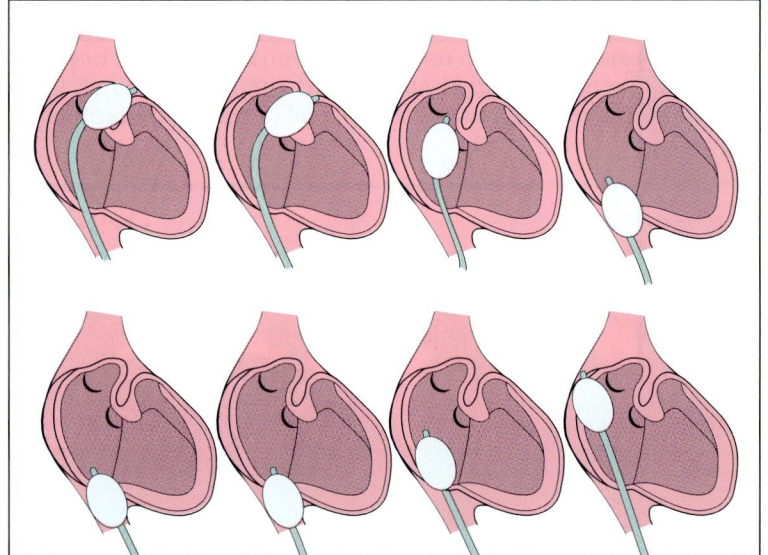

FIGURE 9-27. Sequential diagrams of a balloon atrial septostomy. The indications for this procedure include anatomic situations that have mandated a parallel pulmonary and systemic circulation or cases in which there is no egress for venous return to the concordant ventricle. Whereas these patients initially were destined for an atrial switch repair (Mustard or Senning procedure), today an anatomic correction is performed in the newborn period. Balloon septostomy is still performed frequently at diagnosis to ensure adequate arterial oxygen saturation while awaiting surgery.

PULMONARY VALVE DILATION

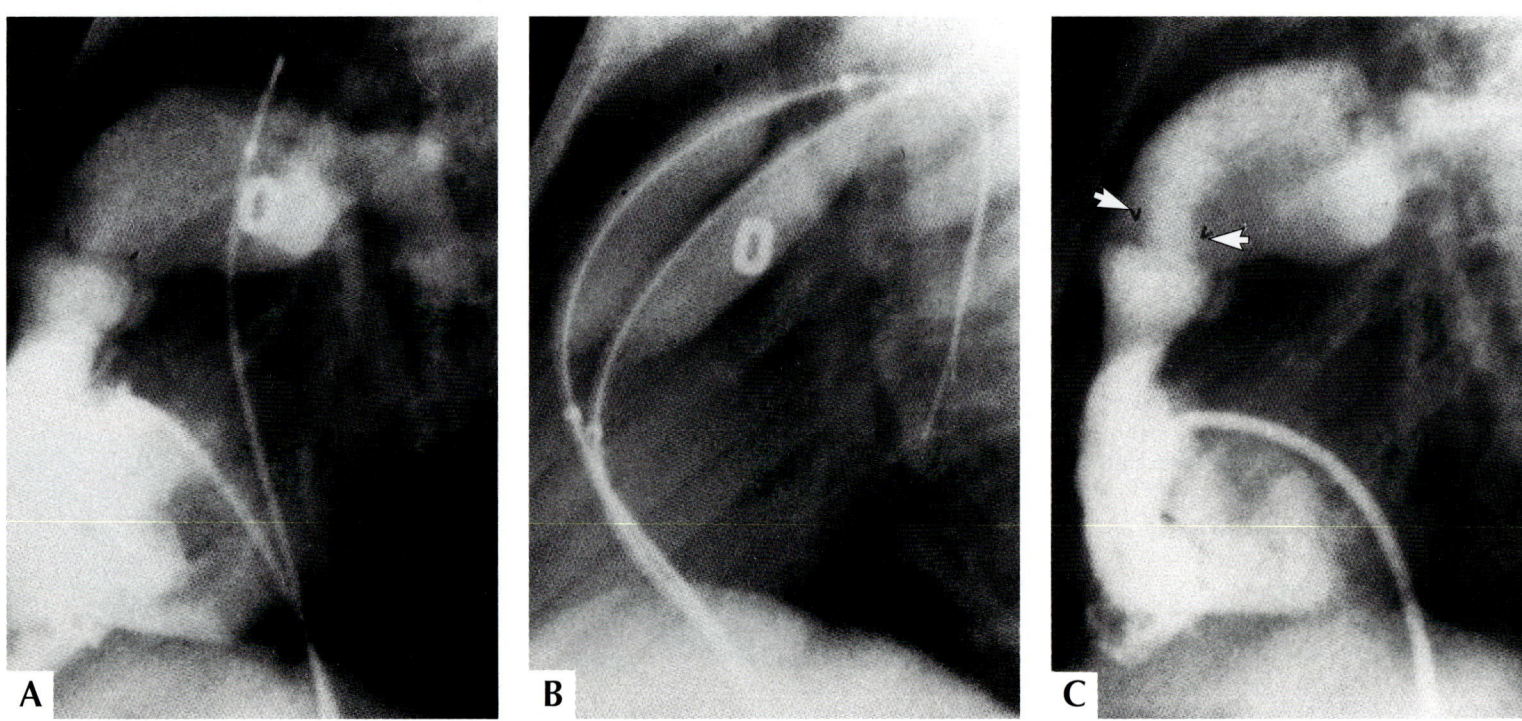

A   **B**   **C**

FIGURE 9-28. Typical pulmonary valve stenosis in a teenager. **A,** Thin doming valve leaflets. **B,** Two balloons inflated across the valve. **C,** Disrupted valve leaflets (*arrowheads*). Indications for pulmonary valve balloon dilation include a peak systolic right ventricular–to–main pulmonary artery gradient greater than 40 mm Hg. Owing to the persistence of the arterial duct in the newborn, tricuspid regurgitation, and pulmonary hypertension, the gradient may be low (<40 mm Hg). Such cases require intervention based on clinical and echocardiographic findings.

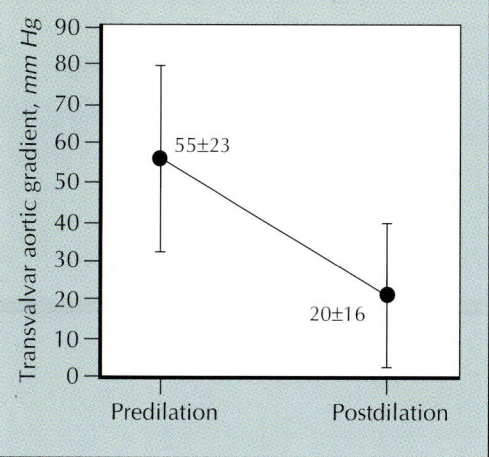

FIGURE 9-29. Results of balloon dilation of the aortic valve in 125 patients (newborns [$n = 20$] through 18 years of age). Although considered a palliative procedure, the recurrence rate requiring reintervention has been surprisingly low over the 8 years of follow-up. Surgical intervention has only been required in cases in which the hemodynamic results were not satisfactory, although a second dilation is attempted first. More often surgery is required to repair the aortic valve in those few patients ($n = 4$) with balloon-induced severe aortic regurgitation. No replacements have yet been required in our patient group due to this complication. Gradient reduction of 60% of predilation values can be achieved. An increase in angiographic grade of aortic regurgitation is frequent, but generally mild.

NATIVE (UNOPERATED) COARCTATION OF THE AORTA

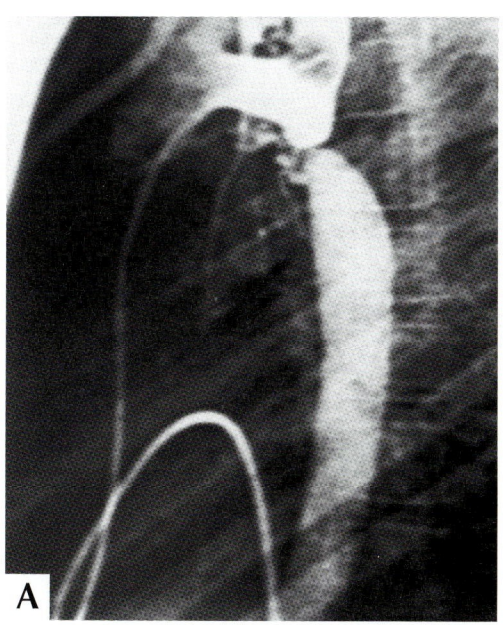
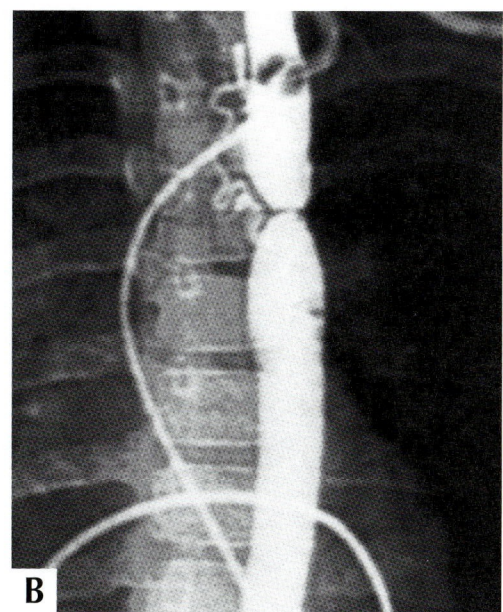
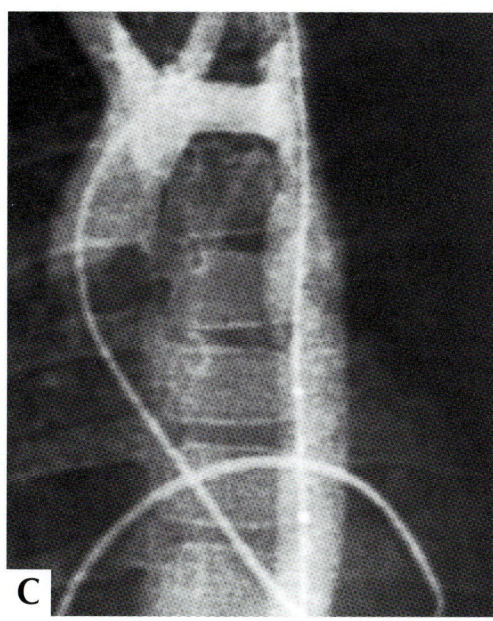

FIGURE 9-30. The indications for intervention for unoperated lesions are the same as those for recurrent coarctation. Early experience has suggested that the response to dilation in the neonatal expression of the disease is transient, and few centers routinely apply this technique in that age group. At the Hospital for Sick Children in Toronto, the technique is offered as initial therapy to all patients older than 1 year of age. A and B, Ascending aortograms from a 5-year-old showing the typical weblike coarctation of the aorta, with the catheter placed from the venous circulation. C, After angioplasty, the stabilizing wire was placed into the left subclavian artery, which guided the balloon catheter to the site of dilation.

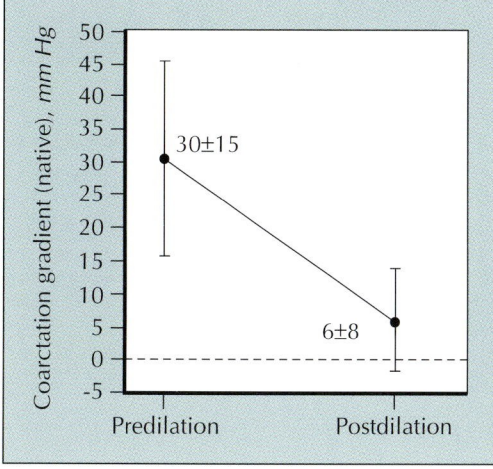

FIGURE 9-31. Results of native coarctation angioplasty at the Hospital for Sick Children, Toronto. A significant reduction in gradient was achieved. Follow-up from this patient group found a persistence of gradient reduction to 11 ± 12 mm Hg [44] over a 2-year period.

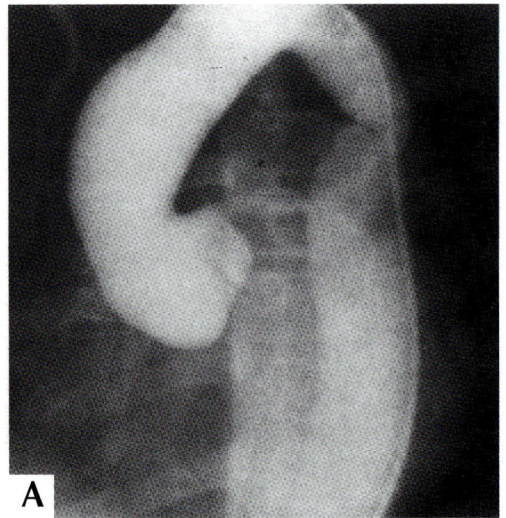
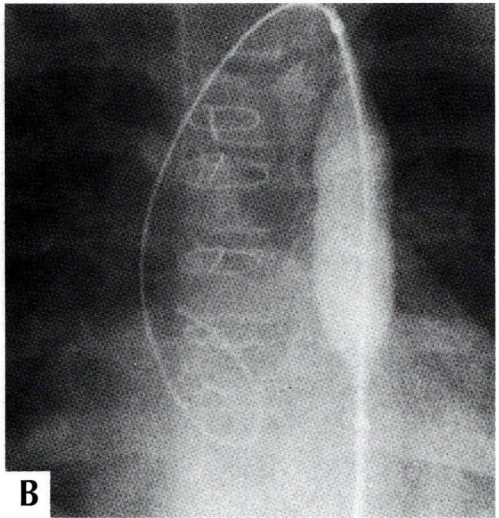
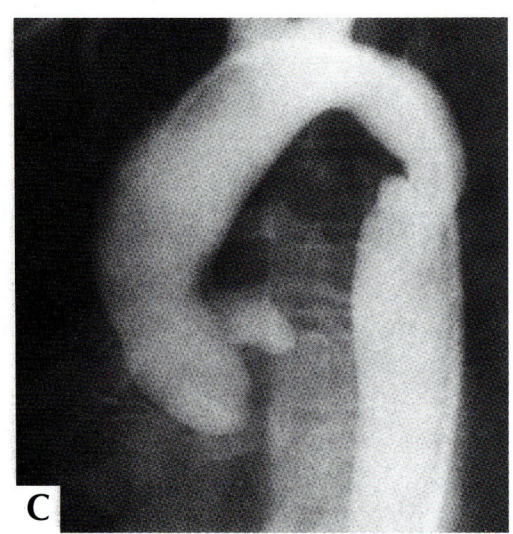

A **B** **C**

FIGURE 9-32. Recurrent coarctation after subclavian flap aortoplasty. **A,** Retrograde aortogram localizing the level and extent of the coarctation. **B,** Balloon dilation (usually inflated for 30 seconds) with guidewires in place in the ascending aorta. **C,** Postdilation aortogram showing marked improvement in stenotic segment. Balloon dilation is the primary treatment choice for postsurgical repair of a recurrent obstruction. Its effectiveness is

not influenced by the type of repair, *ie*, patch, end-to-end, or subclavian flap. Patients generally have systemic hypertension or an arm-leg blood pressure difference of more than 20 mm Hg at rest. As in all angioplasty procedures, catheters should not be maneuvered past dilated segments unless guided over a wire to prevent inadvertent transmural catheter passage.

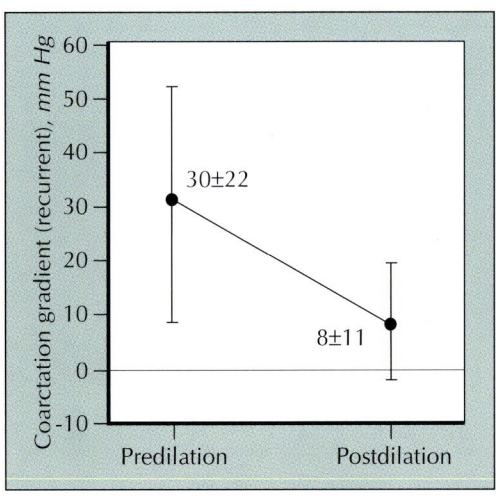

FIGURE 9-33. Results of angioplasty procedures in 89 patients with recurrent coarctation at the Hospital for Sick Children, Toronto, over an 8-year period (1987–1995). These results are similar to those reported by the multicenter Valvuloplasty and Angioplasty of Congenital Anomalies (VACA) Registry [45]. Follow-up data from this population (mean, 3 years) would suggest long-term gradient relief, although surgical reintervention was required when there was an associated hypoplastic transverse arch.

REFERENCES

1. Higgins CB, Silverman NH, Kersting-Sommerhoff BA, *et al.*: Congenital Heart Disease: Echocardiography and Magnetic Resonance Imaging. New York: Raven Press; 1990.

2. Ebels T: Surgery of the left atrioventricular valve and of the left atrioventricular outflow tract in atrioventricular septal defect. *Cardiol Young* 1991, 1:344–355.

3. Silverman NH, Anderson RH, Zuberbuhler JR: Atrioventricular septal defects: cross-sectional echocardiographic and morphologic comparisons. *Int J Cardiol* 1986, 13:309–331.

4. Meijboom EJ, Wyse RK, Ebels T, *et al.*: Doppler mapping of postoperative left atrioventricular valve regurgitation. *Circulation* 1988, 77:311–315.

5. Ebels T, Meijboom EJ, Anderson RH, *et al.*: Anatomic and functional "obstruction" of the outflow tract in atrioventricular septal defects with septal valve orifices ("ostium primum atrial septal defect"): an echocardiographic study. *Am J Cardiol* 1984, 54:843–847.

6. Yoo S-J, Choi Y-H: Ventricular septal defect. In *Angiograms in Congenital Heart Disease*. Edited by Yoo S-J, Choi Y-H. Oxford: Oxford University Press; 1991:29–54.

7. Rastelli GC, Kirklin JW, Titus JL: Anatomic observations on complete form of persistent common atrioventricular canal with septal reference to atrioventricular valves. *Mayo Clin Proc* 1996, 41:296–308.

8. Lipshultz SE, Sanders SP, Mayer JE, *et al.*: Are routine preoperative cardiac catheterization and angiography necessary before repair of ostium primum atrial septal defect? *J Am Coll Cardiol* 1988, 11:373–378.

9. Cabrera A, Pastor E, Galdeano JM, *et al.*: Cross-sectional echocardiography in the diagnosis of atrioventricular septal defect. *Int J Cardiol* 1990, 28:19–23.

10. Sreeram N, Stumper OFW, Kaulitz R, *et al.*: Comparative value of transthoracic and transesophageal echocardiography in the assessment of congenital abnormalities of the atrioventricular junction. *J Am Coll Cardiol* 1990, 16:1205–1214.

11. Davidson WR Jr, Pasqual MJ, Fanelli C: A Doppler echocardiographic examination of the aortic valve and left ventricular outflow tract. *Am J Cardiol* 1991, 67:547–549.

12. Kleinert S, Geva T: Echocardiographic morphometry and geometry of the left ventricular outflow tract in fixed subaortic stenosis. *J Am Coll Cardiol* 1993, 22:1501–1508.

13. Snider AR, Serwer GA: *Echocardiography in Pediatric Heart Disease*, ed 1. Littleton, MA: Year Book Medical Publishers; 1990.

14. Roberson DA, Silverman NH: Ebstein's anomaly: echocardiographic and clinical features in the fetus and neonate. *J Am Coll Cardiol* 1989, 14:1300–1307.

15. Quaegebeur JM, Sreeram N, Fraser AG, *et al.*: Surgery for Ebstein's anomaly: the clinical and echocardiographic evaluation of a new technique. *J Am Coll Cardiol* 1991, 17:722–728.

16. Koike K, Musewe NN, Smallhorn JF, Freedom RM: Distinguishing between anomalous origin of the left coronary artery from the pulmonary trunk and dilated cardiomyopathy: role of echocardiographic measurement of the right coronary artery diameter. *Br Heart J* 1989, 61:192–197.

17. Rowe RD, Vlad P, Keith JD: Atypical tetralogy of Fallot: noncyanotic form with increased lung vascularity. Report of four cases. *Circulation* 1955, 12:230–238.

18. Gasul BM, Dillon RF, Urla V, Hait G: Ventricular septal defects: their natural transformation into those with infundibular stenosis or into the cyanotic or noncyanotic types of tetralogy of Fallot. *JAMA* 1957, 164:847–853.

19. Nadas AS: Hypoxemia. In *Nadas' Pediatric Cardiology*. Edited by Fyler DC. Philadelphia: Hanley & Belfus; 1992:73–82.

20. Collett RW, Edwards JE: Persistent truncus arteriosus: a classification according to anatomic types. *Surg Clin North Am* 1949, 29:1245–1270.

21. VanPraagh R, VanPraagh S: The anatomy of common aorticopulmonary trunk (truncus arteriosus communis) and its embryologic implications: a study of 57 necropsy cases. *Am J Cardiol* 1965, 406–425.

22. Van Mierop LHS, Patterson DF, Schnarr WR: Pathogenesis of persistent truncus arteriosus in light of observations made in a dog embryo with the anomaly. *Am J Cardiol* 1978, 41:755–762.

23. Anderson RH, Thiene G: Categorization and description of hearts with a common arterial trunk. *Eur J Cardiothorac Surg* 1989, 3:481–487.

24. Edwards JE: Persistent truncus arteriosus: a comment [editorial]. *Am Heart J* 1976, 92:1–2.

25. Calder AL, Brandt PWT, Barratt-Boyes BG, Neutze JM: Variant of tetralogy of Fallot with absent pulmonary valve leaflets and origin of one pulmonary artery from the ascending aorta. *Am J Cardiol* 1980, 46:106–116.

26. Kutsche LM, Van Mierop LHS: Anatomy and pathogenesis of aorticopulmonary septal defect. *Am J Cardiol* 1987, 59:443–447.

27. Butto F, Lucas RV, Edwards JE: Persistent truncus arteriosus: pathologic anatomy in 54 cases. *Pediatr Cardiol* 1986, 7:95–101.

28. Rosenquist GC, Bharati S, McAllister HA, Lev M: Truncus arteriosus communis: truncal valve anomalies associated with small conal or truncal septal defects. *Am J Cardiol* 1976, 37:410–412.

29. Carr I, Bharati S, Kusnoor VS, Lev M: Truncus arteriosus communis with intact ventricular septum. *Br Heart J* 1979, 42:97–102.

30. Gatzoulis MA, Shore D, Yacoub M, Shinebourne EA: Complete atrioventricular septal defect with tetralogy of Fallot: diagnosis and management. *Br Heart J* 1994, 71:579–583.

31. Jatene AD, Fontes VF, Paulista PP, *et al.*: Anatomic correction of transposition of the great vessels. *J Thorac Cardiovasc Surg* 1976, 72:364–370.

32. Lecompte Y, Zannini L, Hazan E, *et al.*: Anatomic correction of transposition of the great arteries: new technique without use of a prosthetic conduit. *J Thorac Cardiovasc Surg* 1981, 82:629–631.

33. Piccoli GP, Hamilton DI: Interposition of a modified aortic homograft conduit as main pulmonary trunk in anatomic correction of transposition of the great arteries. *J Thorac Cardiovasc Surg* 1981, 82:429–435.

34. Yacoub MH, Radley-Smith R, Hilton CJ: Anatomical correction of complete transposition of the great arteries and ventricular septal defect in infancy. *BMJ* 1976, May:1112–1114.

35. Yacoub MH, Radley-Smith R, Maclaurin R: Two-stage operation for anatomical correction of transposition of the great arteries with intact interventricular septum. *Lancet* 1977, 1:1275–1278.

36. Castañeda AR: Anatomic correction of transposition of the great arteries at the arterial level. Edited by Sabiston Jr DC, Spencer FC. In *Surgery of the Chest*, ed 5. Philadelphia: W.B. Saunders; 1990:1435–1446.

37. Kirklin JW, Blackstone EH, Tchervenkov CI, Castañeda AR, and the Congenital Heart Surgeons Society: Clinical outcomes after the arterial switch operation for transposition: patient, support, procedural and institutional risk factors. *Circulation* 1992, 86:1501–1515.

38. Wernovsky G, Mayer Jr JE, Jonas RA, *et al.*: Factors influencing early and late outcome of the arterial switch operation for transposition of the great arteries. *J Thorac Cardiovasc Surg* 1995, 109:289–302.

39. Planche C, Bruniaux J, Lacour-Gayet F, *et al.*: Switch operation for transposition of the great arteries in neonates: a study of 120 patients. *J Thorac Cardiovasc Surg* 1988, 96:354–363.

40. Dick M, Fyler DC, Nadas AS: Tricuspid atresia: clinical course in 101 patients. *Am J Cardiol* 1975, 36:327–337.

41. Dick M, Rosenthal A: The clinical profile of tricuspid atresia. In *Tricuspid Atresia*. Edited by Rao PS. Mt Kisco, NY: Futura Publishing Co; 1982:83–111.

42. Taussig HB, Keinonen R, Momberger N, *et al.*: Long-term observations in the Blalock-Taussig operation IV: tricuspid atresia. *Johns Hopkins Med J* 1973, 132:135–142.

43. Dick M II, Rosenthal A: The clinical profile of tricuspid atresia. In *Tricuspid Atresia*, ed 2. Edited by Rao PS. Mt Kisco, NY: Futura Publishing Co; 1992:117–140.

44. Houde C, Zahn EM, Burrows PE, *et al.*: Native coarctation angioplasty, medium-term results. *J Am Coll Cardiol* 1992, 19:25A.

45. Hellenbrand WE, Allen HD, Golinko RJ, *et al.*: Balloon angioplasty for aortic recoarctation: results of valvuloplasty and angioplasty of congenital anomalies registry. *Am J Cardiol* 1990, 117:1157–1158.

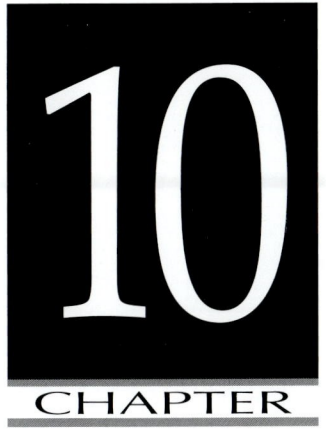

10 CHAPTER

COR PULMONALE, PRIMARY PULMONARY HYPERTENSION, AND CARDIAC TUMORS

Edited by Samuel Z. Goldhaber

Michael F. Allard, Richard N. Channick, Evan Loh,
Bruce M. McManus, Glenn P. Taylor, Janet E. Wilson

COR PULMONALE

The term *cor pulmonale* describes a spectrum of cardiopulmonary syndromes that are characterized by pulmonary hypertension, right ventricular hypertrophy, and right ventricular dilatation. Cor pulmonale includes a diverse range of etiologies, pathophysiologic mechanisms, and clinical characteristics. The common denominator of all these syndromes is pulmonary hypertension.

DEFINITION AND NATURAL HISTORY

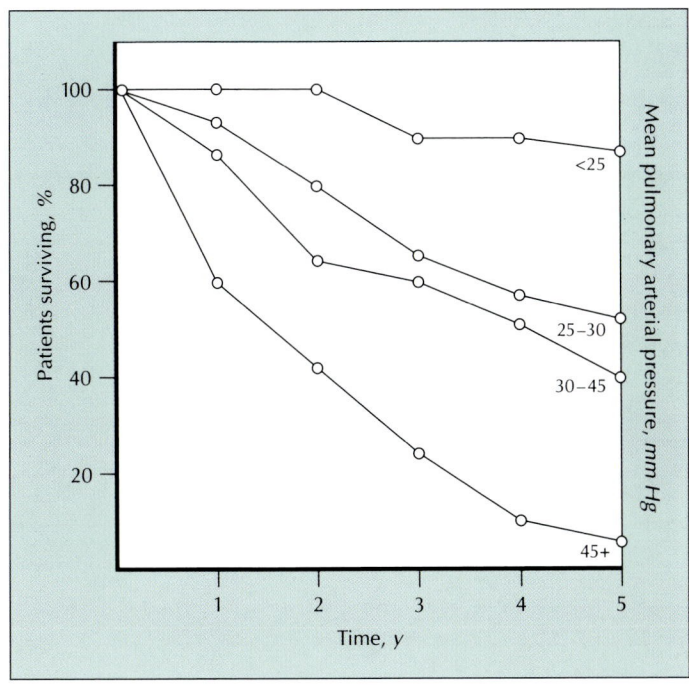

FIGURE 10-1. Correlation between survival (in years) and base-line mean pulmonary arterial pressure in patients with pulmonary hypertension secondary to parenchymal lung disease. A higher initial presenting mean pulmonary artery pressure was associated with significantly higher mortality. These findings suggest that regardless of the etiology of pulmonary hypertension, mean pulmonary artery pressure remains the single best determinant of long-term survival. (*Adapted from* Bishop [1].)

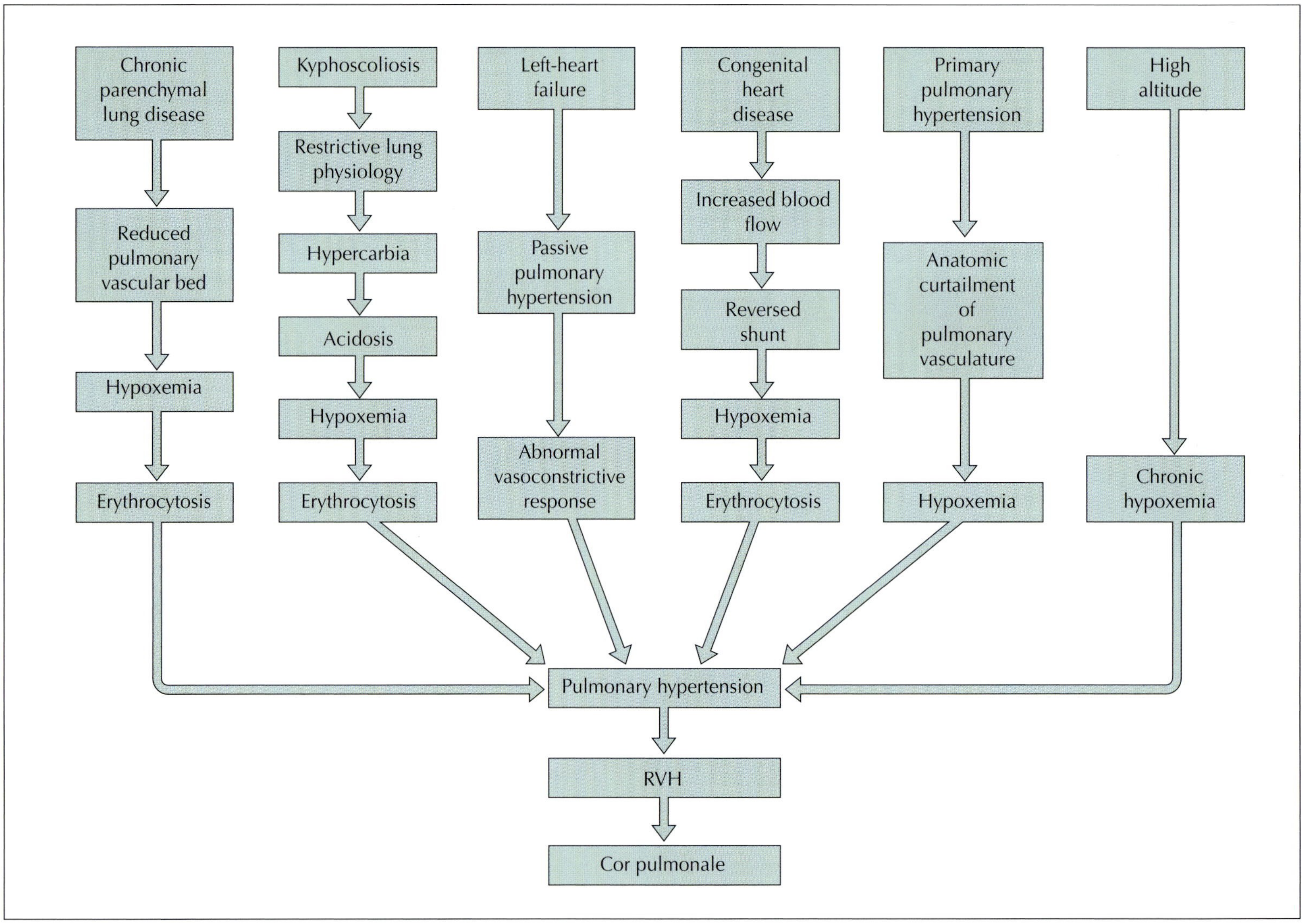

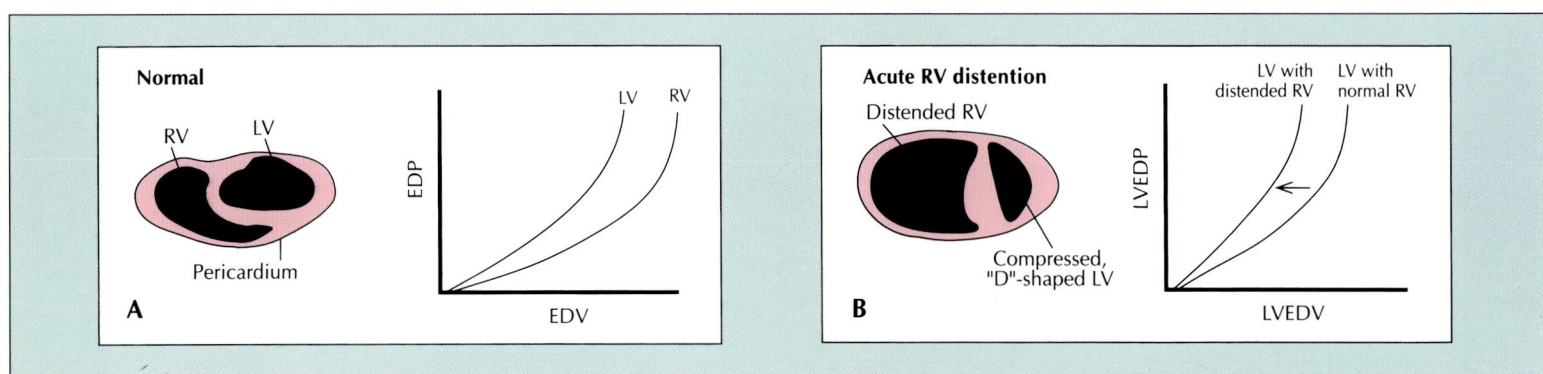

Chronic parenchymal lung disease
Reduced pulmonary vascular bed
Hypoxemia
Erythrocytosis
Kyphoscoliosis
Restrictive lung physiology
Hypercarbia
Acidosis
Hypoxemia
Erythrocytosis
Left-heart failure
Passive pulmonary hypertension
Abnormal vasoconstrictive response
Congenital heart disease
Increased blood flow
Reversed shunt
Hypoxemia
Erythrocytosis
Primary pulmonary hypertension
Anatomic curtailment of pulmonary vasculature
Hypoxemia
High altitude
Chronic hypoxemia
Pulmonary hypertension
RVH
Cor pulmonale

FIGURE 10-2. Flow diagram demonstrating the etiology and pathophysiology of cor pulmonale. General categories of disease states and the various pathophysiologic mechanisms that lead to development of the disorder are shown. Note that the final common pathway for the group of diseases that comprises cor pulmonale is advanced, long-standing pulmonary hypertension. RVH—right ventricular hypertrophy.

PATHOPHYSIOLOGY

Normal
RV
LV
Pericardium
A
EDP
EDV
LV
RV
Acute RV distention
Distended RV
Compressed, "D"-shaped LV
B
LVEDP
LVEDV
LV with distended RV
LV with normal RV

FIGURE 10-3. Interdependence of the right (RV) and left (LV) ventricles. **A,** Under normal conditions, the RV is much more distensible than the LV. **B,** In patients who develop acute cor pulmonale, there is a sudden and large increase in RV volume. Because of space limitations imposed by the pericardium, the distended RV impinges upon and compresses the LV cavity. The increase in RV volume causes the interventricular septum to shift toward the LV, thus causing a decrease in the dimension of the septum to free wall of the LV. The distention of the RV decreases the overall LV end-diastolic volume (LVEDV), even though the LV end-diastolic pressure (LVEDP) remains the same (*arrow*). As the LV becomes progressively less compliant, increases in LVEDP do not normally augment LVEDV. Therefore, the LV is unable to compensate for its loss of volume. Eventually, the LV cavity is obliterated, resulting in low forward cardiac output and hemodynamic collapse. (*Adapted from* Weber *et al.* [2].)

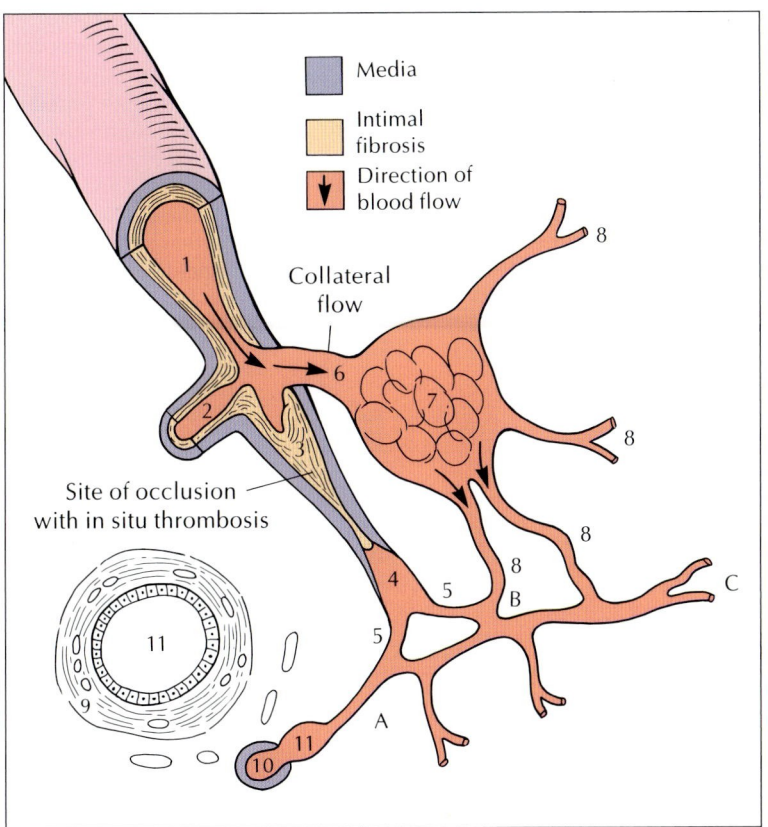

FIGURE 10-4. Diagram demonstrating the origin and probable connections of small, thin-walled collateral blood vessels in the lung in advanced cases of pulmonary hypertension. Such connections create functional arteriovenous fistulae and right-to-left shunting that contribute to the hypoxemia observed in patients with advanced cor pulmonale. 1—Dilated muscular pulmonary artery with thin wall media and intimal fibrosis considered part of the generalized dilatation proximal to the site of vascular occlusion; 2—Hypertrophied muscular pulmonary artery arising as a side branch of the muscular pulmonary artery with an accumulation of intimal fibrous tissue at the site of origin; 3—Terminal muscular pulmonary artery occluded by fibrous tissue and/or thrombosis in situ; 4—Terminal dilated pulmonary arteriole; 5—Capillaries in alveolar walls arising from the pulmonary arteriole; 6—Dilated, thin-walled, veinlike branch of hypertrophied parent muscular pulmonary artery; 7—Localized angiomatoid lesion; 8—Capillaries in alveolar walls arising from dilatation lesions; 9—Dilated thin-walled vessels in submucosa of small bronchus with vascular smooth muscle proliferation; 10—Small bronchial artery in fibrotic coat of a small bronchus giving rise to thin-walled branches; 11—cross-sectional view of the small bronchial artery with medial hyperplasia; A—Bronchopulmonary anastomosis at capillary level; B—Anastomosis between capillaries arising from parent muscular pulmonary artery and dilatation lesions; C—Possible anastomosis between thin-walled vessels of the pulmonary artery and those of the pulmonary vein. (*Adapted from* Harris and Heath [3].)

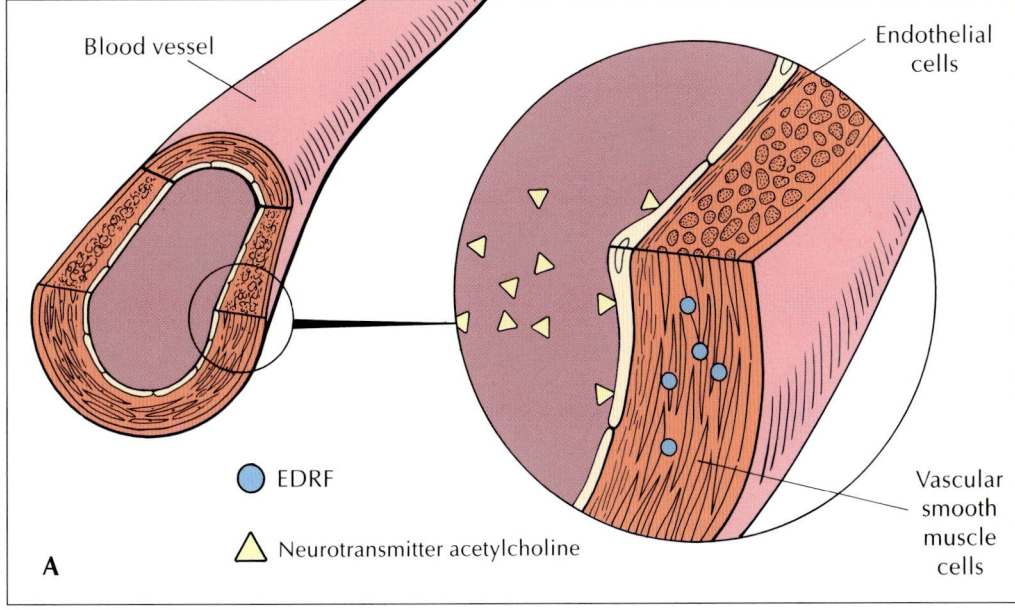

FIGURE 10-5. Endothelial control of pulmonary artery tone.

A, The normal pulmonary artery dilates when a neurotransmitter, such as acetylcholine, binds to endothelial cells on the vessel's inner walls. These cells release endothelium-derived relaxing factor (EDRF), whose active moiety has been identified as nitric oxide, which then diffuses to adjacent vascular smooth muscle cells, causing them to relax. Because acetylcholine stimulates the endothelium to release EDRF and cause vasodilation, the loss of response to acetylcholine can be used as a bioassay of EDRF release and overall endothelial function [4]. Constriction of pulmonary arteries and focal vascular injury are prominent features of pulmonary hypertension. Inhibition of EDRF augments pulmonary hypertension in newborn lambs [5]. In pulmonary arterial rings of patients undergoing heart-lung transplantation for end-stage chronic obstructive lung disease, the endothelium-dependent pulmonary relaxation that is normally achieved in response to acetylcholine is impaired [6]. (*continued*)

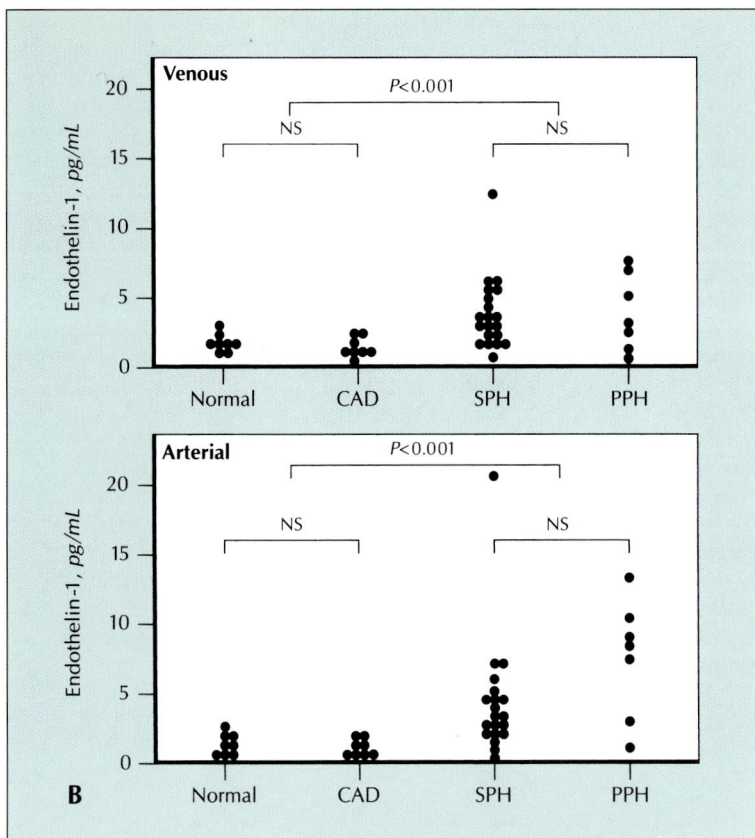

Figure 10-5. (*continued*) **B,** Endothelin, a 21–amino-acid peptide also produced by the endothelium, causes potent vasoconstriction and smooth muscle proliferation. Plasma endothelin-1 levels are normal in patients with coronary artery disease (CAD) but elevated in patients with primary (PPH) and secondary (SPH) pulmonary hypertension [7]. Immunocytochemical analysis has shown that endothelin-1 is localized primarily to endothelial cells of pulmonary arteries with medial thickening and intimal fibrosis [8]. Endothelin-1 mRNA is increased at these same sites in patients with pulmonary hypertension. These findings suggest that local production of endothelin-1 contributes to the vascular abnormalities associated with secondary and primary pulmonary hypertension. (Part A *adapted from* Snyder and Bredt [4]; part B *adapted from* Stewart *et al.* [7].)

PATHOPHYSIOLOGY OF PULMONARY HYPERTENSION

A INCREASED RESISTANCE TO PULMONARY VENOUS DRAINAGE

Elevated left ventricular diastolic pressure
  Left ventricular systolic failure
  Left ventricular diastolic dysfunction
  Constrictive pericarditis
Left atrial hypertension
  Mitral valve disease
  Cor triatriatum
  Left atrial myxoma or thrombus
Pulmonary venous obstruction
  Congenital stenosis of pulmonary veins
  Anomalous pulmonary venous connection with obstruction
  Pulmonary veno-occlusive disease
  Mediastinal fibrosis

C INCREASED RESISTANCE TO FLOW THROUGH LARGE PULMONARY ARTERIES

Pulmonary thromboembolism
Peripheral pulmonic stenosis
Unilateral absence or stenosis of the pulmonary artery

B INCREASED RESISTANCE TO FLOW THROUGH PULMONARY VASCULAR BED

Decreased cross-sectional area of pulmonary vascular bed secondary to parenchymal diseases
  Chronic obstructive pulmonary disease
  Restrictive lung disease
  Collagen-vascular diseases (scleroderma, systemic lupus erythematosus, rheumatoid arthritis)
  Fibrotic reactions (Hamman-Rich syndrome, desquamative interstitial pneumonitis, pulmonary hemosiderosis)
  Sarcoidosis
  Neoplasm
  Pneumonia
  Status after pulmonary resection
  Congenital pulmonary hypoplasia
Decreased cross-sectional area of pulmonary vascular bed secondary to Eisenmenger's syndrome
Other conditions associated with decreased cross-sectional area of the pulmonary vascular bed
  Primary pulmonary hypertension
  Hepatic cirrhosis and/or portal thrombosis
  Chemically induced aminorex fumarate, *Crotalaria* alkaloids
  Persistent fetal circulation in the newborn

Figure 10-6. Clinical causes of pulmonary hypertension that either result in or are associated with cor pulmonale, including (**A**) increased resistance to pulmonary venous drainage; (**B**) increased resistance to flow through pulmonary vascular bed; (**C**) increased resistance to flow through large pulmonary arteries; (*continued*)

D <u>HYPOVENTILATION</u>

Obesity-hypoventilation syndromes
Pharyngeal-tracheal obstruction
Neuromuscular disorders
  Myasthenia gravis
  Poliomyelitis
  Damage to central respiratory center
Disorders of the chest wall
Pulmonary parenchymal disorders associated
  with hypoventilation

E <u>MISCELLANEOUS CAUSES OF PULMONARY HYPERTENSION</u>

Residence at high altitude
Isolated partial anomalous pulmonary venous drainage
Tetralogy of Fallot
Hemoglobinopathies
Intravenous drug abuse
Alveolar proteinosis
Takayasu's disease

FIGURE 10-6. (*continued*) (**D**) hypoventilation; and (**E**) miscellaneous causes [9].

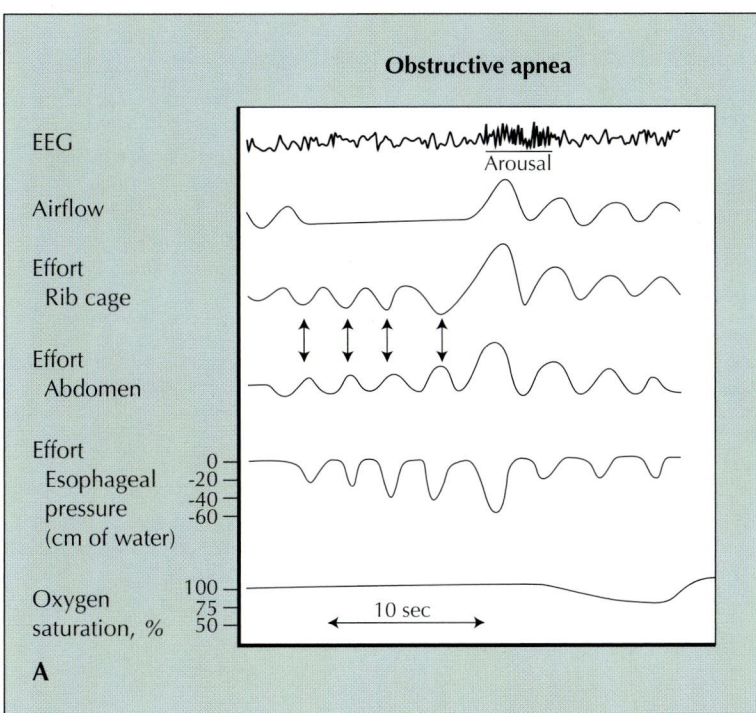

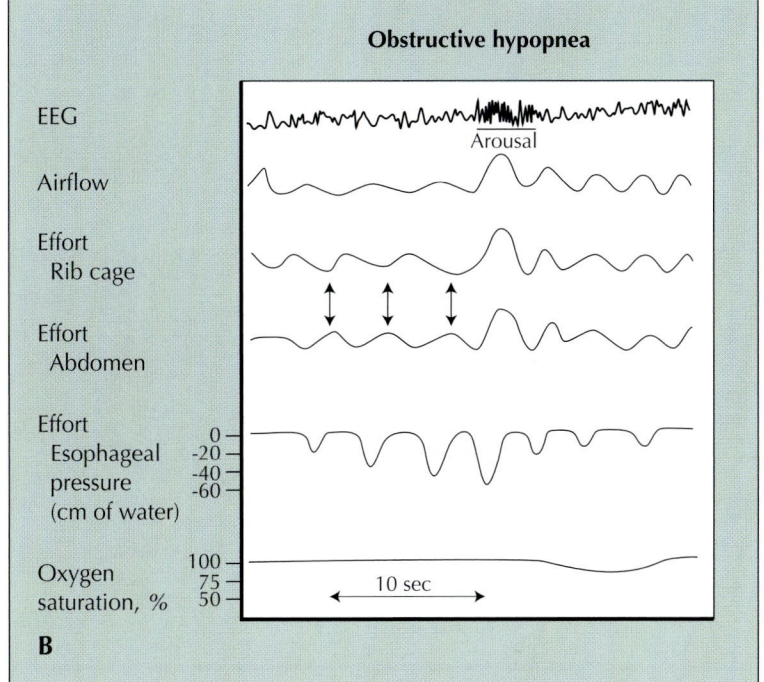

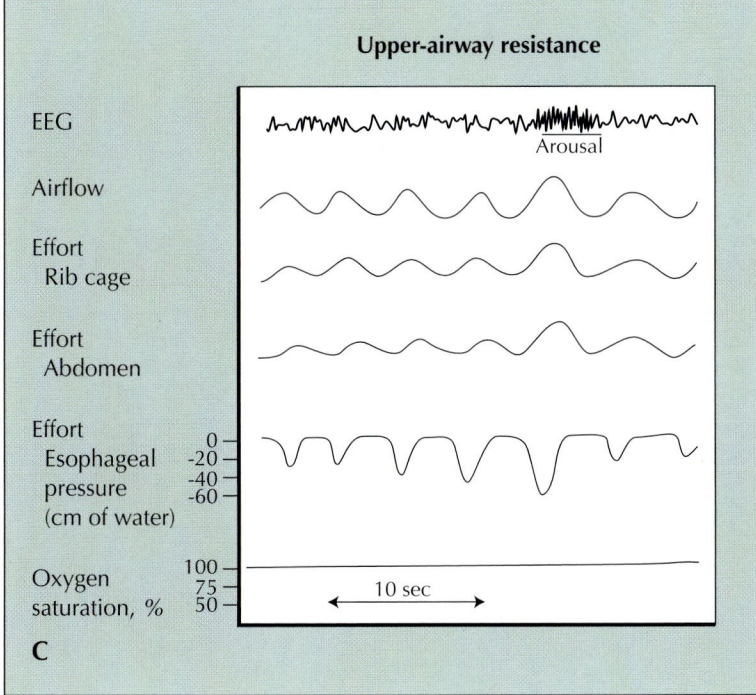

FIGURE 10-7. **A—C**, The sleep apnea syndrome should be suspected after eliciting a history of both daytime sleepiness and snoring while sleeping. Sleep apnea is underdiagnosed even though most patients can be effectively treated with continuous positive airway pressure. Cardiac complications include nocturnal sudden death caused by cardiac arrhythmia (especially bradyarrhythmia), myocardial ischemia, cardiomyopathy, and pulmonary and systemic arterial hypertension [10]. The major societal complication is an increased risk of traffic accidents [11] caused, in part, by lax governmental regulation of affected patients [12]. (*Adapted from* Strollo and Rogers [10].)

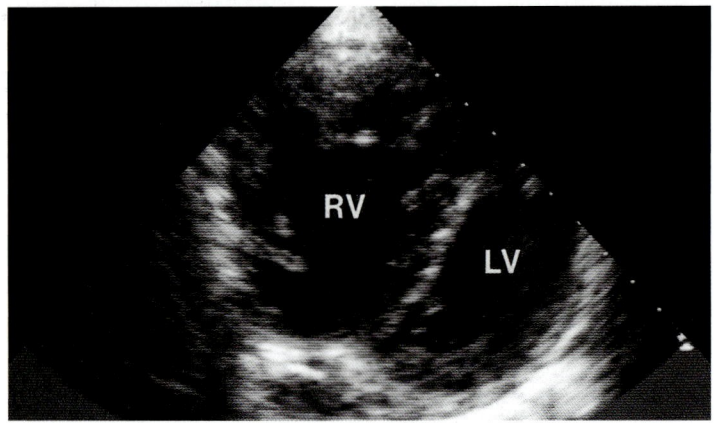

FIGURE 10-8. Echocardiographic features of the heart in a patient with cor pulmonale. Shown here is a short-axis view demonstrating a markedly enlarged RV with RV hypertrophy. Abnormal bowing of the interventricular septum into the LV gives a characteristic *D* configuration of the LV, consistent with volume and pressure overload of the RV.

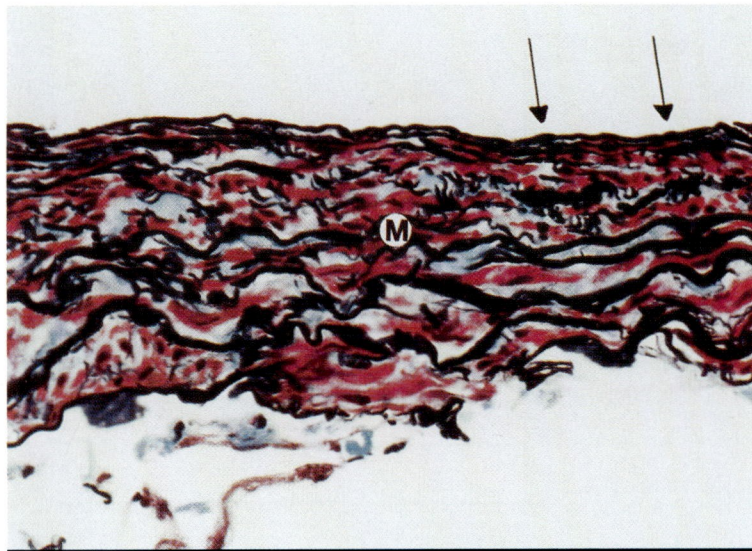

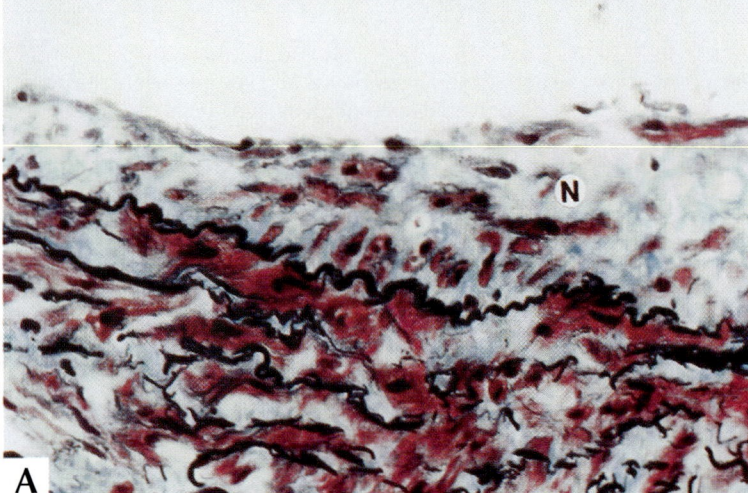

FIGURE 10-9. A—C, Assessing the etiology of pulmonary hypertension has been difficult, in part because of the inaccessibility of pulmonary vascular tissue for analysis. A novel endoarterial biopsy catheter appears successful in obtaining endovascular biopsy samples from distal canine pulmonary arteries that are 2 to 3 mm in luminal diameter [13]. (*From* Rothman *et al.* [13]; with permission.) (*continued*)

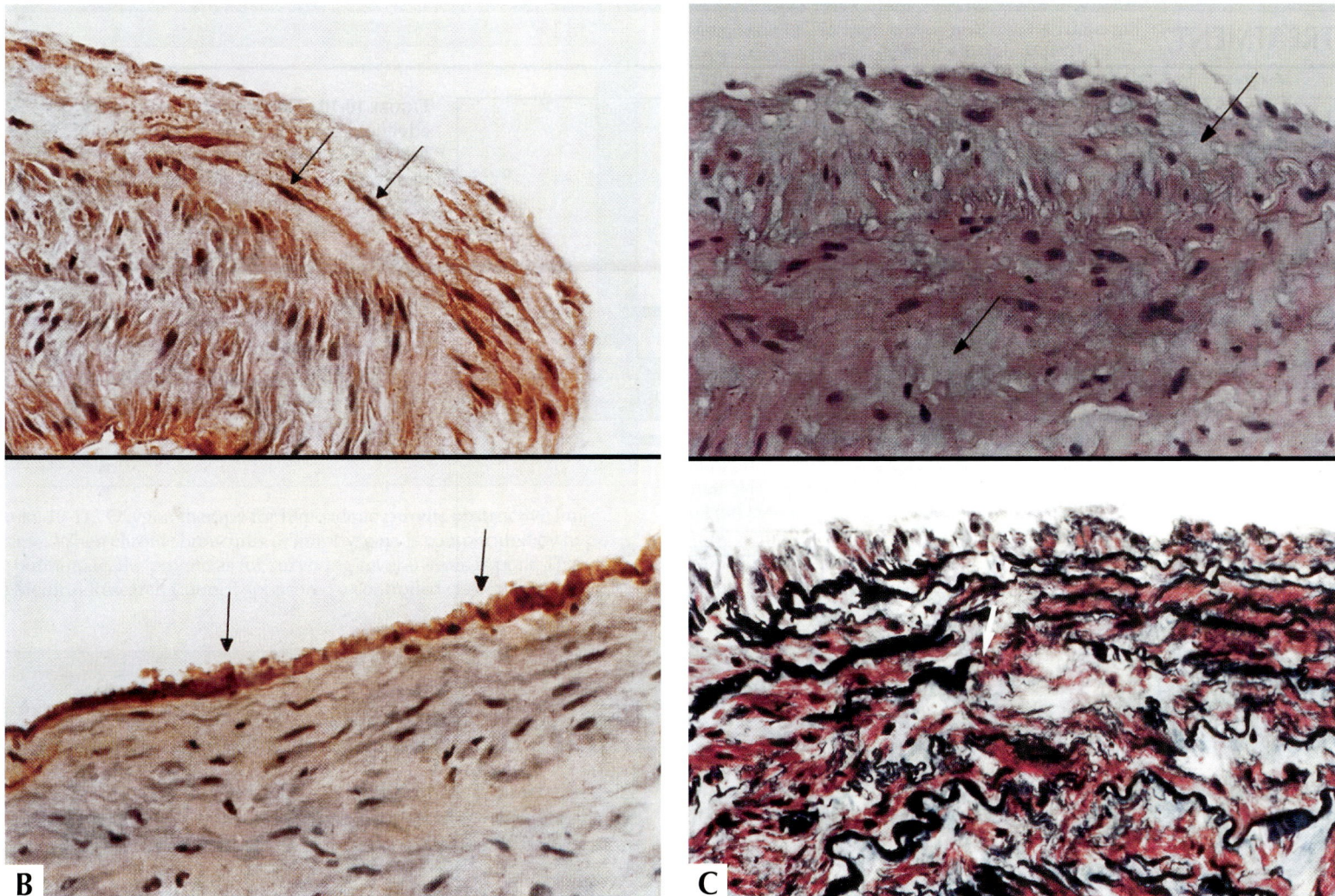

Figure 10-9. (*continued*)

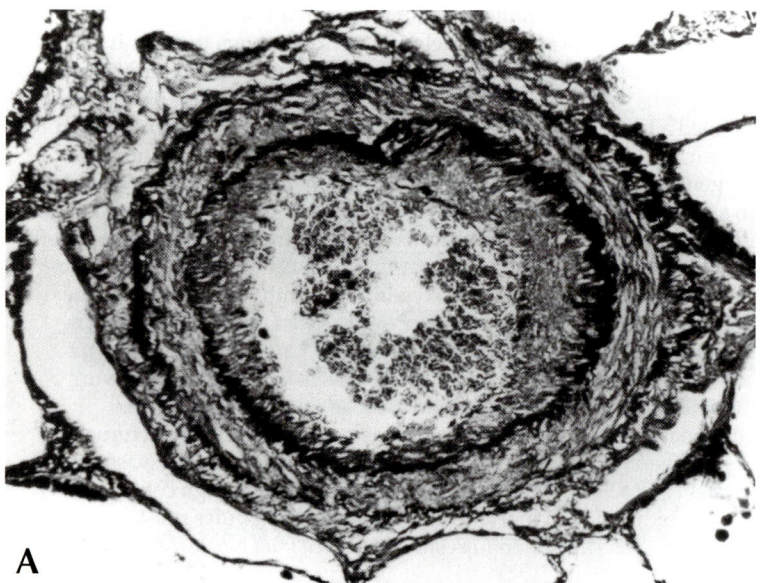

A

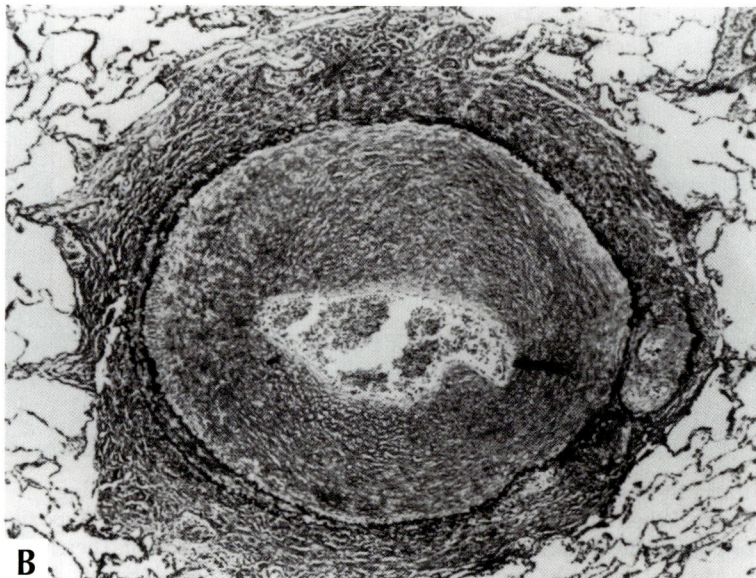

B

FIGURE 10-13. Histopathologic features of PPH. Several lesions have been identified in patients with PPH. **A,** Hypertrophy of the medial layer of muscular arteries is seen to some degree in virtually all cases of PPH. Medial hypertrophy is present in all forms of pulmonary hypertension and probably correlates with the degree of pulmonary arterial pressure elevation. Medial hypertrophy is generally considered a reversible lesion. **B,** Cellular proliferation and concentric fibrosis in the intima. Intimal proliferation may be a primary process or secondary to endothelial cell damage and release of growth factors. Intimal fibrosis may lead to complete obliteration of the vessel lumen.

PATHOGENESIS

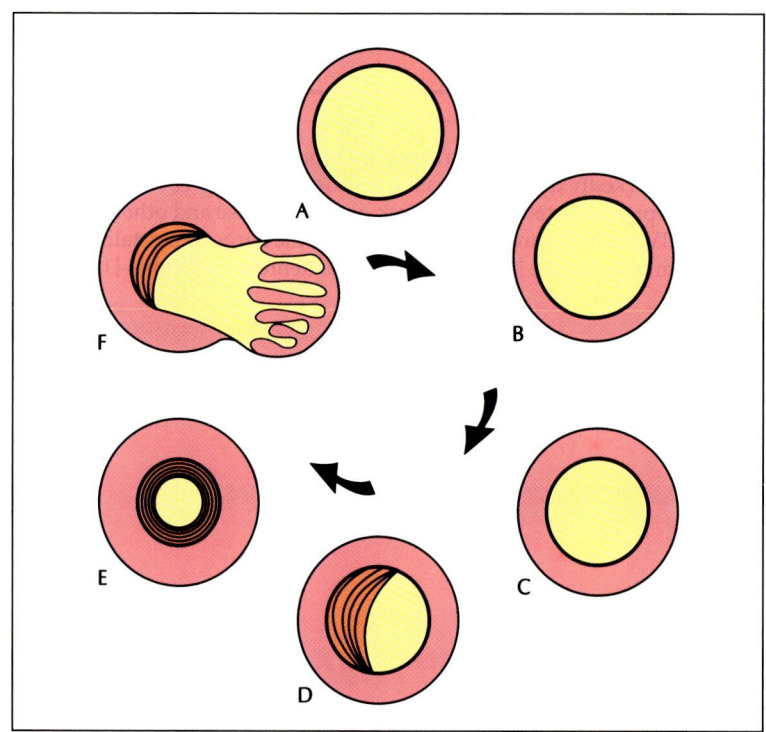

FIGURE 10-14. One potential explanation for the pathogenesis of intimal fibrosis and plexiform lesions is vasoconstriction. Vasoconstriction leads to progressive medial hypertrophy (A, B, C) and elevated pulmonary artery pressure. Elevated pulmonary artery pressure results in endothelial damage and intimal proliferation (D) with concentric fibrosis (E). Plexiform lesions then develop from intimal scarring as part of the repair process (F). A significant role for vasoconstriction in the pathogenesis of PPH is likely in some patients; this group typically responds to vasodilators. The absence of vasoreactivity in the majority of patients with PPH, however, suggests that either 1) PPH can develop as a primary proliferative and fibrotic process without a vasoconstrictive phase or 2) the disease progresses from one of predominantly vasoconstriction and medial hypertrophy to structural lesions that are irreversible. Which of these explanations is most accurate is not known. (*Adapted from* Rich [13].)

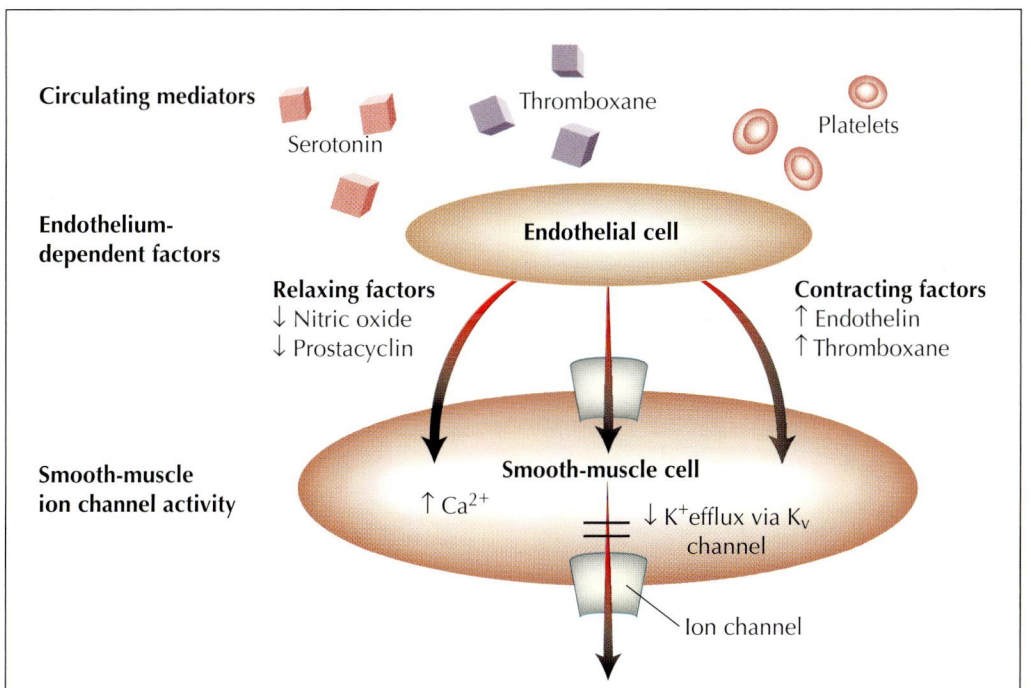

Figure 10-15. Algorithm for investigation of suspected pulmonary hypertension. (*Adapted from* Gaine and Rubin [18].)

Circulating mediators

Serotonin

Thromboxane

Platelets

Endothelium-dependent factors

Endothelial cell

Relaxing factors
↓ Nitric oxide
↓ Prostacyclin

Contracting factors
↑ Endothelin
↑ Thromboxane

Smooth-muscle ion channel activity

Smooth-muscle cell

↑ Ca^{2+}

↓ K^+ efflux via K_v channel

Ion channel

DIAGNOSTIC APPROACH

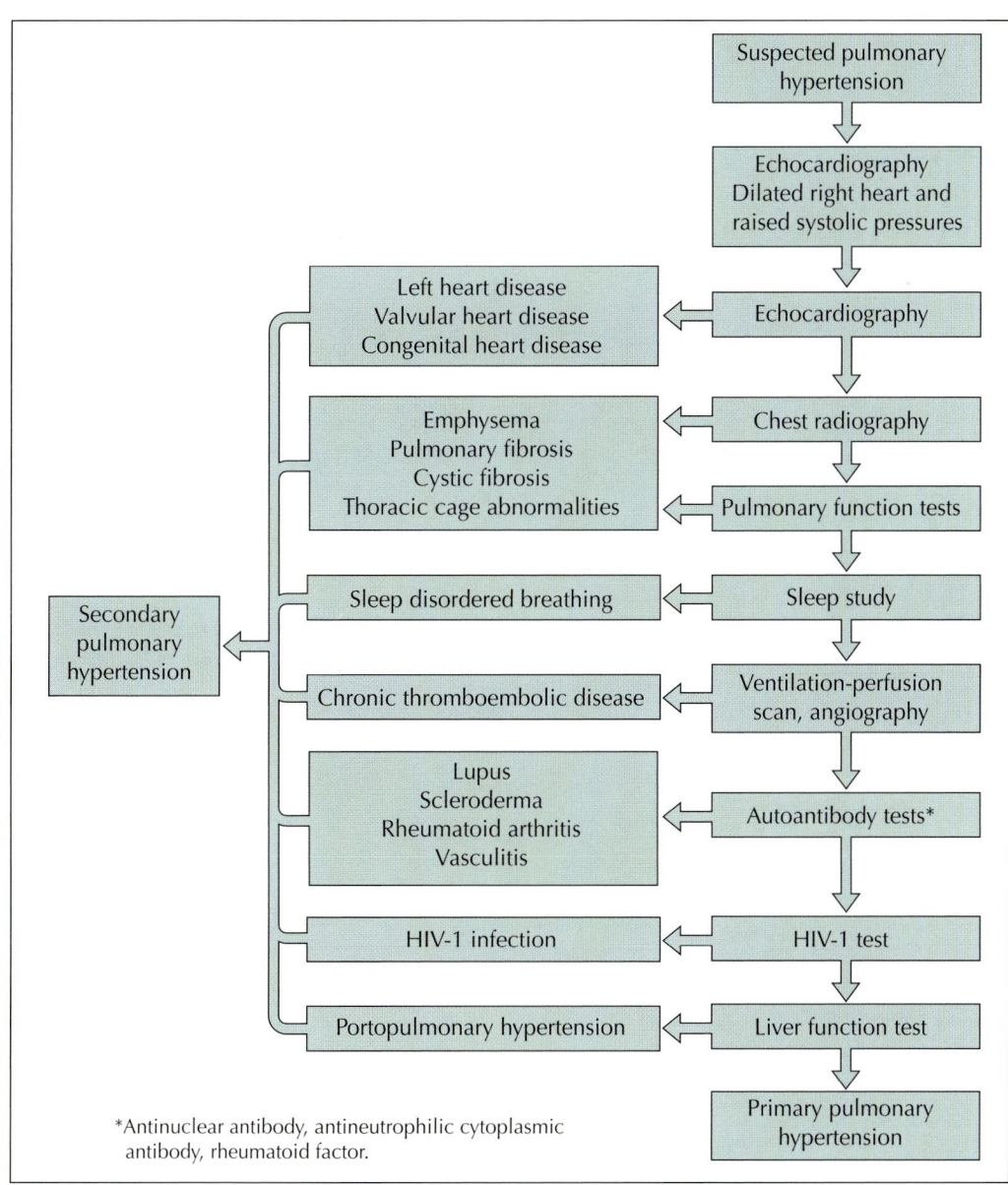

Figure 10-16. Potential mechanism in pathogenesis of primary pulmonary hypertension. (*Adapted from* Gaine and Rubin [18].)

Suspected pulmonary hypertension

Echocardiography
Dilated right heart and raised systolic pressures

Left heart disease
Valvular heart disease
Congenital heart disease

Echocardiography

Emphysema
Pulmonary fibrosis
Cystic fibrosis
Thoracic cage abnormalities

Chest radiography

Pulmonary function tests

Secondary pulmonary hypertension

Sleep disordered breathing

Sleep study

Chronic thromboembolic disease

Ventilation-perfusion scan, angiography

Lupus
Scleroderma
Rheumatoid arthritis
Vasculitis

Autoantibody tests*

HIV-1 infection

HIV-1 test

Portopulmonary hypertension

Liver function test

Primary pulmonary hypertension

*Antinuclear antibody, antineutrophilic cytoplasmic antibody, rheumatoid factor.

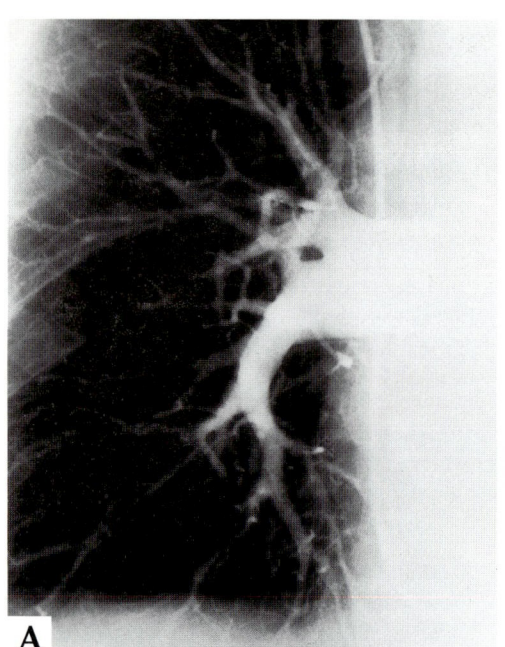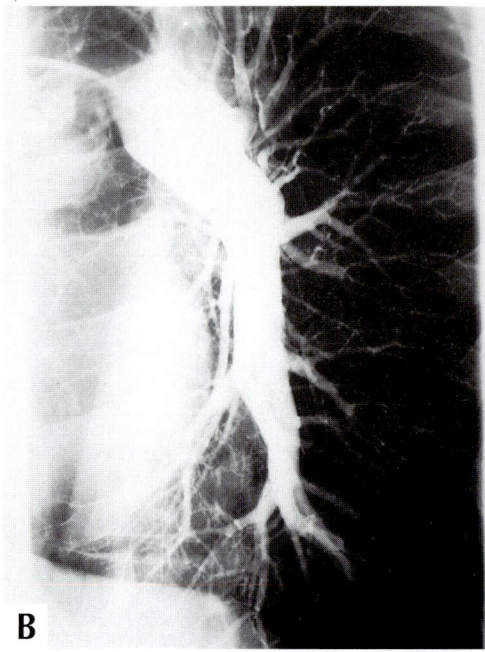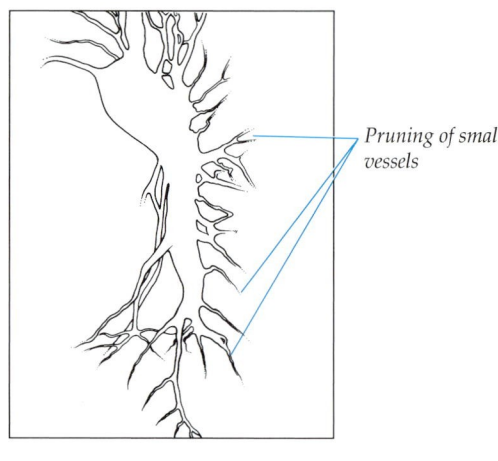

Pruning of small vessels

FIGURE 10-17. Pulmonary angiograms. **A**, The normal angiogram demonstrates a diffuse branching pattern with smoothly tapering vessels and branches leading to the periphery of the lung. **B**, In PPH, pulmonary angiography demonstrates marked "pruning" of small vessels with absent peripheral flow. No segmental or larger vascular abnormalities are noted.

TREATMENT

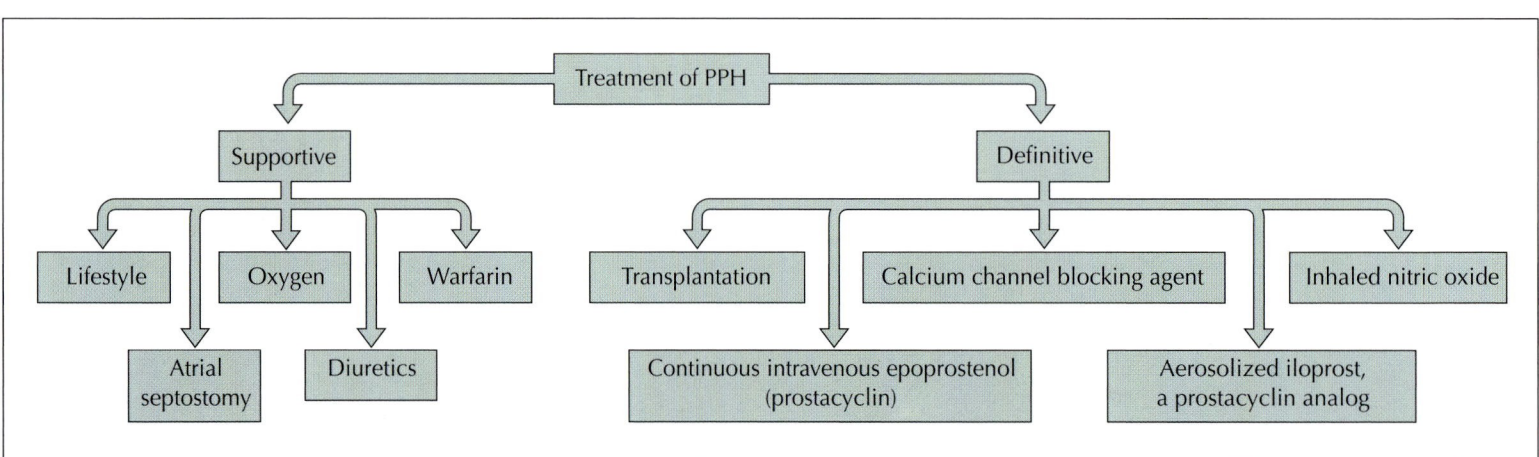

FIGURE 10-18. Treatment options in PPH. Therapeutic interventions may be supportive if aimed at symptomatic relief, or "definitive" if significant survival prolongation is possible; no treatment in PPH is truly curative. Limitation of activity is strongly recommended. Pregnancy is contraindicated. Some patients will demonstrate significant oxygen desaturation upon exercising, due to impaired cardiac reserve. In this group, supplemental oxygen is indicated. Diuretics are useful in relieving symptoms of right-sided heart failure, such as hepatic congestion, ascites, and peripheral edema. These agents, however, must be used with extreme caution, as the right ventricle is quite preload-dependent in these patients and precipitous reductions in intravascular volume can be hazardous. Continuous intravenous prostacyclin infusion (PGI_2) improves exercise tolerance and survival in patients with PPH [19]. It also appears to be effective for patients with pulmonary hypotension caused by the scleroderma spectrum of disease [20]. More recently, inhaled nitric oxide [21] and aerosolized iloprost (an analogue of prostacyclin) [22] have been used in patients with PPH.

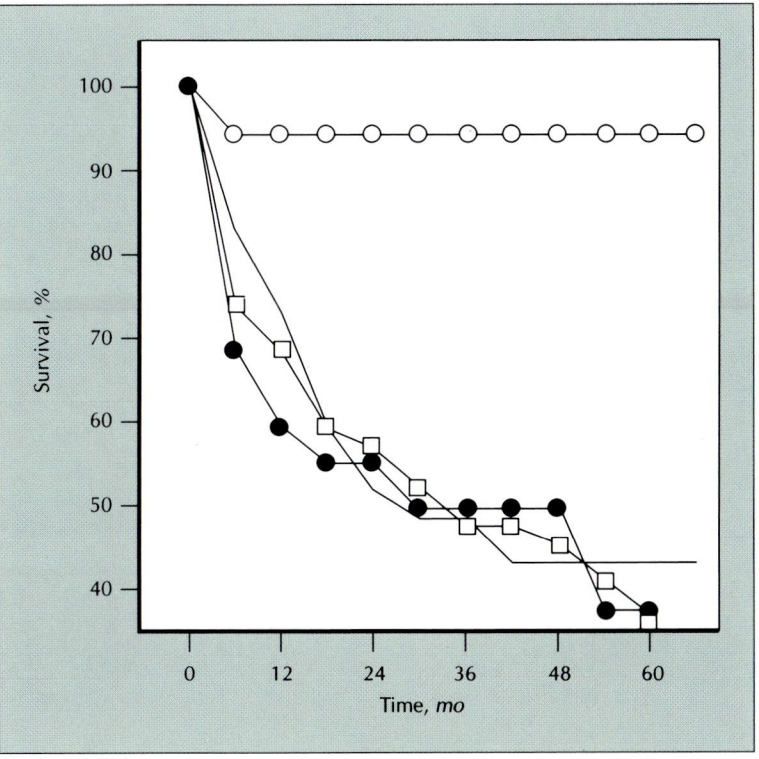

FIGURE 10-19. Survival curves in patients who responded acutely to calcium channel blockers (nifedipine or diltiazem) and were continued on treatment with one of these agents (*open circles*), compared with patients in the same study who did not respond favorably to calcium channel blockers (*solid line*), patients from the NIH Registry treated at the study institution (*solid circles*), and patients in the NIH Registry Cohort (*open squares*). This is the first evidence of improved survival with long-term pharmacologic therapy for PPH. The group that responded to calcium channel blockers also had a sustained reduction in pulmonary arterial pressure, pulmonary vascular resistance, and right ventricular chamber size diameter; symptoms were significantly alleviated. (*Adapted from* Rich *et al*. [23].)

CARDIAC TUMORS

As cardiac imaging becomes more common, with increasing resolution and tissue definition provided by echocardiography, computed tomography, and magnetic resonance imaging, cardiac tumors are being diagnosed with increasing frequency.

Among adults, myxomas account for three quarters of the primary tumors; among children, rhabdomyomas and fibromas account for more than half of the primary tumors.

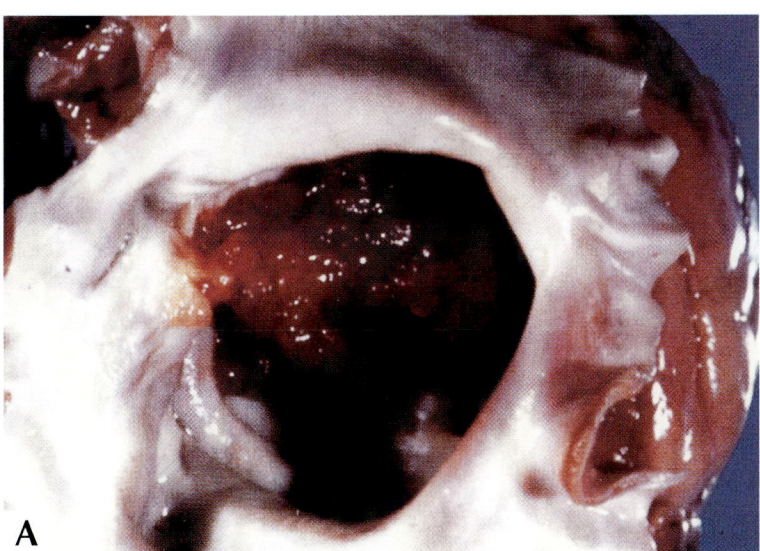

A

FIGURE 10-20. Myxomas. Patients with myxomas present with constitutional symptoms, embolism, or intracardiac obstruction. Fatigue, fever, erythematous rash, arthralgia, myalgia, and weight loss are the most common constitutional symptoms. Common laboratory abnormalities include anemia (usually normochromic and hypochromic) and elevation in the erythrocyte sedimentation rate, C-reactive protein, and globulin levels [24]. Constitutional symptoms mimicking autoimmune and rheumatologic diseases may be caused by the myxoma's production of interleukin 6 [25].

An inherited syndrome with cardiac myxomas and lentiginosis is called the Carney complex. Recently the Carney complex disease gene was identified at the human chromosome 17q2 locus [26].

Most myxomas develop in the left atrium and arise from the interatrial septum. As shown in the gross specimens (**A** to **E**), they may appear gelatinous, irregular, smooth, or calcified [27]. (*From* Burke and Virmani [27]; with permission.) (*continued*)

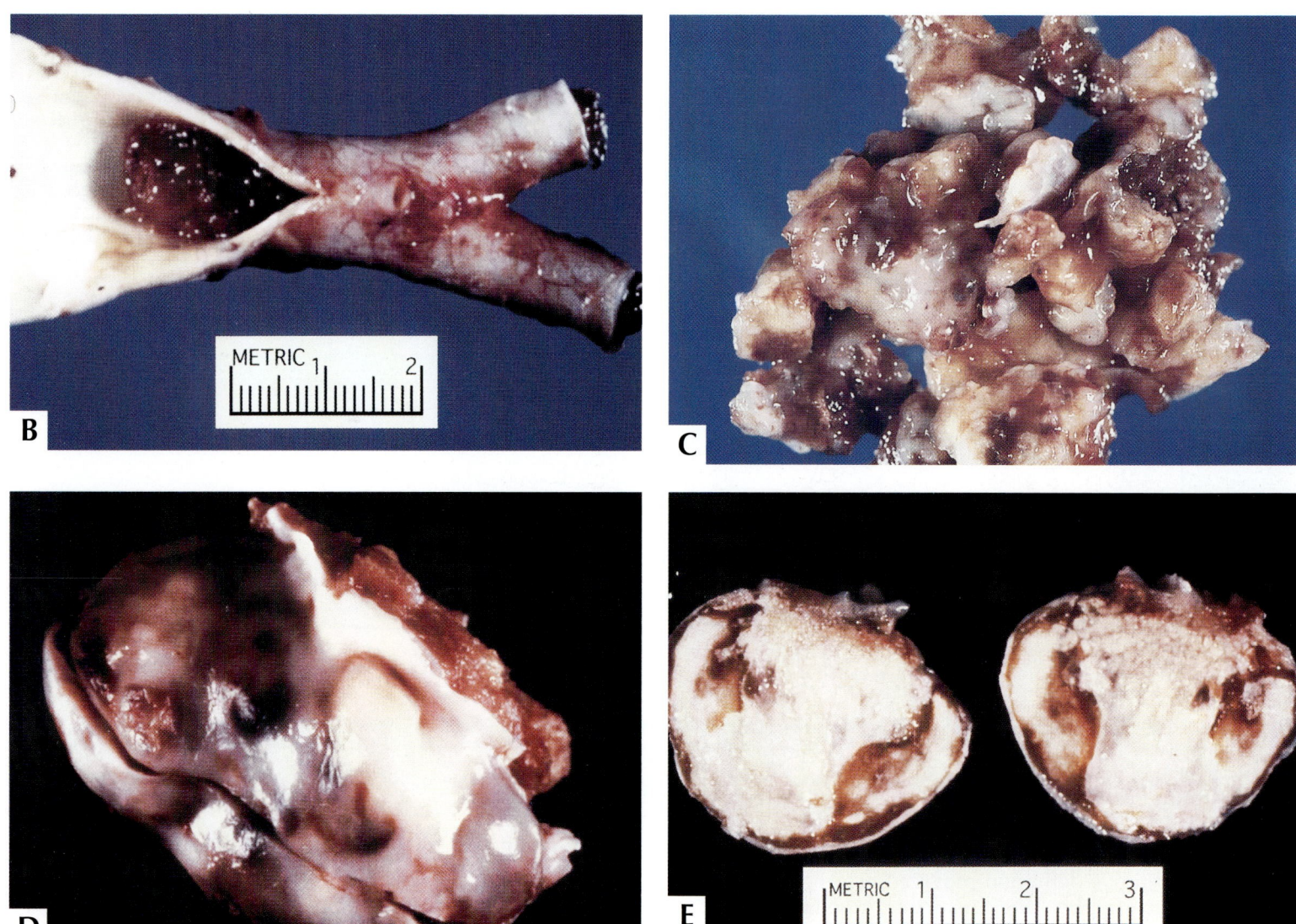

FIGURE 10-20. (*continued*)

SPECIFIC TUMOR PRESENTATIONS

Left Atrial Myxoma

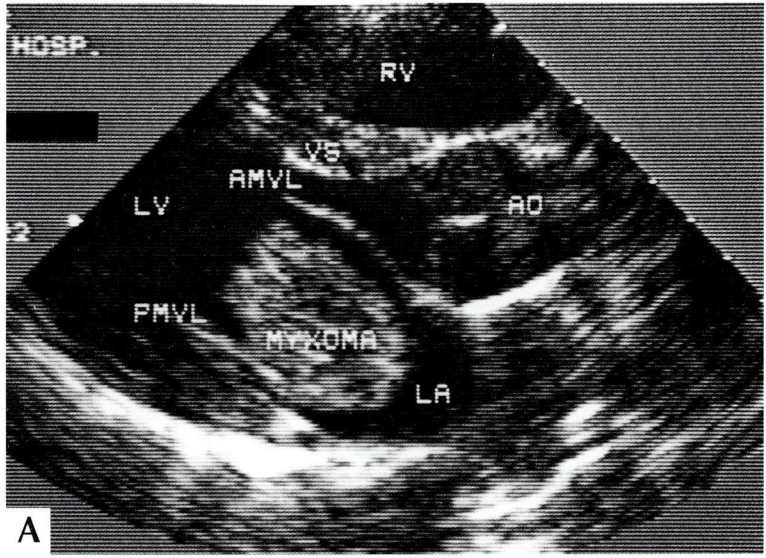

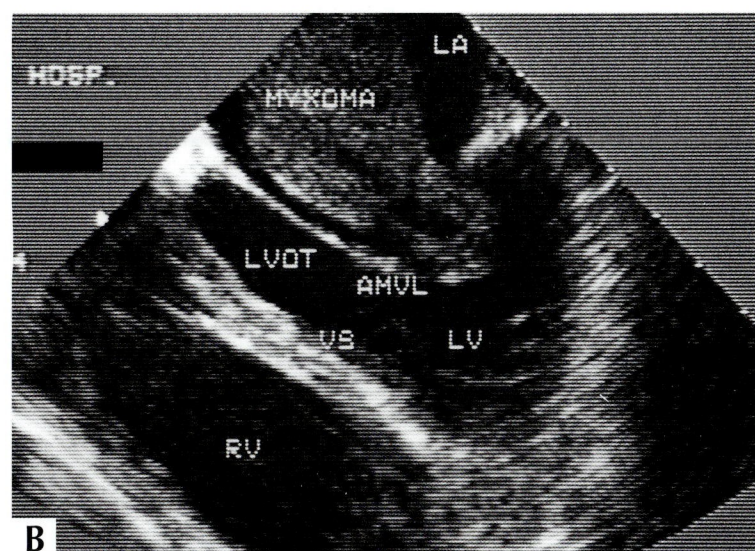

FIGURE 10-21. Transthoracic two-dimensional echocardiogram (**A**) and transesophageal two-dimensional echocardiogram (**B**) showing a left atrial (LA) mass prolapsing into and obstructing the mitral valve orifice. Note the superior resolution of the transesophageal echocardiogram. Although not visible here, the myxoma was attached to the mid-portion of the atrial septum.

Typically, LA myxomas attach to the fossa ovalis; although myxomas are rarely located posteriorly, a mass in this location should arouse suspicion of malignancy. During diastole, an atrial myxoma is visualized on M-mode echocardiography as multiple echoes behind the AMVL on the left and the tricuspid valve on the right. M-mode echocardiography is most useful for intracavitary, pedunculated masses of the LA;

however, it is less effective for visualizing tumors during systole and immobile tumors. Although ventricular myxomas can be seen as multiple intracavitary echoes, they are less frequently detected by this method. Two-dimensional echocardiography provides sufficient information (*ie*, size, attachment, and mobility) for surgical treatment. This imaging modality reveals intracavitary masses with alternating areas of echodensity and lucency and is useful for visualizing small, ventricular, and nonprolapsed tumors. Two-dimensional echocardiography also allows recognition of multiple masses. LV—left ventricle; LVOT—left ventricular outflow tract; PMVL—posterior leaflet of mitral valve; RV—right ventricle; VS—ventricular septum. (*Courtesy of* C.R. Thompson, MD, St. Paul's Hospital, Vancouver, BC.)

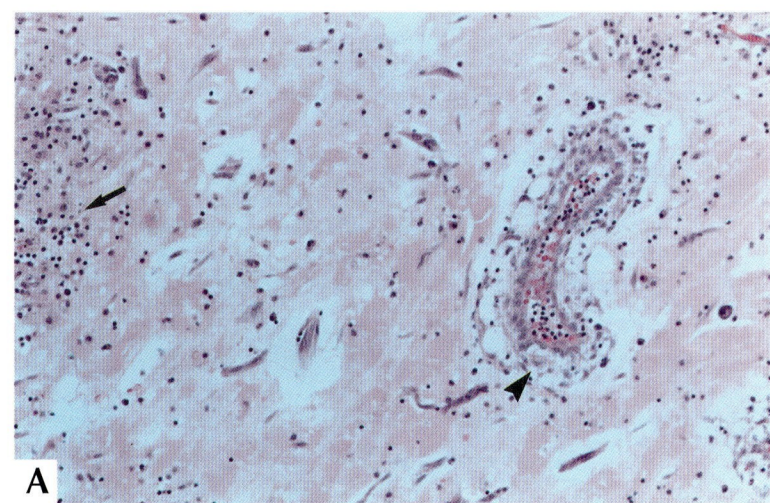

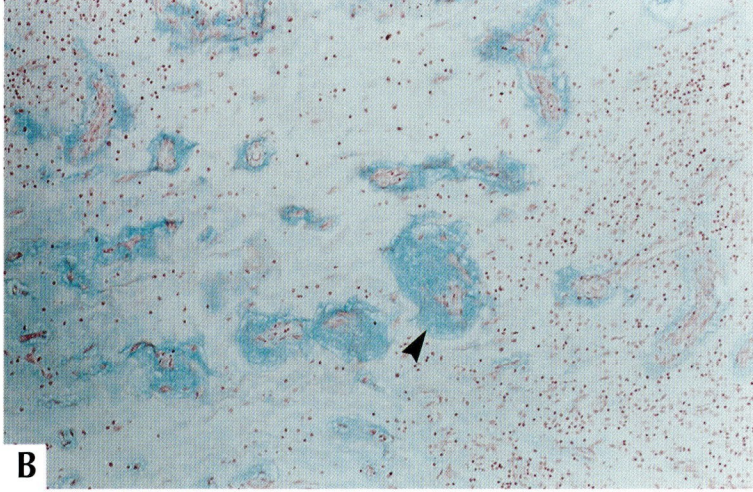

FIGURE 10-22. **A,** Abundant eosinophilic myxoid matrix containing polygonal to stellate myxoma cells distributed singly, in small groups, and around thin-walled vascular channels (*arrowhead*). Focal collections of mononuclear cells (macrophages, lymphocytes, plasma cells) are also seen (*arrow*). Myxomas may also contain glands, areas of recent and old

hemorrhage, as well as calcification and metaplastic bone formation (hematoxylin and eosin, × 200).

B, Large quantities of acid mucopolysaccharide are present in the myxoma matrix, primarily in the vicinity of vascular channels (*arrowhead*) (Alcian blue, × 100).

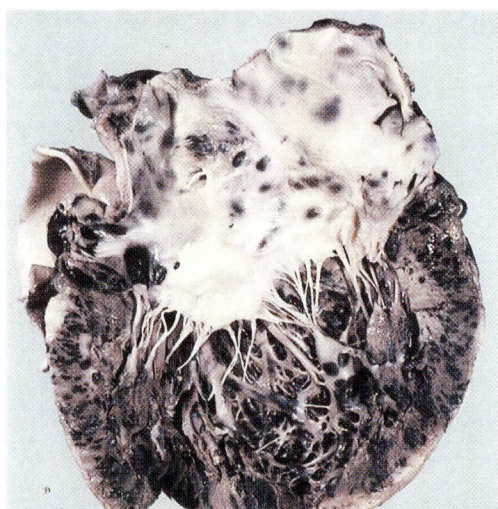

FIGURE 10-23. Malignant melanoma. Tumor metastases to the heart are hundreds of times more common than primary cardiac tumors. They are seen in about 15% of autopsies of patients with disseminated cancer. Some uncommon tumors, such as malignant melanoma [27], involve the heart almost half the time. Lung and breast carcinoma involve the heart and pericardium about 20% to 25% of the time. (*From* Burke and Virmani [27]; with permission.)

REFERENCES

1. Bishop JM: Hypoxia and pulmonary hypertension in chronic bronchitis. *Prog Respir Res* 1975, 9:10.

2. Weber KT, Janicki JS, Shroff S, Fishman AP: Contractile mechanisms and interaction of the right and left ventricles. *Am J Cardiol* 1981, 47:686–695.

3. Harris P, Heath D: Unexplained pulmonary hypertension. In *The Human Pulmonary Circulation*, ed 2. Edited by Harris P, Heath D. Edinburgh: Churchill-Livingstone; 1977:418–440.

4. Snyder SH, Bredt DS: Biological roles of nitric oxide. *Sci Am* 1992:266:68–71, 74–77.

5. Fineman JF, Chang R, Soifer SJ: EDRF inhibition augments pulmonary hypertension in intact newborn lambs. *Am J Physiol* 1992, 262:H1365–H1371.

6. Dinh-Xuan AT, Higenbottam TW, Clelland CA, *et al.*: Impairment of endothelium-dependent pulmonary-artery relaxation in chronic obstruction lung disease. *N Engl J Med* 1991, 324:1539–1547.

7. Stewart DJ, Levy RD, Cernacek P, Langleben D: Increased plasma endothelin-1 in pulmonary hypertension: marker or mediator of disease? *Ann Intern Med* 1991, 114:464–469.

8. Giaid A, Yanagisawa M, Langleben D, *et al.*: Expression of endothelin-1 in the lungs of patients with pulmonary hypertension. *N Engl J Med* 1993, 328:1732–1739.

9. McFadden ER, Braunwald E: Cor pulmonale. In *Heart Disease: A Textbook of Cardiovascular Medicine*, ed 4. Edited by Braunwald E. Philadelphia, WB Saunders, 1992:1581–1601.

10. Strollo PJ Jr, Rogers RM: Obstructive sleep apnea. *N Engl J Med* 1996, 334:99–104.

11. Teran-Santos J, Jimenez-Gomez A, Cordero-Guevara J: The association between sleep apnea and the risk of traffic accidents. *N Engl J Med* 1999, 340:847–851.

12. Suratt PM, Findley LJ: Driving with sleep apnea. *N Engl J Med* 1999, 340:881–883.

13. Rothman A, Mann DM, House MT, *et al.*: Transvenous procurement of pulmonary artery smooth muscle and endothelial cells using a novel endoarterial biopsy catheter in a canine model. *J Am Coll Cardiol* 1996, 27:218–224.

14. Report of the Medical Research Council Working Party: Long term domiciliary oxygen therapy in chronic hypoxic cor pulmonale complicating chronic bronchitis and emphysema. *Lancet* 1981, 1:681–686.

15. Nocturnal Oxygen Therapy Trial Group: Continuous or nocturnal oxygen therapy in hypoxemic chronic obstructive lung disease: a clinical trial. *Ann Intern Med* 1980, 93:391–398.

16. Lilienfeld DE, Rubin LJ: Mortality from primary pulmonary hypertension in the United States. *Chest* 2000, 117:796–800.

17. Rich S: Primary pulmonary hypertension. *Prog Cardiovasc Dis* 1989, 31:205–238.

18. Gaine SP, Rubin LJ: Primary pulmonary hypertension. *Lancet* 1998, 352:719–725.

19. Barst RJ, Rubin LJ, Long WA, *et al.*: A comparison of continuous intravenous epoprostenol (prostacyclin) with conventional therapy for primary pulmonary hypertension. *N Engl J Med* 1996, 334:296–301.

20. Badesch DB, Tapson VF, McGoon MD, *et al.*: Continuous intravenous epoprostenol for pulmonary hypertension due to the scleroderma spectrum of disease: a randomized, controlled trial. *Ann Intern Med* 2000, 132:425–434.

21. Hoeper MM, Olschewski J, Ghofrani HA, *et al.*, and the German PPH Study Group: A comparison of the acute hemodynamic effects of inhaled nitric oxide and aerosolized iloprost in primary pulmnonary hypertension. *J Am Coll Cardiol* 2000, 35:176–182.22.

22. Olschewski H, Ghofrani A, Schemehl T, *et al.*, for the German PPH Study Group: Inhaled iloprost to treat severe pulmonary hypertension: an uncontrolled trial. *Ann Intern Med* 2000, 132:435–443.

23. Rich S, Kaufman E, Levy PS: The effect of high doses of calcium-channel blockers on survival in primary pulmonary hypertension. *N Engl J Med* 1992, 327:76–81.

24. Reynen K: Cardiac myxomas. *N Engl J Med* 1995, 333:1610–1617.

25. Seguin JR, Beigbeder JY, Hvass U, *et al.*: Interleukin 6 production by cardiac myxomas may explain constitutional symptoms. *J Thorac Cardiovasc Surg* 1992, 103:599–600.

26. Casey M, Mah C, Merliss AD, *et al.*: Identification of a novel genetic locus for familial cardiac myxomas and Carney complex. *Circulation* 1998, 98:2560–2566.

27. Burke A, Virmani R: *Tumors of the Heart and Great Vessels: Atlas of Tumor Pathology*, 3rd series, fascicle 16. Washington, DC: Armed Forces Institute of Pathology; 1996.

INDEX

focal origin of, 192
mechanisms of, 190-191
treatment of, 191, 193
Atrial flutter, 191
Atrial flutter circuit, 190
Atrial natriuretic factor (ANF), in heart failure, 117
Atrial premature beats, 175
Atrial premature complexes, focal, 191
Atrial septal defect, 287-288
left and right heart structures in, 288
regurgitation jets in, 288
sites of communication between atria and, 287
Atrial septostomy, balloon, 302
Atrioventricular node reentrant tachycardia (AVNRT), 188
Atrioventricular septal defect (AVSD), 289-290
classification of, 289
echocardiography in, 290
Atropine, for sinus node dysfunction evaluation, 183
Automaticity, 176
Autonomic nervous system, conditions associated with, 180
AVID (Arrhythmic Drug Versus Implanted Defibrillator) Trial, 199, 200
AVNRT (atrioventricular node reentrant tachycardia), 188
AVR. *See* Aortic valve replacement (AVR)
AVSD (atrioventricular septal defect), 289-290
classification of, 289
echocardiography in, 290
Azimilide, for atrial supraventricular tachycardia, 193

Bacterial endocarditis (BE)
bioprosthetic valves and, 282
prophylaxis for, in mitral valve prolapse, 267
Balloon atrial septostomy, 302
Balloon commissurotomy, for mitral stenosis, 257-258
Balloon mitral valvotomy, 259
Balloon valvuloplasty
aortic, indications for, 272
mitral, survival after, 259
Baroreceptor dysfunction, heart failure and, 114
BE (bacterial endocarditis)
bioprosthetic valves and, 282
prophylaxis for, in mitral valve prolapse, 267
Becker muscular dystrophy, 159, 161
Benestent Trial, 100
Beta blockers
antiarrhythmic efficacy of, 179
coronary risk factors and, 238
for heart failure, 129-130
for hypertension, 233
hemodynamic response to, 234
norepinephrine release and, 234
mechanism of action of, 49
for stable angina, 90
Bile acid sequestrants, 28-29
combination therapy using, 33, 34
mechanism of action of, 29
Bioprosthetic valves. *See* Prosthetic valves, bioprosthetic
Biopsy
endoarterial, in cor pulmonale, 312-313
endomyocardial. *See* Endomyocardial biopsy
Blacks, hypertension in, 215
Blalock-Taussig (B-T) shunt, for tetralogy of Fallot, 296
Blood pressure. *See also* Hypertension
automated noninvasive ambulatory monitoring of, 242
classification of, 240
Brugada's syndrome, 196
B-T (Blalock-Taussig) shunt, for tetralogy of Fallot, 296

CABG. *See* Coronary artery bypass grafting (CABG)
Calcification, annular, of mitral valve, 259
Calcium
excitation-contraction coupling and, 107
handling of, in heart failure, 112-113
Calcium-channel blockers. *See also specific drugs*
for acute coronary syndromes, results of therapy with, 50
coronary risk factors and, 238
for hypertension, 233
mechanism of action of, 235
for isolated systolic hypertension, 247
mechanisms of action of, 91
for prevention of myocardial infarction, meta-analysis of trials of, 48
for primary pulmonary hypertension, survival and, 319
for stable angina, 90, 91
Canadian Implantable Defibrillator Study (CIDS), 200
Captopril, for hypertensive emergencies, 246
Captopril test, in renovascular hypertension, 224
CAPTURE trial, 65, 66
Cardiac Arrest Hamburg Study (CASH), 200
Cardiac Arrhythmia Suppression Trial (CAST), 51-52
Cardiac contraction, normal, 105-108
contractile protein interactions and, 105
determinants of, 108
excitation-contraction coupling and, 107
structure of heart and, 106
Cardiac glycosides, for heart failure, 127-128
Cardiac pacing, 201-206
dual-chamber timing cycle for, 203
for hypertrophic cardiomyopathy, 146
indications for, 203-204
modes of, 202
pacemaker syndrome and, 205
pulse generator design for, 201
rate-adaptive, 206
sensing and, 201-202
sequence of ventricular activation and, 205
survival and, 206
Cardiac rupture
infarct-related, 47
predisposition to, atherosclerotic plaque and, 42
types of, 72
vulnerability to, consistency of atherosclerotic plaque and, 43
Cardiac tamponade, 167-168
echocardiography in, 167, 168
hemodynamic changes in, 167, 168
respiration and, 168
Cardiac transplantation
contraindications to, 135, 136
for heart failure, 134-140
patient management and, 137-139
selection of candidates for, 134-135
surgery for, 136-137
survival and, 139-140
Cardiac tumors, 319-322
metastatic, 322
Cardiogenic shock
diagnosis of, 70
left ventricular, 69-71
pathophysiology of, 69-70
treatment of, 70-71
Cardiomegaly, congestive heart failure with, 121
Cardiomyopathy. *See* Dilated cardiomyopathy; Hypertrophic cardiomyopathy (HCM); Restrictive cardiomyopathy
Cardiovascular risk factors, 21

Fibric acids, 32-33
  clinical trials with, 33
  mechanism of action of, 32
Fibrinogen, platelet aggregation and, 63
Fibroblast growth factor (FGF), endothelial response to vascular
    injury and, 2
Fish oils, effects on plasma lipids, 24
Flecainide
  for acute coronary syndromes, results of therapy with, 51
  antiarrhythmic efficacy of, 179
4P trial, 65
Framingham Heart Study, 13, 119
Friedreich's ataxia, 159

G proteins, adrenergic receptor types and functional
    relationships to, 216
Gemfibrozil, clinical trials of, 19, 20
Genetic dyslipoproteinemias, frequency in patients with coronary
    heart disease, 9
Genetic mutations, dilated cardiomyopathy caused by, 161
Genetics, of hypertension, 213
GISSI (Gruppo Italiano per lo Studio della Streptochinasi
    nell'Infarti Miocardico) trials
  GISSI-1, 60
  GISSI-3, 50
Glycoprotein IIB/IIIA inhibitors, 65-66
GM-CSF (granulocyte-macrophage colony-stimulating factor),
    endothelial response to vascular injury and, 2
Granulocyte-macrophage colony-stimulating factor (GM-CSF),
    endothelial response to vascular injury and, 2
Granulomas, sarcoid, in sarcoid heart disease, 152-153
Great arteries, complete transposition of, 299
Gruppo Italiano per lo Studio della Streptochinasi nell'Infarti
    Miocardico (GISSI) trials
  GISSI-1, 60
  GISSI-3, 50
GUSTO trials, 57, 59, 60
  GUSTO I, 59
  GUSTO III, 59
Gynecoid obesity, 24

H ancock stented porcine valves, 281
HBNP (human brain natriuretic peptide), for heart failure, 133
HCM. See Hypertrophic cardiomyopathy (HCM)
HDFP (Hypertension Detection and Follow-up Program), 236,
    238-239
HDL. See High-density lipoproteins (HDL)
Heart, structure of, 106
Heart block
  cardiac pacing and, 206
  in Lyme disease, 151
Heart failure, 105-142
  adrenergic nervous system and, 113-115
  assessment of, 120
  atrial natriuretic factor and, 117
  cardiac transplantation for. See Cardiac transplantation, for
    heart failure
  with cardiomegaly, 121
  clinical features of, 119-122
  diastolic, 108-109, 121
  dilated cardiomyopathy in, 150
  endothelin and, 118-119
  epidemiology of, 120
  initial management of, 131
  with left ventricular hypertrophy, 121

  myocardial remodeling and. See Myocardial remodeling
  normal contraction and. See Cardiac contraction, normal
  pharmacologic management of, 122-133
    for acute, severe heart failure, 131-133
    angiotensin-converting enzyme inhibitors for, 124-125
    beta blockers for, 129-130
    digitalis glycosides for, 127-128
    diuretics for, 123
    physiologic response to, 122
    positive inotropic agents for, 126
    vasodilators for, 126
  renin-angiotensin-aldosterone system and, 116
  restrictive cardiomyopathy and, 154
  systolic, 108-109, 121
  ventricular remodeling and, 110-111
Heart rate, adapting to activity, 206
Heart valves. See also Valvular heart disease; specific valves
  prosthetic
    bioprosthetic, 281-284
    mechanical, 280-281
Helsinki Heart Study, 19
Hemodynamic overload, ventricular remodeling and, 110
Hemodynamics
  in aortic regurgitation, 273-274
  beta blocker effects on, 234
  in chronic aortic regurgitation, 276-277
  hypertension autonomic nervous system, 216
Heparin
  clinical use of, 53
  mortality reduction with, 60
High-density Lipoprotein Cholesterol Intervention Trial (VA-HIT), 20
High-density lipoproteins (HDL), 13-15
  coronary heart disease endpoints related to, 13
  metabolism of
    drug effects on, 28
    reverse cholesterol transport and atherosclerosis related to, 13
  myocardial infarction risk related to, 35
  nascent, 14
  raising levels of, 15
  reverse cholesterol transport and, 13, 14
  structure of, 14
Hormonal therapy, for coronary heart disease prevention, 33
Human brain natriuretic peptide (hBNP), for heart failure, 133
Hydralazine, for hypertensive emergencies, 246
Hydrochlorothiazide, race and efficacy of, 238-239
Hygienic therapy, in hypertension, 233
Hypereosinophilic heart disease, 156-157
  biopsy in, 157
  clinical manifestations of, 157
  pathogenesis of, 156
Hyperlipidemia, familial, combined, 18
Hyperlipoproteinemias, 7-9
  frequency in patients with established coronary heart disease, 9
  lipoproteins in development of atherosclerotic lesion and, 8
  oil-drop (mixed micelle) model of lipoprotein structure and, 7
Hypertension, 213-250
  in children, 244
  in elderly people, 244
  pathogenesis of, 213-223
    adrenergic nervous system and. See Adrenergic nervous
      system, hypertension and
    genetic and environmental factors in, 213-215
    renin-angiotensin system and, 217-223
  pheochromocytoma and. See Pheochromocytomas
  in pregnancy, 243-244
    classification of, 243

Plexiform lesions, vasoconstriction and, 316
PMVT (polymorphic ventricular tachycardia), mechanisms for, 200
Polymorphic ventricular tachycardia (PMVT), mechanisms for, 200
Potassium
    intake of, hypertension and, 214
    in primary aldosteronism, 228
Potassium-sparing diuretics, for heart failure, 123
Potts shunt, for tetralogy of Fallot, 296
Pregnancy, hypertension in. *See* Hypertension, in pregnancy
Preload reserve, 108
PRISM PLUS trial, 66
Procainamide, antiarrhythmic efficacy of, 179
Programmed cell death, in heart failure, 112-113
    neurohumoral systems in, 115
Programmed electrical stimulation (PES), for ventricular
        tachycardia, 197
Propafenone, antiarrhythmic efficacy of, 179
Propranolol
    race and efficacy of, 238-239
    for sinus node dysfunction evaluation, 183
Prosthetic valves, 280-284
    bioprosthetic, 281-284
        auscultatory characteristics of, 284
        degenerative changes of, 282
        endocarditis and, 282
        selection for individual patients, 283
        structural deterioration of, 283
    mechanical, 280-281
Proteinuria, in diabetes mellitus, antihypertensive effect on, 238-239
PSVT (paroxysmal supraventricular tachycardia), 190
PTCA. *See* Percutaneous transluminal coronary angioplasty (PTCA)
Pulmonary angiograms, 318
Pulmonary artery, endothelial control of tone in, 309-310
Pulmonary hypertension. *See also* Cor pulmonale
    primary, 315-319
    algorithm for investigation of, 317
    diagnostic approach for, 317-318
    epidemiology of, 315
    histopathology of, 316
    pathogenesis of, 316-317, 317
    treatment of, 318-319
Pulmonary stenosis, 302-303
Pulmonary valve atresia, tetralogy of Fallot with, 294-295
Pulmonary valve stenosis, 302
PURSUIT trial, 66

Q
Quinidine, antiarrhythmic efficacy of, 179

R
Race, hypertension and, 215
Ramipril, for heart failure, 124
Randomized Interventional Treatment of Angina (RITA) trial, 102
Recainam, antiarrhythmic efficacy of, 179
Reentrant tachycardia, implantable cardioverter-defibrillator for, 208
Reentry
    antiarrhythmic drug effects on, 178, 179
    arrhythmias and, 177-178
        mechanism for, 178
        sequence of activation within reentry circuit and, 177
    random, atrial fibrillation and, 190
    sinus node, therapeutic options for, 184
Renal function, in diabetes mellitus, antihypertensive effect on, 238-239
Renin, 217
    mechanisms governing release of, 218
    urinary sodium excretion and, 218
Renin-angiotensin system. *See also* Angiotensin I; Angiotensin II

angiotensin-converting enzyme inhibitor effects on, 235
circulating components of, 221
in heart failure, 116
hypertension and, 217-221
    angiotensin-converting enzyme actions and, 218
    juxtaglomerular apparatus and, 217
    mechanisms of renin release and, 218
    renin activity related to urinary sodium excretion and, 218
Renovascular hypertension, 223-226
    atherosclerotic post-stenotic dilatation and, 225
    causes of, 223, 225
    Cushing's syndrome and. *See* Cushing's syndrome
    diagnosis of, 224
Reperfusion, for cardiogenic shock, 70
Reperfusion therapy, time to
    infarct size and, 57
    mortality reduction and, 58
Restrictive cardiomyopathy, 154-156
    heart failure and, 154
    myocytes in, 155
    pathophysiology of, 155
    signs and symptoms of, 156
Reteplase
    characteristics of, 58
    comparison with other thrombolytic agents, 59
Revascularization, for cardiogenic shock, 70
Right ventricular outflow tract ventricular tachycardia (RVOT VT),
    194-195
Risk factors. *See* Cardiovascular risk factors
RITA (Randomized Interventional Treatment of Angina) trial, 102
RVOT VT (right ventricular outflow tract ventricular tachycardia),
    194-195

S
St. Jude bileaflet valve, 281
SAJ (sinoatrial junction) block, 181
Salt sensitivity, among blacks, 215
Sarcoidosis, cardiac, 152-153
Saruplase, characteristics of, 58
SAVE (Survival and Ventricular Enlargement) study, 124
Septostomy, atrial, balloon, 302
Seven Countries Study, 22
SHEP (Systolic Hypertension in the Elderly Program), 238-239, 247
SHOCK trial, 71
Shunts, for tetralogy of Fallot, 296
Silent ischemia, 92-93
    detection of, 93
    myocardial perfusion imaging in, 92
    significance of, 92
Single-photon emission computed tomography (SPECT),
    myocardial perfusion imaging on, 83
Sinoatrial junction (SAJ) block, 181
Sinus node, autonomic nervous system inputs to, 180
Sinus node ablation, for tachycardia, 182
Sinus node dysfunction (SND), 180-185
    evaluation of, 183
    impulse generation abnormalities and, 181-182
    management of, 184-185
        diagnostic and treatment approach for, 185
        therapeutic options for, 184
    types of, 180-182
Sinus node recovery time (SRT), 183
Sinus node reentry, therapeutic options for, 184
Sinus rhythm, auscultatory signs of mitral stenosis in, 255
Sinus tachycardia
    therapeutic options for, 184
    treatment of, 182

Tissue-type plasminogen activator (t-PA)
    comparison with other thrombolytic agents, 59
    mortality reduction with, 60
Tocainide, antiarrhythmic efficacy of, 179
ToF. See Tetralogy of Fallot (ToF)
Torsades de pointes, 200
t-PA (tissue-type plasminogen activator)
    comparison with other thrombolytic agents, 59
    mortality reduction with, 60
Transannular flow patch, for tetralogy of Fallot, 296
Transesophageal echocardiography (TEE), in chronic aortic
        regurgitation, 276
Transforming growth factors (TGFs), endothelial response to
        vascular injury and, 2
Transplantation. See Cardiac transplantation
Transplantation coronary allograft disease (TCAD), 139
Transposition of the great arteries, 299
Tricuspid atresia, 300-301
    imaging in, 300
    natural history of, 301
Tricuspid stenosis, echocardiography in, 280
Triggered arrhythmias, 177
Triglyceride lipase, hepatic, 16
Triglycerides, 15-20
    chylomicron metabolism and, 16
    coronary heart disease risk related to, 15
        plasma triglyceride levels and, 16
        specific risk factors and, 15
    elevation of
        dysbetalipoproteinemia and, 17-18
        familial combined hyperlipidemia and, 18
        familial hypertriglyceridemia and, 18
    reduction of, clinical trials of drugs for, 19-20
Trimethaphan camsylate, for hypertensive emergencies, 246
Truncus arteriosus communis (TAC), 297-298
    classification of, 297
    imaging in, 298
    pathophysiology of, 298
Tubero-eruptive xanthomas, in dysbetalipoproteinemia, 18
Tumors. See also Malignancies; Pheochromocytomas
    adrenal, in primary aldosteronism, 228
    cardiac, 319-322
        metastatic, 322
24-hour urinary free cortisol test, in renovascular
        hypertension, 226

United States Carvedilol Heart Failure Trials Program, 129

VA-HIT (High-density Lipoprotein Cholesterol Intervention
        Trial), 20
Valve replacement, for mitral stenosis, 259
Valvotomy, for mitral stenosis, 259
Valvular heart disease, 253-285. See also specific disorders
Valvuloplasty
    aortic, indications for, 272
    mitral, survival after, 259

Vascular endothelial growth factor (VEGF), endothelial
        response to vascular injury and, 2
Vascular injury, endothelial response to, 2
Vascular occlusion, in atherosclerosis, 6
Vasoconstriction
    angiotensin II receptors and, 219
    endothelium-dependent mechanism of, hypertension and, 222
    intimal fibrosis and plexiform lesions and, 316
Vasodilator in Heart Failure Trial (VHeFT), 122, 126
Vasodilator mechanism, endothelium-dependent,
        hypertension and, 221-222
Vasodilators
    for heart failure, 126
    for hypertensive emergencies, 246
Vasopressors
    for cardiogenic shock, 70
    for heart failure, 132
VEGF (vascular endothelial growth factor), endothelial
        response to vascular injury and, 2
Vena cava, superior, biopsies from, in transplant patients, 137
Ventricles. See also Left ventricular entries
    interdependence of, 308
Ventricular assist devices, 140
Ventricular fibrillation (VF), thrombolytic therapy and, 52
Ventricular hypertrophy, patterns of, 110
Ventricular remodeling, 110-111
    drug therapy to improve, 124
    early, after myocardial infarction and infarct expansion, 111
Ventricular septal defect, 288-289
Ventricular septal rupture (VSR), 71
Verapamil, antiarrhythmic efficacy of, 179
Very low density lipoproteins (VLDL), metabolism of, 17
Vesnarinone, for heart failure, 126
Veterans Administration Study, 236
Veterans Administration Vasodilator in Heart Failure Trial
        (VHeFT), 122, 126
Veterans Affairs Cooperative Studies Program, 20
VF (ventricular fibrillation), thrombolytic therapy and, 52
VHeFT (Veterans Administration Vasodilator in Heart Failure
        Trial), 122, 126
Visceral obesity, central, 24
VLDL (very low density lipoproteins), metabolism of, 17
VSR (ventricular septal rupture), 71

Wall motion abnormalities
    on echocardiography, 85
    natural history of, 85-86
Warfarin, for acute coronary syndromes, results of therapy
        with, 51
Warfarin Reinfarction Study (WARIS), 51
WARIS (Warfarin Reinfarction Study), 51
Waterston shunt, for tetralogy of Fallot, 296
Wenckebach block, 181
Wide complex tachycardia, diagnosis of, 193-194